MEDICAL EMERGENCIES: DIAGNOSTIC AND MANAGEMENT PROCEDURES FROM BOSTON CITY HOSPITAL

medical emergencies

DIAGNOSTIC AND MANAGEMENT PROCEDURES FROM BOSTON CITY HOSPITAL

edited by

ALAN S. COHEN, M.D.

Chief of Medicine, Boston City Hospital; Director, Thorndike Memorial Laboratory; Conrad Wesselhoeft Professor of Medicine, Boston University School of Medicine

RALPH B. FREIDIN, M.D.

Director, Primary Care Center, Boston City Hospital; Assistant Visiting Physician, Boston City Hospital and Thorndike Memorial Laboratory; Assistant Professor of Medicine, Boston University School of Medicine; formerly Chief Resident in Medicine, Boston City Hospital

MARTIN A. SAMUELS, M.D.

Senior Resident in Neurology, Massachusetts General Hospital; Clinical Fellow in Neurology, Harvard Medical School; formerly Chief Resident in Medicine, Boston City Hospital

LITTLE, BROWN AND COMPANY
BOSTON

THE DIAGNOSIS AND TREATMENT of medical emergencies is an important part of the experience of all house officers. At the Boston City Hospital, interns, assistant residents, and residents in medicine are all intimately involved with patients not only in the triage procedures but in the immediate problems of diagnosis and management. Increasing attention is being directed toward the broad aspects of emergency medicine.

We feel that ideas originally stimulated by a series of thought-provoking lectures by the attending faculty for the orientation of incoming house officers at Boston City Hospital will be of interest to a large number of physicians. This book is therefore intended to provide for the interested physician detailed discussion of the diagnosis and treatment of a broad spectrum of emergency problems especially relevant to internal medicine. It is hoped that these chapters will give the reader an understanding of the decision-making process involved in the handling of medical emergencies.

We thank Ms. Carolyn Whalen for her patient efforts in the preparation of this manuscript.

A. S. C.
R. B. F.
M. A. S.

CONTRIBUTING AUTHORS

EDWARD A. ALEXANDER, M.D.
Chief, Renal Section, and Associate Director, Medical Service, Boston City Hospital; Visiting Physician, Boston City Hospital and Thorndike Memorial Laboratory; Associate Professor of Medicine, Boston University School of Medicine

CHARLES MICHAEL BLISS, M.D.
Chief, Gastroenterology Section, Boston City Hospital; Associate Visiting Physician, Boston City Hospital and Thorndike Memorial Laboratory; Assistant Professor of Medicine, Boston University School of Medicine

MARK J. BRAUER, M.D.
Director, Blood Bank, Boston City Hospital; Associate Visiting Physician, Boston City Hospital and Thorndike Memorial Laboratory; Assistant Professor of Medicine, Boston University School of Medicine

JEROME S. BRODY, M.D.
Chief, Pulmonary Section, Boston City Hospital; Visiting Physician, Boston City Hospital and Thorndike Memorial Laboratory; Associate Professor of Medicine, Boston University School of Medicine

ARAM V. CHOBANIAN, M.D.
Director, Cardiovascular Institute, Boston University Medical Center; Visiting Physician, Boston City Hospital and Thorndike Memorial Laboratory; Professor of Medicine, Boston University School of Medicine

ALAN S. COHEN, M.D.
Chief of Medicine, Boston City Hospital; Director, Thorndike Memorial Laboratory; Conrad Wesselhoeft Professor of Medicine, Boston University School of Medicine

ENOBONG A. EKONG, M.D.
Director, Coronary Care Unit, Martin Luther King, Jr. Hospital; Assistant Professor of Medicine, Drew Medical Center, Los Angeles, California; formerly Assistant Visiting Physician, Boston City Hospital and Thorndike Memorial Laboratory; Assistant Professor of Medicine, Boston University School of Medicine

S. Edwin Fineberg, M.D.
Director, Diabetes Clinic, Boston City Hospital; Co-Program Director, General Clinical Research Center, Thorndike Memorial Laboratory; Assistant Visiting Physician, Boston City Hospital; Assistant Professor of Medicine, Boston University School of Medicine

Ralph B. Freidin, M.D.
Director, Primary Care Center, Boston City Hospital; Assistant Visiting Physician, Boston City Hospital and Thorndike Memorial Laboratory; Assistant Professor of Medicine, Boston University School of Medicine; formerly Chief Resident in Medicine, Boston City Hospital

Nelson M. Gantz, M.D.
Assistant Director, Outpatient Department, Boston City Hospital; Assistant Visiting Physician, Boston City Hospital and Thorndike Memorial Laboratory; Assistant Professor of Medicine, Boston University School of Medicine

Don L. Goldenberg, M.D.
Assistant Director, Medical Service, Boston City Hospital; Assistant Visiting Physician, Boston City Hospital and Thorndike Memorial Laboratory; Assistant Professor of Medicine, Boston University School of Medicine

William B. Hood, Jr., M.D.
Chief, Cardiology Section, Boston City Hospital; Visiting Physician, Boston City Hospital and Thorndike Memorial Laboratory; Professor of Medicine, Boston University School of Medicine

Raymond S. Koff, M.D.
Chief, Hepatology Section, Boston Veterans Administration Hospital; Assistant Visiting Physician, Boston City Hospital; Associate Professor of Medicine, Boston University School of Medicine

Robert M. Levin, M.D.
Associate Director, Medical Service, Boston City Hospital; Visiting Physician, Boston City Hospital and Thorndike Memorial Laboratory; Associate Professor of Medicine, Boston University School of Medicine

Leah M. Lowenstein, M.D.
Visiting Physician, Boston City Hospital and Thorndike Memorial Laboratory; Associate Professor of Medicine, Boston University School of Medicine

Michael W. Pozen, M.D.
Assistant Visiting Physician, Boston City Hospital and Thorndike Memorial Laboratory; Assistant Professor of Medicine, Boston University School of Medicine

Ethan Samuel Rofman, M.D.
Chief of Psychiatry, Veterans Administration Hospital, Bedford, Massachusetts; formerly Liaison Psychiatrist, Boston City Hospital

Martin A. Samuels, M.D.
Senior Resident in Neurology, Massachusetts General Hospital; Clinical Fellow in Neurology, Harvard Medical School; formerly Chief Resident in Medicine, Boston City Hospital

PANTEL S. VOKONAS, M.D.
Assistant Visiting Physician, Boston City Hospital and Thorndike Memorial Laboratory; Assistant Professor of Medicine, Boston University School of Medicine

MICHAEL E. WHITCOMB, M.D.
Chief, Pulmonary Section, University Hospital; Assistant Visiting Physician, Boston City Hospital; Assistant Professor of Medicine, Boston University School of Medicine; formerly Associate Director, Pulmonary Section, Boston City Hospital

CONTENTS

MEDICAL EMERGENCIES: DIAGNOSTIC AND MANAGEMENT PROCEDURES FROM BOSTON CITY HOSPITAL

1   DRUG OVERDOSES AND POISONINGS

Ralph B. Freidin

Methyl Alcohol
Ethylene Glycol
Salicylates
Phenothiazines
Minor Tranquilizers
Tricyclic Antidepressants
Opioids

DRUG OVERDOSAGE and poison ingestion are medical emergencies frequently seen at the Boston City Hospital. Because it is not possible to maintain familiarity with all the potential toxins, and because in most clinical poisonings the responsible agent is either unknown or one for which there is no specific antidote, this chapter will describe a systematic management plan for these emergencies and then describe the clinical presentation and specific therapy for several major poisonings. The psychiatric problems surrounding these intoxications as well as dysfunction of specific organ systems complicating them are discussed in greater detail in separate chapters (7, Acute Respiratory Failure; 8, Management of Acute Fluid and Electrolyte Problems; and 16, Psychiatric Emergencies).

The manifestations of most overdoses and poisonings are very similar: lethargy, coma, seizures, hypoxia, blood volume depletion, respiratory depression, cardiac depression, renal failure, and electrolyte disturbances. Because these complications are common to many other medical emergencies, it is more important to establish that one is dealing with an intoxication than to identify the specific drug or toxin.

Diagnosis sometimes is easy because a patient may tell a friend or the physician that he has taken an overdose, and he may even say what drug or poison he has taken. Other patients may be reluctant to admit what they have done and instead offer only vague complaints of abdominal pain, behave strangely, or evidence metabolic disturbances. Other patients may be acutely confused, agitated, or stuporous, and may be having seizures or be in coma. In all of these patients showing such clinical states, drug toxicity and poisoning should be considered as part of the differential diagnosis.

Patients who have taken an unknown quantity of medicine in the presence of a family member in order to attract attention frequently dramatize and tend to overestimate the amount they have ingested. On the other hand, patients who try to minimize what they have done may have taken much larger quantities than they are willing to admit.

To assist in the diagnosis, one should question family members or friends who accompanied the patient or the ambulance service which brought the patient to the accident floor. Were there any empty medicine bottles or containers of commercial products found with the patient? Is the patient currently under the care of a physician, and has he prescribed any medications? Has the patient ever taken an overdose or poisoned himself before? Does the patient have evidence of old scars from previous suicide attempts or signs of intravenous injections?

Once a diagnosis of drug overdose or poisoning has been established, the physician should immediately institute the following sequence:

(1) provide general supportive care, (2) estimate severity, (3) prevent further absorption of ingested material, and (4) initiate removal of absorbed toxin. To spend time searching for a specific drug and its antidote, and thus delay basic supportive measures, is an error. *There are very few specific antidotes.* One needs to recognize that most morbidity and mortality from drug overdosage are due to excitation or depression of the central nervous system with depression or loss of normal reflexes (e.g., gag reflex), depression of respiratory drive, cardiac arrhythmias, and loss of vascular tone. Individually, or in combination, these may result in aspiration of gastric contents, respiratory failure, and cardiovascular collapse. Thus, the essence of managing a patient with an overdose or ingestion is to anticipate and prevent these complications. By observing a few basic principles, modified by special maneuvers (e.g., alkalinizing the urine, peritoneal dialysis, or hemodialysis) for special overdoses, most morbidity and mortality from *all* overdosage or ingestion can be avoided.

GENERAL PRINCIPLES OF MANAGEMENT

SUPPORTIVE CARE

1. *Evaluate carefully but speedily the status of the cardiovascular, respiratory, and central nervous systems.* A large-bore (no. 18 or no. 19) intravenous catheter should be installed and firmly secured. Because acute thiamine deficiency and hypoglycemia can mimic many intoxications, all stuporous, comatose, or hypotensive patients should receive immediately (1) thiamine, 50 mg I.V., (2) glucose, 50 to 100 ml of 50% solution I.V. In addition, patients with pinpoint pupils, hypoventilation, and depressed mental status should be treated with naloxone, 0.4 to 1.2 mg I.V. because of a possible narcotic overdose. Naloxone will not cause respiratory depression or interfere with a toxicology screen.

2. *Establish the rate, depth, and pattern of the patient's respirations.* Is the patient able to maintain adequate ventilation on his own? If he is breathing slowly (less than 10 times/min), with shallow respirations, an endotracheal tube should be inserted and connected to humidified compressed air, or 24% oxygen (i.e., use T-tube adaptor). However, the rate of breathing per se is not a very reliable index of adequate ventilation, because slow rates may be associated with either hypo- or hyperventilation. Studies of arterial blood gases, particularly the Pa_{CO_2}, drawn on room air will help define the situation. Hypercapnia indicates that the patient is unable to maintain adequate gas exchange with this means, and a mechanically assisted ventilator (preferably a patient-triggered volume respirator with a control to take over if the patient stops breathing) will be necessary. Patients with severe glutethimide overdose, characterized by fluctuating levels of consciousness and sudden apnea, should be managed only with a mechanical respirator which will automatically breathe for the patient if he becomes apneic.

The level of consciousness must be determined. If the patient is comatose, stuporous, drowsy, or has a depressed gag reflex, an endotracheal tube should be placed to keep his airway patent and prevent aspiration. The decision to intubate because of the patient's depressed mental status should be made without reference to his respiratory status. However, the usual situation is that a drowsy or stuporous patient also has poor ventilation. If intubation is done for neurological reasons, a T-tube adaptor is all that is necessary.

3. *Stabilize the circulation.* Exposure to toxic substances can result in two types of circulatory disturbances: (1) faulty vasomotor tone or altered capillary permeability, and (2) depressed cardiac output. Both of these disorders are manifested as clinical hypotension.

Faulty vasomotor tone results from depression of vasomotor centers of the brain stem and usually occurs in association with generalized central nervous system depressants (e.g., barbiturates, glutethimide, ethanol). This category of hypotension is best treated by expanding the intravascular space with intravenous saline solution (1,000 ml normal saline solution with 20 mEq KCl). If the systolic blood pressure does not stabilize at 90 mHg after 500 to 1,000 ml of this fluid has been given in 30 minutes, one should add levarterenol (2 ml or 4 mg/liter of saline solution) and administer at a rate sufficient to stabilize the systolic pressure at 90 to 100 mHg. Epinephrine should not be used to restore the blood pressure in patients with overdoses, because it will worsen the hypotension associated with ingestion of phenothiazines and tricyclic antidepressants. In large doses, dopamine may produce the same paradoxical hypotension, and thus should be avoided.

Patients who are hypotensive because of loss of intra- or extravascular fluid (i.e., blood loss, diarrhea, vomiting, and leakage of plasma into lungs, serous cavities, or gastrointestinal tract) should be treated by volume expansion. They may not be hypotensive when lying flat, but will become so when caused to sit up or stand. To avoid the risk of hepatitis, one should not give whole blood or fresh frozen plasma unless the patient is actively hemorrhaging. Instead, mannitol or dextran should be given in conjunction with normal saline solution. Vasopressor drugs usually are not necessary except in the very late stages of this type of shock.

Some patients are hypotensive because of suppression of cardiac contractility (e.g., from diphenylhydantoin) rather than altered vascular tone or loss of intravascular volume. Before administering fluids to hypotensive patients, one must determine if the hypotension is due to low cardiac output. These patients may be in congestive heart failure as well as hypotensive and require treatment for heart failure by removal of intravascular volume to restore blood pressure.

Elderly patients and those whose cardiovascular status is unknown should have their central venous pressure monitored while large volumes of saline are infused rapidly.

4. *Position the patient.* If the patient is alert with intact gag reflex, and properly oriented, he should be positioned in a semierect posture. On the other hand, if he has any of the following: (1) stupor, (2) coma, (3) disorientation, or (4) depressed gag reflex, and it is decided not to use endotracheal intubation, he should be placed in the Sims' (semi-prone) position with his left side down, right knee and thigh drawn up under him, and left arm along his back. A "reversed" Trendelenburg's position with the patient prone and his head lowered 30 to 40 degrees

below his hips is also acceptable. Both of these positions minimize the chance of aspirating oral secretions.

5. *Diagnose and correct any electrolyte disturbance.* Respiratory acidosis (elevated P_{CO_2}, low P_{O_2}, low pH, and normal serum HCO_3^-) and metabolic acidosis (low P_{CO_2}, normal or elevated P_{O_2}, low pH, and low serum HCO_3^-) are the most frequently encountered acid-base disturbances requiring specific treatment. Primary respiratory alkalosis (low P_{CO_2}, elevated pH, normal or elevated P_{O_2}, and normal serum HCO_3^-) is occasionally seen, particularly with ingestion of salicylates, but it almost never requires treatment. Serum electrolytes should be monitored carefully when osmotic or alkaline diuresis is used, because large quantities of Na^+, K^+, and Ca^{++} can be removed by these therapies. Refer to Chapter 8, Management of Acute Fluid and Electrolyte Problems, for detailed discussion of these problems.

6. *Treat generalized convulsions.* These should be treated by giving 1,000 to 1,200 mg of diphenylhydantoin intravenously slowly over 20 to 30 minutes. This should be administered by a 250 mg bolus injected intravenously over 5 minutes and repeated four times. It should not be given with 5% dextrose in water (D/W) infusing, because this will cause the diphenylhydantoin to precipitate. Drugs which suppress the central nervous system—barbiturates and diazepam—should *never* be used initially in cases of overdose, because they are likely to sedate further a patient who already has an altered mental status. If use of Dilantin does not control the seizures, and they are judged to be a risk for the patient (compromised respiration, aspiration, metabolic acidosis, hyperthermia), the patient should be paralyzed with pancuronium (Pavulon), 0.04 to 0.1 mg/kg, or diazepam, 5 to 10 mg I.V. Simultaneously, he should undergo endotracheal intubation, and his respiration should be controlled on a volume respirator.

7. *Obtain laboratory tests.* The initial laboratory tests will be determined by the severity of the clinical situation. However, in all patients suspected of having an overdose or poisoning one or two large tubes of clotted blood and a urine specimen (preferably before diuresis has been started) should be obtained and sent for qualitative and quantitative toxicological examination. In patients with metabolic acidosis the urine sediment should be examined for oxalate crystals (ethylene glycol is metabolized to oxalic acid) and a ferric chloride test performed (several drops of 10% solution of $FeCl_3$ to urine turn violet or purple in presence of salicylic acid). If the patient is alert or only minimally sedated or agitated (and appears to be improving), further blood tests may not be needed. On the other hand, if the patient is considered to have a serious overdose, emergency determination of electrolytes, blood sugar, urea, and arterial blood gases (on room air) should be obtained.

ESTIMATING THE DEGREE OF INTOXICATION

1. *Attempt to judge the severity of an overdose or poisoning.* This is one of the most difficult aspects of managing an overdosed patient, but it is crucial. This estimate, based on clinical assessment of the patient, will have to be made and acted upon before the results of any toxicologic

tests are available. Obviously, if the patient's neurological status or vital signs are severely altered, the estimate is easy. However, if the patient is only moderately somnolent or agitated and his vital signs are "acceptable," the physician must decide if he will improve or may possibly develop more serious manifestations of his overdose. One should try to determine how long ago the ingestion occurred, how many pills were taken, and whether the patient vomited after the overdose. A rapid physical examination should be done to establish baseline values of vital signs: skin color and temperature; mental status, muscle tone, deep tendon reflexes, and abnormal movements; pupils, fundi, extraocular movements; cardiovascular status; lungs; and abdomen. In performing this examination one should be alert for physical signs which may suggest specific toxins. Some of the more important signs are listed in Table 1-1.

Table 1-2 shows a classification scheme developed for patients with barbiturate poisoning [1], but it is applicable for any overdose from a

TABLE 1-1 Physical Signs Suggesting Various Toxins

Physical Signs or Symptoms	Toxins To Be Considered
Vomiting, nausea, diarrhea	Heavy metals (lead, arsenic); alcohols (ethanol, methanol, ethylene glycol); salicylates; digitalis; morphine and its analogs
Coma	Barbiturates; chloral hydrate; paraldehyde; bromide; ethchlorvynol; carbon monoxide; salicylates; atropine; scopolamine; ethanol
Delirium, agitation	Atropine; scopolamine; alcohol; amphetamine; barbiturates; physostigmine
Convulsions	Phenothiazines; strychnine; propoxyphene; amphetamines; alcohols (ethanol, methanol, ethylene glycol); salicylates; carbon monoxide; cholinesterase inhibitors; hydrocarbons
Dilated pupils	Amphetamines; glutethimide; alcohols; belladonna group; meperidine; cocaine; ephedrine; sympathomimetics; parasympatholytics; cyanide; botulin toxin
Constricted pupils	Morphine; propoxyphene; barbiturates; chloral hydrate
Partial or total blindness	Methanol
Pink skin	Carbon monoxide; cyanide; atropine (skin flushed and dry); phenothiazine
Kussmaul respiration	Salicylates; methanol; ethanol; ethylene glycol
Dry mouth	Belladonna group; botulin toxin; antihistamines; morphine; phenothiazines; tricyclic antidepressants
Hematemesis	Mercuric chloride; salicylates; phosphorus; fluoride
Diaphoresis	Alcohol; insulin; fluoride; salicylates; physostigmine
Extrapyramidal tremor	Phenothiazines

TABLE 1-2 Classification of Effects of Central Nervous System Depressants

Class	Characteristics
0	Asleep, but can be aroused and can answer questions
I	Comatose, but will withdraw from painful stimuli; reflexes intact
II	Comatose; does not withdraw from painful stimuli; no respiratory or circulatory depression. Most reflexes intact
III	Comatose; most or all reflexes absent, but without depression of respiration or circulation
IV	Comatose, reflexes absent. Respiratory depression with cyanosis or circulatory failure and shock, or both

Modified from Reed, Driggs, and Foote [1].

central nervous system depressant. As one might expect, patients in classes III and IV have the highest mortality rates.

Interpretation of toxicologic reports is difficult. Because of the large variation in individual susceptibility, such reports are more important in establishing the presence of a toxin than in predicting the severity of the intoxication. The latter is more accurately determined by repeated clinical assessment of the patient. Furthermore, many patients ingest more than one toxin, and they may be synergistic. Patients who abuse drugs may develop tolerance to them so that their response to the drug is altered. This is particularly true of narcotics and amphetamines. Long-term use of alcohol, barbiturates, and glutethimide also produces tolerance and lessens the correlation of the blood level with the extent of toxicity. Table 1-3 lists toxic and lethal levels for major toxins.

2. *Observe all clinical signs carefully.* Careful clinical observation is the most crucial aspect of supportive care and the best means of evaluating the severity of the overdose. The patient should be under constant observation. Serial measurements of blood pressure, pulse, and respiration, and observation of lungs, pupils, mental status, and neurological reflexes should be made and recorded on a flow chart by the same observer at 15- to 30-minute intervals. This type of clinical monitoring is essential to evaluate the progress of the intoxication, response to therapy, and the necessity for additional therapy.

Once support of the patient's vital systems has been established (or if the patient is asymptomatic with stable vital signs initially), attention can be directed to reducing the quantity of drug which the patient has in his body. The methods of accomplishing this are: (1) gastric emptying to prevent further absorption, and (2) increasing the rate of excretion to reduce the toxic level. One must recognize that these measures are adjuncts to basic support and at no time should they receive more attention than conscientious supportive care.

PREVENTION OF FURTHER ABSORPTION OF INGESTED MATERIAL

REMOVAL OF GASTRIC CONTENTS Further absorption of the ingested drug may be terminated by inducing vomiting or by gastric lavage. This

TABLE 1-3 Toxic and Lethal Blood Levels for Major Toxins

Compound	Toxic Level (mg/100 ml)	Lethal Level (mg/100 ml)
Amitriptyline	0.04	0.5–2.0
Amphetamine	>0.01	0.05–0.2*
Barbiturates		
Short-acting	0.7	1–3†
Intermediate	1–3	3–5†
Phenobarbitol	4–6	8–15†
Barbitol	6–8	10
Chlordiazepoxide	0.55	2–3
Chlorpromazine	0.1–0.2	0.3–1.2
Diazepam	0.5–2	2
Ethanol	150	400
Ethchlorvynol	2	10–15
Ethylene glycol	150	200–400
Glutethimide	1–8	3–10*
Imipramine	0.06	0.2–0.4
Meperidine	0.2	0.5–3*
Meprobamate		5–20†
Methadone		0.1–0.4
Methanol	20	89
Methaqualone	1–3	2–3
Morphine	—	0.05–0.4*
Paraldehyde	20–40	50
Propoxyphene	0.1	0.1–3‡
Salicylate‡	6 hr: 50	90–120
	12 hr: 40	70–100§
	24 hr: 25	50–65§
	48 hr: 10	20–30§

* Higher figure is for tolerant users.
† Lower figure applies in presence of alcohol.
‡ All levels given are for single acute ingestion.
§ Lower figure indicates severe poisoning, higher figure almost certain lethality.
Source: Modified from Done, A. K. *Emergency Medicine.* May, 1975. Pp. 193–201.

should be done without delay except for emergency supportive measures. Fortunately, most toxins provoke vomiting spontaneously. However, when there is a doubtful history, emesis should be induced if there are no contraindications. The absolute contraindications for inducing vomiting are: (1) stupor or coma, (2) evidence of ingestion of caustic alkalis, corrosive acids, petroleum distillates, and strychnine (once hyperexcitability has occurred). The length of time after ingestion beyond which gastric emptying will be of little benefit has not been determined. However, small but probably insignificant quantities of barbiturates can be recovered from gastric contents 4 hours after ingestion [2]. The same is probably true of salicylates. Hence, a conservative estimate is that 6 hours after the ingestion, gastric emptying is ineffective.

To induce vomiting with syrup of ipecac (10 to 15 ml followed by 1 or 2 glasses of warm water) is easy and entails minimal risk to the patient. It produces vomiting in about 60% of patients in 15 minutes and in about 90% of them within 30 minutes [3]. Vomiting is a normal neuro-logical reflex and as such produces emptying of most of the stomach con-tents. The vomitus frequently consists of both duodenal and gastric contents. Ipecac is particularly effective when the stomach contains particulate matter such as capsules or food which cannot be removed by a nasogastric tube. In salicylate poisoning, induced vomiting has been shown to be more effective in emptying stomach than gastric lavage [4].

The disadvantage of ipecac is the delay in onset of emesis. During this time, the patient's level of consciousness may change from alert to stu-porous, and thus he may be at risk of aspirating when he vomits. Thus, after administering ipecac, one must carefully observe the patient until he has finished vomiting in order to prevent complications. The patient should be placed in the Sims' position after the emetic is given. If his level of consciousness decreases before he vomits, the stomach should be emptied via a nasogastric tube. Last, if ipecac does not result in vom-iting, it must be removed, for it is a gastric irritant and when absorbed is a myocardial toxin (causing arrhythmias and myocarditis). Despite these drawbacks, ipecac is the recommended method for gastric empty-ing (except where specifically contraindicated) for all ingestions occur-ring 5 to 6 hours before arrival of the patient on the accident floor.

GASTRIC LAVAGE This treatment should be reserved for patients in whom vomiting cannot be induced or is contraindicated. The major advantage of lavage is that results are obtained immediately. However, it is very uncomfortable to the patient, and one may seriously traumatize him as well as cause him to aspirate during the procedure. Placing a nasogastric tube in the oropharynx has been reported to induce apnea. Furthermore, lavaging does not completely empty the stomach, and in fact, the vol-ume of fluid used may actually force the drug beyond the pylorus.

PREFERENCE FOR GASTRIC LAVAGE The two circumstances for which gastric lavage is preferred to induced vomiting are: (1) depressed central nervous system, (2) ingestion of large quantities of petroleum distillates.

DEPRESSED CENTRAL NERVOUS SYSTEM Patients who are stuporous or comatose, or who have a suppressed gag reflex, are unable to protect their airway via the normal reflex. The airway must be protected with an en-dotracheal tube *before* the stomach is mechanically emptied. After the endotracheal tube has been placed, the nasogastric tube can easily and safely be inserted.

LARGE QUANTITIES OF PETROLEUM DISTILLATES Although a person (most often an infant) will usually take only one swallow of kerosene or similar substance, sometimes large amounts are ingested. It is dan-gerous to allow such quantities to remain in the stomach because they will become absorbed, with resultant depression of central nervous sys-tem and heart. Vomiting may also occur, with pulmonary aspiration of the hydrocarbons, resulting in acute, fulminating, hemorrhagic broncho-pneumonia. Hence, if the amount ingested is unknown, the risk of gas-tric lavage must be weighed against leaving the material in the stomach.

Some authorities recommend cautious lavage, whereas others believe that the outcome of petroleum product ingestion is more related to vomiting than to leaving material in the stomach [5].

In most instances, the specific composition of lavage fluid is of less importance than its volume. Table 1-4 gives a list of several antidotes which can be employed as lavaging fluids. Although this is not a complete list, it illustrates the point that gastric lavage should not be delayed in an attempt to locate the "proper" fluid. One should use large quantities of tap water or normal saline solution, making sure that the return is equal to what is put into the stomach.

ACTIVATED CHARCOAL This substance is a rapidly effective absorbent with a broad spectrum of activity. It is essentially capable of binding, and hence inactivating, all organic and inorganic chemicals, with the exception of cyanide. Its absorptive potency is not significantly affected by the acidity or alkalinity of the chemical. Although the pH range of the gastrointestinal tract does not seem to influence the permanency of the chemical inactivation, it is recommended that the charcoal and its attached poison be removed from the stomach as soon as possible, rather than be passed per rectum.

The customary dose of activated charcoal for children and adults is 10 gm of a powder stirred into enough water to produce a thick slurry. It should not be used simultaneously with ipecac because it effectively binds and inactivates the emetic. Hence its use is essentially limited to the cases in which gastric lavage is indicated. In such cases, it becomes the initial lavage fluid and is subsequently replaced by tap water or normal saline solution. Table 1-5 shows the approximate amount of substance absorbed by 1 gm of activated charcoal.

TABLE 1-4 Composition of Antidote as Lavage Fluid

Antidote	Dose (gm/1,000 ml H_2O)	Poison*	Complications
Tannic acid	30–50	Strychnine, quinine, lead, silver	Hepatotoxin
Potassium permanganate	0.1	Strychnine, nicotine, physostigmine, quinine	Strong irritant; undissolved particles may cause gastric erosion
Sodium bicarbonate	50 (5% solution)	$FeSO_4$	Gastric distension; possible gastric perforation if wall partially eroded
Magnesium oxide Magnesium hydroxide	25	Acetylsalicylic acid, H_2SO_4, oxalic acid	CNS depression if excessive amounts allowed to remain in stomach

* Partial list; includes only those poisons occurring with significant frequency.

TABLE 1-5 Amount of Substance Removed by 1 Gram of Activated Charcoal

Substance	Maximum Absorption (mg)
Mercuric chloride	1,800
Sulfanilamide	1,000
Strychnine nitrate	950
Morphine hydrochloride	800
Atropine sulfate	700
Nicotine	700
Salicylic acid	550
Phenol	400
Phenobarbital	350
Alcohol	300

Source: Anderson, A. H. *Acta Pharmacol. Toxicol.* 2:69, 1946.

ENHANCING EXCRETION OF ABSORBED MATERIAL

Increasing the rate of excretion of the drug, and thus reducing the duration of toxicity, may be accomplished by (1) forced water or osmotic diuresis, (2) alkalinizing the urine to decrease tubular reabsorption by increasing the fraction of the drug remaining in the ionized form in the renal tubular fluid, and (3) peritoneal dialysis or hemodialysis. Each of these measures has possible serious complications (e.g., fluid overload, electrolyte disturbances) and thus they should be used only in those circumstances for which their benefit is clearly greater than their risk.

FORCED DIURESIS Only those drugs which are excreted unchanged in the urine will be affected by increasing the rate of glomerular filtration (water diuresis) or by preventing passive solute reabsorption in the proximal tubules (osmotic diuresis).

1. Water diuresis exerts its principal effect by increasing volume and flow in all segments of the nephron. However, it has no effect on passive solute resorption, which occurs in the proximal tubules and is the major mechanism of tubular resorption of toxic materials. Although water diuresis may increase renal clearance of some materials, its effect on most toxins is minimal. In barbiturate poisoning, frequently diuresis may not be produced by water alone because of the drug's stimulation of antidiuretic hormone. Renal clearance of salicylates is not increased by increasing glomerular filtration rate with water diuresis.

2. Osmotic diuresis increases the excretion of some toxins by reducing passive solute resorption, and hence water resorption, in the proximal tubule. This prevents the tubular concentration of the toxin and its inactive resorption (from an area of higher to lower concentration) which would follow.

Of the drugs involved in intoxication only salicylates, barbiturates, methanol, and ethchlorvynol (Placidyl) have been shown to have an increased rate of removal during an osmotic diuresis with glucose, urea, or mannitol. This response has been reasonably well documented for long-acting barbiturates (phenobarbital and barbital) but is equivocal for short-acting barbiturates (secobarbital and pentobarbital). However, the clinical studies which suggest that osmotic diuresis can reduce by one-third the duration of coma from long-acting barbiturates were performed in conjunction with alkalinization of the urine [6, 7]. Thus, it is not possible to discern the individual benefits of these therapies. The rate of decline of the plasma level for short-acting barbiturates is about 4.5%/hr with, and 4.0%/hr without, forced diuresis [8]. This demonstrates that although the renal clearance of short-acting barbiturates can be increased significantly with osmotic diuresis, this increased excretion is clinically insignificant when compared to the total amount of barbiturate in the body and is insufficient to alter the length of coma, which is more related to the rate of hepatic metabolism of these barbiturates.

Opinions vary concerning the role of forced diuresis in the treatment of salicylate poisoning. Some feel that it is of limited value by itself and can find no physiological explanation why it should be effective when water diuresis is not [4, 9]. Others believe that forced diuresis will increase renal clearance of free salicylate and reduce the half-life from 20 to 24 hours to 12 hours. They feel that osmotic diuresis should be used when dialysis is not readily accessible [10].

In practice, osmotic diuresis has a clinically significant role in the management of overdoses from long-acting barbiturates, salicylates, methanol, and ethchlorvynol. Infusion should be employed in these types of intoxication as long as there are no contraindications such as cardiac, renal, or pulmonary insufficiency. Great care should be taken to avoid complications of fluid overload and electrolyte disturbance, particularly hypokalemia. One should be particularly cautious in using osmotic diuresis in any patient over the age of 40 years because of the possibility of asymptomatic heart disease.

PROTOCOL FOR OSMOTIC DIURESIS To increase the excretion of drugs by osmotic diuresis:

1. Replace any fluid deficit and stabilize cardiovascular system
2. Place indwelling Foley catheter in bladder
3. Give a primary dose of 0.5 gm/kg body weight of 25% mannitol
4. Give maintenance infusion of 1.25 to 2.5% mannitol in 5% dextrose in water solution with 40 mEq KCl/liter alternating similar concentration of mannitol in normal saline solution with 40 mEq of KCl at 500 ml/hr
5. Adjust infusion rate to produce urine output of 6 to 8 ml/min

Despite the excellent results achieved with conservative management alone, osmotic diuresis is capable of reducing the duration of coma, and thus its complications, in patients poisoned with long-acting barbiturates. This is particularly important when constant observation and supportive care are not available (i.e., a medical ward rather than an intensive care unit), and in those patients who have a class II or greater

phenobarbital or ethchlorvynol intoxication and are likely to have prolonged coma of 5 to 7 days.

ALKALINE DIURESIS An alkaline urine facilitates the excretion of those
chemicals whose pKa (the pH at which the ionized fraction equals the
nonionized fraction) is below 8.0, which is the physiologic upper limit
of urinary pH. Alkalinization of the tubular fluid enhances excretion of
such compounds by increasing its ionized fraction, which is impermeable
to the lipid cellular membrane of the renal tubule cells. This concept is
depicted in Figure 1-1.

With respect to drug overdoses, this concept is clinically applicable
to intoxication from long-acting barbiturates and salicylates. Phenobarbital has a pKa of 7.24, and barbital has a pKa of 7.8. Pentobarbital and
secobarbital, the short-acting barbiturates, have pKa of 7.96 and 7.90, respectively, which fall outside the maximum urinary pH, and their excretion cannot be clinically affected by attempts to alkalinize the urine.

Salicylic acid has a pKa of 3.0, and its excretion is increased in an alkaline urine. When the urine pH is below 6.0, renal clearance of salicylates is 5 to 15 ml/min and their half-life (t½) is about 20 to 24 hours.
Osmotic diuresis can reduce half-life to 12 hours [10]. With an alkaline
urine flowing at 6 to 8 ml/min, salicylate clearance will be in the range of
30 to 50 ml/min, and the half-life reduced to 6 to 8 hours [11, 12]. However, most adults with salicylate poisoning will have a primary respiratory alkalosis, and administering alkali to these patients is considered to
be harmful [4]. Nevertheless, some patients have been successfully
treated with alkalinization of the urine without serious complications
[11]. Although acetazolamide has been used to rapidly alkalinize the
urine, it causes systemic acidosis, which favors the intracellular movement of salicylates. This drug leads to a notable increase in mortality in
salicylate-poisoned experimental animals, and some believe it to be dangerous in treating patients [9]. In children, who usually have a metabolic
acidosis with salicylate ingestion, it is not possible to administer sufficient
quantities of alkali to raise the urinary pH. Because of the inherent dangers and alternate methods of accelerating excretion, alkalinization of
the urine with lactate, bicarbonate, or acetazolamide is not recommended in treating salicylate poisoning.

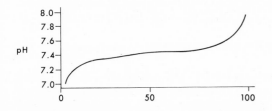

FIGURE 1-1   Titration curve of weak acid against base.

Glutethimide has a pKa of 11.0, so that its excretion is not influenced by alkalinization of the urine. Finally, ethchlorvynol is unaffected, because it is a neutral molecule and does not ionize. Thus, *attempts to alkalinize the urine should be used only for patients with known phenobarbital intoxication.*

DIALYSIS

For a toxin to be removed by dialysis, it must have certain qualities. Its molecule must be small enough to diffuse through the dialyzing membrane, be it peritoneum or cellophane, and approach equilibrium at a reasonable rate. It must be distributed in the body water in a freely diffusable, or readily dissociable, form. The normal mechanisms for its metabolism and inactivation must be sufficiently slow so that dialysis will significantly contribute to its elimination. In general, peritoneal dialysis is only ⅛ to ¼ as efficient as hemodialysis. Furthermore, because the delivery of the toxin to the peritoneal surface is dependent on blood flow, the efficiency of peritoneal dialysis is significantly reduced in hypotensive patients. Thus, peritoneal dialysis should be used only when hemodialysis is not immediately practical. There are many drugs which fulfill these criteria and which are known to be dialyzable across the peritoneum or the blood. Table 1-6 lists those drugs of major clinical importance.

The fact that a drug is dialyzable is not an automatic indication for dialysis in all intoxicated patients. Most patients will recover completely if attentive, supportive care is maintained until they regain full consciousness. Special procedures, such as dialysis, have their own morbidity and mortality rates, and in an overdosed patient they may distract from or interfere with essential supportive measures [14]. Table 1-7 lists several considerations which should figure in the decision to institute emergency dialysis. Table 1-8 compares the effectiveness of various

TABLE 1-6 Dialyzable Poisons of Major Clinical Importance

Barbiturates
   Long-acting
   Intermediate-acting
   Short-acting

Glutethimide

Depressants, Sedatives, and Tranquilizers
   Ethchlorvynol (Placidyl)

Alcohols
   Ethanol
   Methanol
   Ethylene glycol

Analgesics
   Acetylsalicylic acid

Modified from Krepshield, J. H., et al. *Trans. Am. Soc. Artif. Intern. Organs* 19: 590–633, 1973.

TABLE 1-7 Clinical Guidelines for Emergency Dialysis

1. Severe clinical intoxication with abnormal or widely fluctuating vital signs, including hypotension or hypertension despite appropriate therapy, apnea, severe hypothermia or hyperthermia, or any combination of these.
2. An underlying disease compromising the function of an organ with a major role in metabolism and excretion of the particular drug. Essentially this will include chronic hepatic and renal disease.
3. A significant quantity of a circulating chemical whose metabolites are of equal or greater toxicity than the parent compound. Major examples are the conversion of methanol to formaldehyde and ethylene glycol to oxalic acid.
4. Progressive clinical deterioration despite aggressive supportive care.
5. The presence of an underlying disease which adds significant co-morbidity to the hazards of coma. Chronic lung disease would be the most important example.

Modified from Krepshield, et al. *Trans. Am. Soc. Artif. Intern. Organs* 19:590–633, 1973 [13].

methods of accelerating the removal of toxins of major clinical importance.

BARBITURATES Because of their protein-binding and lipid solubility, peritoneal dialysis can only minimally increase the rate of elimination of short-acting barbiturates. This increment (from 12 to 15 mg/hr to 20 to 40 mg/hr) is not sufficient to reduce the duration of coma or improve the condition of the patient clinically [8, 15]. Hemodialysis, however, is capable of removing short-acting barbiturates about 8 to 10 times faster than peritoneal dialysis or osmotic diuresis and has a therapeutic role in the treatment of severe overdoses from these drugs [16, 17].

Excretion of long-acting barbiturates can be accelerated by both methods of dialysis. However, hemodialysis is capable of removing 300 to 400 mg/hr compared to about 90 to 100 mg/hr by peritoneal dialysis [14]. Although patients have been shown to benefit from both types of dialysis, hemodialysis is clearly the procedure of choice for those patients fitting the criteria set out in Table 1-7.

GLUTETHIMIDE (DORIDEN) Peritoneal dialysis is not capable of removing significantly greater amounts of glutethimide than osmotic diuresis or alkalinization of the urine, neither of which seems to be very effective [18]. Hemodialysis can eliminate large quantities of the toxin, and at rates 30 to 200 times faster than by the urine, and 20 times faster than by peritoneal dialysis [19]. Despite these pharmokinetics, the total amount of drug removed by hemodialysis may constitute only 10 to 20% of the total quantity ingested. Whether the removal of this small fraction actually results in falling blood levels, decreased duration of coma, and reduced morbidity is not clear. Some physicians believe that there is a cause and effect relation and that hemodialysis is an important therapeutic modality in treating patients with glutethimide overdoses

TABLE 1-8 Effectiveness of Methods to Increase Removal of Toxins

Drug	Water Diuresis	Osmotic Diuresis	Alkalinization of Urine	Peritoneal Dialysis	Hemodialysis
Barbiturates					
Short-acting	0	0	0	+ (clearance 20–40 mg/hr)	+++ (clearance 150–350 mg/hr)
Long-acting	0	+ (clearance 15 mg/min)	++	++ (clearance 90–100 mg/hr)	++++ (clearance 300–400 mg/hr)
Salicylates	0 ($t\frac{1}{2}$ 20–24 hr)	+ ($t\frac{1}{2}$ 12 hr)	++ ($t\frac{1}{2}$ 6–8 hr)*	+	++++ ($t\frac{1}{2}$ 4–6 hr)
Ethchlorvynol	?	+ (clearance 50–75 mg/hr)	0	+ (clearance 50–75 mg/hr)	+++ (clearance 200–250 mg/hr)
Methanol	0	+ (clearance 5 ml/min)	0	++ (clearance 25 ml/min)	++++ (clearance 125–200 ml/min)
Glutethimide	0	0	0	+	++++ (clearance 150–850 mg/hr)
Ethylene glycol	?	?	0	++	++++
Chlorpromazine	+	+	0	0	0
Meprobamate	+	++	0	++	++++
Tricyclic antidepressants	0	0	0	0	0

* Although capable of increasing excretion of salicylates, alkalinization of the urine is potentially dangerous in these patients unless the patient is undergoing hemodialysis, which will prevent a severe metabolic alkalosis from occurring.

whose blood level is above 3 mg/100 ml, or when the amount ingested is more than 0.15 gm/kg (about 10 gm for a 70-kg person), or when the patient is first seen in profound coma with signs of cerebral or pulmonary edema [13]. The experience of others indicates that hemodialysis does not reduce the length of coma or accelerate the decrease of blood levels, nor does it change the mortality rate. In fact, they suggest that aggressive supporting care alone can reduce the mortality rate to 2 to 3%, so that there is no place for hemodialysis in treating glutethimide intoxication [20].

On balance, the presently available clinical data do not seem to justify a major role for hemodialysis in the management of patients with glutethimide overdoses. It may, however, be of benefit to those patients who fit the criteria set out in Table 1-7.

ETHCHLORVYNOL (PLACIDYL) When peritoneal dialysis has been used in the treatment of ethchlorvynol intoxication, the rate of elimination of the drug is no greater than by an osmotic diuresis through normally functioning kidneys. At most, both of these methods remove no more than 100 mg/hr, whereas the total amount of drug ingested for an overdose is in the range of 15 to 25 gm. Peritoneal dialysis does not have a place in the treatment of such overdoses if urine output can be maintained around 5 to 7 ml/min [21, 22]. However, in the face of renal impairment, and when hemodialysis cannot be performed, peritoneal dialysis would be beneficial.

Hemodialysis, on the other hand, appears to be capable of eliminating clinically significant quantities of this drug. Somewhere between 25 and 40% of the ingested dose can be removed by this method. Furthermore, the rate of removal is 2 to 2.5 times faster than by forced diuresis or peritoneal dialysis [22, 23]. Clearly, hemodialysis is a significant contribution to the management of patients who have consumed more than 10 gm of the drug or who have a serum level above 7.0 mg/100 ml [13].

METHYL ALCOHOL (METHANOL OR WOOD ALCOHOL) Prior to the use of dialysis, severe methanol poisoning had a mortality rate of 20 to 50% [24], and many of the survivors had significant loss of vision. Dialysis, in particular hemodialysis, has greatly reduced the rates of morbidity and mortality. Emergency dialysis is a treatment ideally suited for methanol poisoning for the following reasons: (1) methanol has a small molecule which diffuses well across the peritoneum or a cellophane coil; (2) dialysis removes the primary substrate and prevents its conversion into the toxic metabolites; (3) the toxic metabolites, formic acid and formaldehyde, are also dialyzable; (4) dialysis facilitates the management of metabolic acidosis.

In an untreated patient, methanol slowly disappears from the blood over 48 to 72 hours, depending on the initial concentration. Osmotic diuresis can produce a methanol clearance of about 5 ml/min. Peritoneal dialysis is about four to five times as effective and will raise the clearance to 20 to 25 ml/min. Hemodialysis increases the clearance to 125 to 200 ml/min (depending on the type of coil used), which is about 20 to 25 times more *efficient* than forced diuresis [13, 25, 26]. Because the rate of removal of methanol is critical to the mortality and morbidity of this intoxication, dialysis has an undisputed role in its management.

Although the degree of acidosis determined at presentation correlates with the mortality, the speed of its correction seems to have little influence on the length of coma and visual disturbances. These manifestations are instead related to the rapidity of methanol removal. Both types of dialysis correct the acidosis with equal speed. However, hemodialysis causes a much more abrupt decline in blood methanol levels. This rapid removal of the primary substrate prevents the production of the toxic metabolites and can be shown to result in less morbidity and mortality [27, 28]. Thus the earlier hemodialysis can be started, the sooner methanol is removed, and the better the therapeutic outcome.

ETHYLENE GLYCOL Emergency dialysis, both peritoneal and hemodialysis, have been used successfully in treatment of ethylene glycol poisoning. The immediate mortality rate and chronic renal failure appear to be significantly reduced by dialysis [29]. However, the clinical data are insufficient to compare the relative effectiveness and clearances of hemodialysis and peritoneal dialysis.

Dialysis is effective in this type of poisoning because it (1) facilitates the management of metabolic acidosis; (2) removes ethylene glycol and prevents its metabolism to toxic substrates; (3) removes oxalic acid, thus preventing its deposit in soft tissues, and probably removes glycoaldehyde, glycolate, and glyoxalate; (4) treats renal failure.

SALICYLATES Because 70 to 80% of ingested salicylates are recoverable in the urine, proper renal function is necessary for their elimination. They are slowly excreted in an acid urine and rapidly eliminated in an alkaline urine. However, as mentioned above, alkalinization of urine is not recommended for adults, and is ineffectual in children, with salicylate intoxication.

Peritoneal dialysis has been used effectively in treating salicylate toxicity in adults and children. It is moderately more efficient than the normal kidney and osmotic diuresis, but only ¼ as efficient as hemodialysis. However, if repeated 2 or 3 times, allowing 2 hours for equilibration and with 5% albumin in the dialysate, significant quantities of salicylates can be removed [30]. Peritoneal dialysis with 5% albumin in the dialysate solution is a safe and effective means of removing salicylates when hemodialysis is unavailable [13, 31].

Adult patients who have serum salicylate levels in excess of 100 mg/100 ml should undergo emergency hemodialysis. A salicylate level in this range obtained at any time indicates life-threatening intoxication. Emergency hemodialysis also should be considered in any patient who (1) has a serum level of 90 mg/100 ml; (2) may have taken a second toxin; (3) is clinically deteriorating; (4) has a profound acid-base disturbance; or (5) has rising salicylate levels despite treatment [32].

The rate of salicylate removal by hemodialysis is from 5 to 7 times, and may reach 20 times [33], that of the normal kidney. It is 2 to 5 times more effective than osmotic diuresis and twice as effective as alkaline diuresis [9].

CLINICAL MANIFESTATIONS AND THERAPEUTIC OUTLINE FOR IMPORTANT INTOXICANTS

BARBITURATES

The clinical picture of barbiturate intoxication is one of progressive central nervous system depression. The first symptom is usually drowsiness. Occasionally, patients are confused; and excitement, delirium, and hallucinations are not uncommon. The patient may complain of headache, blurred vision, parathesias, or vertigo. Ataxia and slurred speech can be present. The central nervous system depression progresses through suppression and finally loss of deep reflexes. Response to painful stimuli may cease and the Babinski sign may be elicited. Depression of brain stem function may progress until extraocular movements show the doll's eye sign or are unresponsive to cold-water stimulation. Pupils are usually slightly constricted but remain responsive to light. Brain stem dysfunction is also manifested by suppression of the pontine-medullary respiratory center. Respirations are usually shallow and slowed. Occasionally, the patient may be breathing rapidly, but minute volume is always reduced. Alterations in vasomotor tone lead to a "relative hypovolemia" and hypotension. This hypotension is aggravated by hypoxia from respiratory depression and can progress to cardiovascular collapse.

Most deaths occur in the first 24 to 48 hours as a result of respiratory arrest. Deaths occurring as late as 4 to 5 days after ingestion of poison are usually due to complications of coma or cardiovascular collapse: bronchopneumonia, renal failure, or cerebral edema.

Frequently patients taking an overdose of barbiturates will simultaneously ingest other central nervous system depressants such as ethanol, diazepam, chlordiazepoxide, meprobamate, or tricyclic antidepressants. These have a potentiating effect on barbiturates, and one should be alert to this possibility when the clinical picture is disproportionate to the barbiturate level.

TREATMENT Treatment of barbiturate intoxication includes the following:

1. General supportive care
2. Careful attention to respiratory function; drawing of arterial blood gases
   a. 24 to 28% oxygen mask if P_{CO_2} is less than 40 mHg
   b. Endotracheal intubation if P_{CO_2} is greater than 40 mHg
3. Emptying of stomach if ingestion has occurred within six hours
   a. Ipecac if clinical judgment is that patient will remain alert for 30 to 45 minutes
   b. Gastric lavage, after endotracheal intubation, if patient is stuporous or comatose

4. If ingestion of phenobarbital is suspected, osmotic diuresis (6 to 8 ml/min) with mannitol and alkalinization of urine
5. Hemodialysis if criteria in Table 1-7 are present

GLUTETHIMIDE (DORIDEN)

The clinical picture of glutethimide intoxication is very similar to that of barbiturate intoxication. The major differences are (1) a more protracted coma (average 45 to 55 hours) interrupted by spontaneous variations in the depth of central nervous system depression; (2) dilated and slowly reactive or nonreactive pupils rather than the constricted, reactive pupils which are seen with barbiturate poisoning; and (3) hypotension unresponsive to fluids. Other nonspecific findings are paralytic ileus and bladder atony from anticholinergic activity of glutethimide.

The blood levels correlate poorly with the severity of the intoxication. In fact, some patients awaken from coma with a blood level greater than that initially recorded at the onset of coma [20]. In the past, this has been explained by the protein binding of the drug and its concentration in body fat. However, recent evidence suggests that the degree of central nervous system depression correlates well with an active metabolite (4-hydroxy-2-phenylglutarimide) of glutethimide [34].

TREATMENT The treatment is the same as that outlined for barbiturates, with dialysis reserved for those patients fulfilling the criteria of Table 1-7.

ETHCHLORVYNOL (PLACIDYL)

The clinical picture of ethchlorvynol intoxication is similar to that of other hypnotics and sedatives. It can result in protracted deep coma, hypothermia, hypotension, bradycardia, apnea, and cardiac arrest. The duration of coma appears to correlate well with the initial serum level on a milligram per kilogram basis. Coma from ethchlorvynol not infrequently lasts 5 to 7 days, which is significantly longer than that from barbiturates (around 40 hours) or glutethimide (around 50 hours) [19, 21].

The only finding on initial examination which may be indicative of this drug is the pungent aromatic odor which may be noted on the patient's breath.

TREATMENT The treatment consists of

1. Supportive care with attention to respiratory function and cardiovascular status
2. Maintaining mannitol-induced osmotic diuresis at 6 to 8 ml/min
3. Hemodialysis for patients fulfilling the criteria in Table 1-7

METHYL ALCOHOL (METHANOL OR WOOD ALCOHOL)

Methanol is a common ingredient of cleaning agents, paint and shellac solvents, canned heat, antifreeze, and illegal whiskey. Most frequently, methanol poisoning occurs in patients desperately addicted to ethanol. However, since it is also rapidly absorbed from the skin and lungs, industrial poisonings are also possible.

The metabolites (formic acid and formaldehyde), rather than the substrate, produce the toxicity, and hence the clinical picture begins to be seen 12 to 24 hours after the ingestion has occurred. Formic acid and other organic acids resulting from the uncoupling of oxidative phosphorylation cause a severe metabolic acidosis. Formaldehyde has a direct toxic effect on retinal cells.

The typical first symptoms are visual disturbances (blurred or dim vision or photophobia), minimal to moderate inebriation, headache, and abdominal pain (pancreatitis). Vital signs are usually normal except for some hyperventilation. Examination of the eyes shows dilated, poorly reactive pupils with hyperemic optic discs and retinal edema. Laboratory studies reveal an unexplained metabolic acidosis with appropriate anion gap.

The actual quantity of methyl alcohol which will be fatal or result in loss of vision is poorly established. Three teaspoons (15 ml) have proved fatal in some cases, whereas other patients have survived ingestion of 500 ml. In general, 80 gm of methanol is usually lethal if the patient is untreated, and a blood level of 100 mg/100 ml places the patient at significant risk for permanent loss of vision [24]. The minimal ingestion of 2 teaspoons (10 ml) should be considered toxic. There appears to be a great variation in individual susceptibility. Patients with long-term addiction to ethanol are less sensitive than those not addicted.

Methanol and ethanol are both oxidized by hepatic alcohol dehydrogenase. Because methanol is metabolized at $\frac{1}{5}$ the rate of ethanol, its oxidation can be effectively blocked by competitive inhibition of the enzyme system with ethanol. Equimolar concentrations of ethanol have been shown to completely halt the oxidation of methanol, and ratios as high as 1 : 16 are probably sufficient to accomplish this [25]. Thus, *infusion of ethyl alcohol* at a rate to maintain a blood ethanol level of at least 100 mg/100 ml can prevent the production of toxic metabolites and is a vital part of managing methanol poisoning. This should be initiated as soon as the diagnosis is established. To achieve blood ethanol levels of 100 mg/100 ml, the average 70-kg person will require a loading dose of 50 gm of ethanol I.V. given over one hour, and 10 to 12 gm hourly thereafter. Ethanol does not interfere with hemodialysis of methanol, but the rate of ethanol infusion must be increased to compensate for that removed during dialysis. An alternative method would be to use a hemodialysis fluid with an ethanol concentration of 100 mg/100 ml.

TREATMENT   Management of methanol ingestion should thus include

1. Basic supportive measures
2. Correction of acidosis with bicarbonate
3. Infusion of ethyl alcohol (loading dose of 50 gm I.V. and then 8 to 10 gm hourly to maintain blood level of 100 to 200 mg/100 ml)
4. Emergency dialysis—hemodialysis if available and peritoneal dialysis as a substitute. The minimum degree of toxicity for which dialysis is

indicated is unsettled. However, a blood level of 50 to 100 mg/100 ml is generally accepted as an indication for dialysis

ETHYLENE GLYCOL

Ethylene glycol is a colorless, odorless polyalcohol that occurs in many industrial products: detergents, paints, lacquers, cosmetics, polishes, and pharmaceuticals. It is most commonly known as a deicer and antifreeze. Because of its easy availability and sweet taste, ethylene glycol is a significant cause of poisoning. The lethal dose for adults (when untreated) is about 100 ml, or 1.5 to 2.0 ml/kg.

Ethylene glycol, per se, is nontoxic, but its metabolism yields toxic products. The major pathway for its degradation is as follows:

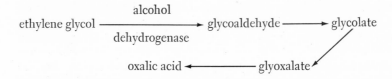

The aldehyde production has been experimentally shown to have a specific depressive effect on the central nervous system. These aldehydes also uncouple oxidative phosphorylation, which results in accumulation of organic acids. Like other alcohols, ethylene glycol metabolism proceeds through hepatic alcohol dehydrogenase. This alters the NADH : NAD ratio in favor of NADH and produces lactic acid [35]. Oxalic acid, although accounting for only 2 to 3% of the metabolism of the parent compound, contributes significantly to the metabolic acidosis. It also has a specific toxic effect on the renal tubular cells [36], and results first in renal failure and later in interstitial nephritis. Glycoaldehyde and other ethylene glycol metabolites may also be nephrotoxic.

The clinical picture of ethylene glycol poisoning has three distinct stages. The first stage has its onset about 6 to 12 hours after ingestion. This correlates well with the maximum concentration of the aldehyde metabolites. Central nervous system depression predominates in the initial stage. A transient exhilaration may occur followed by evidence of alcoholic intoxication progressing to stupor and coma with or without a period of convulsions. Nausea, vomiting, and hematemesis may be present. The second stage is characterized by cardiopulmonary symptoms of rapidly progressive tachypnea, cyanosis, pulmonary edema, and death within one to three days. If the patient survives the first two stages, the renal, or third stage will predominate. Flank pain, costovertebral angle tenderness, and renal dysfunction from proteinuria to anuria occur [35, 37]. In contradistinction to ethanol intoxication, there will be no alcoholic odor on the breath. The fundoscopic exam will *not* show the hyperemic optic discs (although papilledema is occasionally seen) characteristic of methanol poisoning.

Laboratory tests show moderate polymorphonuclear leukocytosis and a normal hematocrit. A severe metabolic acidosis (HCO_3^- 8–10 mEq/liter) with an appropriate anion gap will be present. Hypocalcemia, caused by the chelating effect of oxalic acid, is also frequent. This can produce clinical tetany and cardiac dysfunction. The urine will have a low specific gravity, with proteinuria, microscopic hematuria, pyuria, cylindrinuria, and numerous calcium oxalate crystals.

Because measurements of serum ethylene glycol and oxalic acid are not readily available, these clinical and laboratory findings should lead to the diagnosis of ethylene glycol poisoning, and treatment should be started. Before the use of dialysis, treatment consisted of support and correcting the acidosis with alkali. In about 85% of the severe cases, the patient died of direct central nervous system toxicity or pulmonary edema and the survivors developed chronic renal failure [37]. Emergency dialysis has greatly improved the clinical outcome of this intoxication.

Because ethylene glycol is an alcohol and is degraded by alcohol dehydrogenase, its metabolism can be competitively inhibited by infusion of ethyl alcohol, which has greater affinity for the enzyme. This appears to have a clinical role in ethylene glycol poisoning. If used immediately, ethanol can block the conversion to the toxic metabolites and allow excretion (or removal by dialysis) of the parent compound [29].

TREATMENT Management of ethylene glycol poisoning should include

1. Basic supportive measures
2. Correction of acidosis with bicarbonate
3. Correction of hypocalcemia with calcium gluconate
4. Infusion of ethanol (loading dose of 50 gm I.V. followed by 8 to 10 gm/hr to maintain blood alcohol level of 100 to 200 mg/100 ml)
5. Emergency dialysis—hemodialysis if possible, peritoneal as a substitute. Any patient who has consumed 60 ml in the preceding 48 hours or 15 ml for the preceding 5 days should have dialysis [38]

SALICYLATES

Poisoning from salicylates usually results from ingestion of acetylsalicylate (aspirin) or methylsalicylate (oil of wintergreen). In adults, salicylate ingestion is most often a suicide attempt, whereas in children it is an accident. Although the rate of absorption following oral ingestion varies with the type of aspirin preparation, peak salicylate levels generally are reached in 30 to 90 minutes [9]. Because salicylates have direct toxic effects on the central nervous system, intermediate metabolism, and blood clotting elements, the clinical manifestations occur almost directly following the ingestion. Although it is highly variable, severe toxicity does not occur in a healthy adult if less than 10 to 15 gm (200 to 300 mg/kg) is consumed [4].

Patients with salicylate poisoning initially show central nervous system stimulation in the form of hyperventilation, tinnitus, vomiting, confusion, delirium, bizarre behavior, and occasionally seizures. The late effects on the nervous system are lethargy and coma, followed by cardiovascular collapse or respiratory arrest. The hyperventilation characteristically occurs by increased depth of respiration rather than increased rate.

This is a dose-related phenomenon, occurring in adults and children, and results in a primary respiratory alkalosis. An increased peripheral production of carbon dioxide caused by the uncoupling of oxidative phosphorylation by the salicylates, renal excretion of HCO_3^- with Na^+ and K^+, and an exchange of intracellular H^+ for extracellular K^+ all act to offset the initial respiratory alkalosis. The uncoupling of oxidative phosphorylation also can result in profound hyperthermia, which can produce brain damage and hepatic necrosis. Salicylates also inhibit dehydrogenase and aminotransferase systems, thus causing inorganic acids (acetoacetate, β-hydroxybutyrate, pyruvate, and glutamate) to build up. Because much of the buffering capacity is lost in compensating for the respiratory alkalosis, the accumulation of these organic acids can result in severe metabolic acidosis. Salicylic acid contributes very little directly to this acidosis. Children are most susceptible to this acidosis. Adults appear resistant to this action of salicylates and are rarely seen with a significant metabolic acidosis. However, when adults do become acidotic from salicylates, the prognosis is grave [30].

Salicylates cause clotting dyscrasias by lowering factor VII levels and altering platelet function. By producing a rapid fall in hepatic glycogen and antagonizing the effect of cortisone on liver gluconeogenesis, they can precipitate hypoglycemia.

DIAGNOSIS Although salicylate intoxication should be considered in any patient who is seen with hyperventilation, vomiting, confusion, lethargy, fever, and coma, a serum salicylate level greater than 40 mg/100 ml will confirm the diagnosis. While awaiting the results of this quantitative test, the urine can be screened for the presence of salicylates by mixing a few drops of 10% ferric chloride with a urine sample. The urine turns violet to purple in the presence of salicylates. A false positive test can result from ketonuria, but acidifying and heating the urine will remove the ketones. Phenothiazine gives a more pinkish color.

A random serum salicylate level assists in the diagnosis, but it does not predict the severity of intoxication, which correlates better with the peak salicylate level. Furthermore, the initial salicylate level may not be the highest, and a second level should be obtained about 2 hours later to check for delayed absorption. The peak level and the severity of the intoxication can be calculated from the nomogram in Figure 1-2 by knowing (1) the number of hours since ingestion and (2) the serum salicylate level. Table 1-9 can be used to predict the severity and major symptoms of salicylate intoxication.

TREATMENT Treatment of salicylate poisoning should include

1. General supportive care
2. I.V. fluids to correct water and electrolyte losses
3. Osmotic diuresis with mannitol to achieve urine flow of 6 to 8 ml/min
4. Measurement of serum salicylate level and calculation of peak level (repeat in 2 hours to check for delayed absorption)
5. Dialysis—hemodialysis if possible, peritoneal if not, if

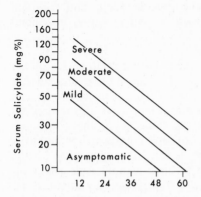

Figure 1-2   Nomogram for estimating the severity of poisoning from the serum salicylate level at varying intervals after ingestion of a single dose. From Done, A. K. *Pediatrics* 26:800–807, 1960.

a. Serum salicylate level is in excess of 100 mg/100 ml
b. Serum salicylate level is 90 mg/100 ml if patient has taken second drug
c. Patient is deteriorating clinically
d. Severe acid-base disturbance is present
e. Salicylate level rises despite therapy

Respiratory alkalosis should not be treated.

PHENOTHIAZINES

Phenothiazines are commonly prescribed drugs and thus are a common overdose. Because of their high therapeutic ratio, intoxication with these drugs rarely results in death. The average daily antipsychotic dose for chlorpromazine (Thorazine) is 300 to 800 mg, whereas the average overdose among 100 patients intoxicated with this drug was 6.25 gm [39]. Despite this wide margin of safety, there was still one death in this series. Because these major tranquilizers potentiate barbiturates, alcohol,

TABLE 1-9 Approximate Limits for Estimating Severity of Salicylate Intoxication

Peak Level (mg/100 ml)	Predicted Degree of Intoxication	Major Symptoms
<50	Not intoxicated	None
50–80	Mild	Mild to moderate hyperpnea
80–100	Moderate	Severe hyperpnea, lethargy, and/or excitability
100	Severe	Severe hyperpnea, coma or semicoma with or without convulsions
>160	Usually lethal	

minor tranquilizers, and narcotics, multiple drug intoxication must be considered when managing a patient with such an overdose.

The initial manifestations of phenothiazine intoxication reflect cortical stimulation. The patient may be confused, agitated, or delirious. The seizure threshold is lowered, and patients may have generalized convulsions. Because of the alpha-adrenergic blocking effect of phenothiazines, severe orthostatic hypotension with a strong reflex tachycardia is part of the initial clinical picture. Extrapyramidal symptoms usually affect the head and neck muscles as an acute dystonic reaction. The patient has involuntary spasms of tongue and mouth leading to difficulty in speaking or swallowing. Contraction of the masseter muscles may prevent the mouth from opening. Facial grimacing is prominent. Effect on the neck muscles leads to opisthotonus or torticollis, either of which may be associated with oculogyric crisis (spasm of external ocular muscles with painful upward gaze). Hyperkinesis with hyperreflexia may also be present. Back and leg muscles may be affected, with a resultant bizarre gait.

The initial stimulated phase may progress to central nervous system depression, with drowsiness, somnolence, and coma. Respiratory depression results from a direct brain stem effect of the phenothiazines. The action of the drug on the hypothalamus causes loss of temperature control. The patient becomes poikilothermic, and usually later shows hypothermia. The initial strong tachycardia compensating for the hypotension gives way to a rapid, weak pulse and more profound hypotension, shock, and cyanosis.

TREATMENT Treatment consists of

1. General supportive care
2. Stabilization of blood pressure with I.V. normal saline solution (do not use epinephrine or dopamine, which will cause further hypotension in face of an alpha blockade)
3. Careful watching for respiratory failure
4. Use of nasogastric suction to remove drug from stomach (inducing emesis is not possible because of the antiemetic action of phenothiazines)
5. Treatment of seizures with I.V. diphenylhydantoin
6. Diphenhydramine (Benadryl), 50 to 100 mg I.V., for acute dystonic reaction
7. Forced diuresis is moderately helpful for chlorpromazine (Thorazine) but not for trifluoperazine (Stelazine)

MINOR TRANQUILIZERS: MEPROBAMATE AND
BENZODIAZEPAM DERIVATIVES

These antianxiety drugs are all less toxic than barbiturates. Nevertheless, meprobamate carries some hazard (about 4 to 5 times less than barbiturates), whereas the benzodiazepam derivatives (chlordiazepoxide and diazepam) are extremely safe. The intoxicating dose for meprobamate ranges between 10 and 40 gm, which is 5 to 10 times the usual daily dose. Doses of 2.25 gm of chlordiazepoxide, 20 to 150 times greater than the daily dose, have been taken without fatality [40]. However, because of the prevalence of their use, these drugs are frequently part of a multiple drug intoxication. Furthermore, they potentiate the depressant effect of barbiturates, alcohol, phenothiazines, and narcotics.

MEPROBAMATE Meprobamate intoxication resembles that with barbiturates, with drowsiness progressing to coma, flaccidity, areflexia, hypotension, hypothermia, bradycardia, and respiratory depression. The most important aspect of meprobamate intoxication is the severe hypotension. A precipitous drop in blood pressure can occur in a patient who is only slightly comatose. Because of the suddenness with which this may occur, it is important not to confuse meprobamate with barbiturate overdose. The drug seems to depress cardiac contractibility, and thus these patients are likely to develop congestive heart failure when large volumes of intravenous fluids are used to raise the blood pressure. The second major problem of meprobamate overdose is a relapse, with coma and shock, about 12 hours after the patient has improved. This may be due to a secondary absorption of the drug from the intestine following restoration of blood pressure. Hence, care must be taken to monitor these patients carefully for 72 hours after the ingestion. Respiratory depression occurs, but it does not influence the prognosis; however, the excessive secretions in the oropharynx and relaxation of the muscles of the pharyngeal wall can lead to significant respiratory complications.

Meprobamate is degraded in the liver and disappears from the blood at about 10%/hr. Thus, the coma is not prolonged and respiratory complications are uncommon.

TREATMENT Treatment of meprobamate intoxication includes

1. General supportive care
2. Stabilization of blood pressure with I.V. saline solution while monitoring for early signs of congestive heart failure with central venous pressure measurements
3. Osmotic diuresis for urine flow of 6 to 8 ml/min
4. Hemodialysis if patient does not improve with this regimen

Because meprobamate is not water soluble and it is rapidly absorbed from the stomach, gastric lavage is minimally helpful. Relapse of coma and hypotension should be watched for.

BENZODIAZEPAM DERIVATIVES Clinically, intoxication with chlordiazepoxide (Librium) and diazepam (Valium) is seen as oversedation and muscle relaxation. Coma and hyporeflexia may occur, but alterations of blood pressure and respiration are rare.

TREATMENT Treatment of chlordiazepoxide or diazepam overdose consists of

1. General supportive measures
2. Emptying the stomach by inducing vomiting if possible. Gastric

lavage is helpful for chlordiazepoxide poisoning but not for diazepam, because the latter drug is not water soluble

TRICYCLIC ANTIDEPRESSANTS: IMIPRAMINE AND AMITRIPTYLINE

Despite their wide margin of safety, tricyclic antidepressants are prescribed for severely depressed patients, who may be determined enough to take a sufficient amount of these drugs to commit suicide. A review of such poisonings showed that of 126 amitriptyline overdoses, 6 were fatal. The average lethal dose was 2.2 gm, which is about 10 to 20 times the average daily dose. The same study reported 14 fatalities among 66 imipramine overdoses, with an average lethal dose of 3.6 gm [41].

The clinical manifestations of such an overdose occur about 1 to 4 hours after ingestion. It is characterized by restlessness, agitation, delirium, twitching, clonic movements, hyperreflexia, and generalized seizures. Simultaneously there is a depressed level of consciousness progressing to stupor, coma, and respiratory depression. The anticholinergic effects of these drugs lead to tachycardia, dilated pupils, bowel and bladder paralysis, and decreased sweating. The inhibition of sweating leads to loss of temperature control and results in hyperpyrexia severe enough to cause hepatic, renal, and neurological damage. Ventricular and atrial cardiac arrhythmias are produced by the atropine-like effect of these drugs. Congestive heart failure and acute myocardial infarction may occur.

These drugs are rapidly detoxified in the liver, so that their toxicity lasts only about 24 hours. No free drug is excreted in the urine, so that neither osmotic diuresis nor dialysis is effective.

TREATMENT Treatment for tricyclic antidepressant overdose includes

1. General supportive measures
2. Monitoring for cardiac arrhythmia. Ventricular premature contractions (VPC) should be treated with I.V. lidocaine. Superventricular tachycardia resulting in hypotension or myocardial ischemia may be treated with physostigmine, 2 mg I.M. or slowly I.V.
3. Treatment of congestive heart failure with digitalis
4. Treatment of hypertension with phentolamine, 5 mg I.V.
5. Control of hypotension with I.V. normal saline solution if central venous pressure is monitored. If this does not work, norepinephrine may be used. Epinephrine will cause further fall in blood pressure, for the same reason it does in phenothiazine intoxication
6. Control hyperthermia with an ice blanket
7. Gastric lavage may be helpful because these drugs delay gastric emptying
8. Physostigmine, 2 mg intramuscularly, may be necessary to control severe agitation or cardiac arrhythmias. The peripheral effects of physostigmine can be reversed by atropine, 0.5 mg

Forced diuresis and hemodialysis are ineffective.

Opioids

Poisoning from opioids (heroin, morphine, meperidine, methadone, and propoxyphene) may result from clinical overdosage, accidental overdosage in addicts, or suicidal attempts. The clinical presentation on the accident floor ranges from mild stupor to profound coma. The triad of coma, pinpoint pupils, and depressed respiration should alert one to a possible overdose of these drugs. Fresh or old needle marks over the forearms or lower legs are supportive evidence for the diagnosis. The respiratory rate is slowed, and the patient may be cyanotic. Blood pressure is maintained until respiratory failure occurs, at which time it falls progressively. Proper oxygenation, if initiated early in the course, frequently will reverse the hypotension. After the patient has been hypoxic for a considerable period, capillary damage occurs and intravenous fluids and vasopressors may be necessary. The pupils are symmetrically constricted to pinpoint size. However, if hypoxia has been present for a sufficient time, the pupils may dilate. There may be hypothermia or hyperthermia, and sinus bradycardias or ventricular arrhythmias can occur.

TREATMENT Patients suspected of having an opioid overdose should be treated initially by stabilizing their pulmonary and cardiovascular systems. Once this is done, they should be given naloxone hydrochloride (Narcan) 0.2 mg to 0.4 mg I.V. If the patient's clinical state is caused by opioids, the respiratory rate and depressed mental function will usually respond to the first dose. If there is no clinical change within 3 to 5 minutes, 0.4 mg of naloxone can be given again and repeated a third time if necessary. If after a total of 1.2 mg of naloxone has been administered the patient has shown no response, one must consider other possibilities to explain the central nervous system depression. Patients who have an opioid overdose may have taken more than one drug and thus have only a partial response to naloxone.

Naloxone, as an opioid antagonist, has a pharmacologic effect for 30 to 120 minutes. If the patient initially responded to the drug, and then slowly shows signs of depressed respiration and mental status, the antagonist should be given again. The narcotic effect of morphine and heroin lasts about 4 to 5 hours. However, the effect of methadone may last for 20 to 24 hours. When administering naloxone, it is important to remember that any dosage of this drug can precipitate narcotic withdrawal symptoms depending on the amount of narcotic taken by the patient. These symptoms include lacrimation, rhinorrhea, yawning, perspiration, restlessness, irritability, gooseflesh, abdominal cramps, and bone pain. Although withdrawal symptoms may occur after naloxone is given, the risk to the patient is much greater from a narcotic overdose than from a narcotic withdrawal, which is rarely, if ever, fatal.

TREATMENT Management of opioid overdose includes

1. Basic supportive measures
2. Administration of oxygen at 3 to 5 liters/min

3. Naloxone given in 0.2-mg increments every 3 to 5 minutes until there is a clinical response or a maximum of 1.2 mg is administered

REFERENCES

1. Reed, C. E., Driggs, M. F., and Foote, C. C. Acute barbiturate intoxication: A study of 300 cases based on a physiological classification of the severity of the intoxication. *Ann. Intern. Med.* 37:290–303, 1952.
2. Hadden, J., Johnson, K., Smith, S., Price, L., and Giardena, E. Acute barbiturate intoxication. Concepts in management. *J.A.M.A.* 209:895–900, 1969.
3. Robertson, W. O. Syrup of ipecac—A slow or fast emetic. *Am. J. Dis. Child.* 103:136–139, 1962.
4. Done, A. K., and Temple, A. R. Treatment of salicylate poisoning. *Mod. Treat.* 8:528–551, 1971.
5. Gleason, M. N., Gosselin, R. R., Hodge, H. C., and Smith, R. P. *Clinical Toxicology of Commercial Products: Acute Poisoning.* Baltimore: Williams & Wilkins, 1969. P. 155.
6. Myschetsky, A., and Lassen, N. A. Urea-induced, osmotic diuresis and alkalinization of urine in acute barbiturate intoxication. *J.A.M.A.* 185:936–942, 1963.
7. Lassen, N. A. Treatment of severe acute barbiturate poisoning by forced diuresis and alkalinization of the urine. *Lancet* 2:338–342, 1960.
8. Bloomer, H. A. Limited usefulness of alkaline diuresis and peritoneal dialysis of pentobarbital intoxication. *N. Engl. J. Med.* 272:1309–1313, 1965.
9. Smith, M. J. H., and Smith, P. K. *The Salicylates: A Critical Bibliographic Review.* New York: Interscience, 1966. P. 279.
10. Lawson, A. H. H., Proudfoot, A. T., Brown, S. S., MacDonald, R. H., Fraser, A. G., Cameron, J. C., and Matthew, H. Forced diuresis in the treatment of acute salicylate poisoning in adults. *Q. J. Med.* 38:31–45, 1969.
11. Morgan, A. G., and Polak, A. The excretion of salicylate in salicylate poisoning. *Clin. Sci.* 41:475–484, 1971.
12. Prowse, K., Pain, M., Marsten, A. D., and Cunning, G. The treatment of salicylate poisoning using mannitol and forced alkaline diuresis. *Clin. Sci.* 38:327–337, 1970.
13. Krepshield, J. H., Schreiner, G. E., Lowenthal, D. T., and Gelfand, M. C. Dialysis of poisons and drugs—Annual review. *Trans. Am. Soc. Artif. Intern. Organs* 19:590–633, 1973.
14. Henderson, L. W., and Merrill, J. P. Treatment of barbiturate intoxication. *Ann. Intern. Med.* 64:876–891, 1966.
15. Berman, L. B., and Vogelsang, P. Removal rates for barbiturates using two types of peritoneal dialysis. *N. Engl. J. Med.* 270:77–80, 1964.
16. Setter, J. G., Maher, J. F., and Schreiner, G. E. Barbiturate intoxication: Evaluation of therapy including dialysis in a large series selectively referred because of severity. *Arch. Intern. Med.* 117:224–236, 1966.
17. Lee, H. A., and Ames, A. C. Hemodialysis in severe barbiturate poisoning. *Br. Med. J.* 1:1217–1219, 1965.
18. DeMyttenaere, M., Schoenfeld, L., and Maher, J. F. Treatment of glutethimide poisoning: A comparison of forced diuresis and dialysis. *J.A.M.A.* 203:885–887, 1968.
19. Maher, J. F., Schreiner, G. E., and Westervelt, F. B. Acute glutethi-

mide intoxication: Clinical experience (twenty-two patients) compared to acute barbiturate intoxication (sixty-three patients). *Am. J. Med.* 33: 70–82, 1962.

20. Chazan, J. A., and Garella, S.   Glutethimide intoxication: A perspective study of 70 patients treated conservatively without hemodialysis. *Arch. Intern. Med.* 128:215–219, 1971.

21. Schultz, J. C., Crowder, D. G., and Medart, W. S.   Excretion studies in ethchlorvynol (Placidyl) intoxication. *Arch. Intern. Med.* 117:409–411, 1966.

22. Teehan, B. P., Maher, J. F., Carey, J. J. H., Flynn, P. D., and Schreiner, G. E.   Acute ethchlorvynol (Placidyl) intoxication. *Ann. Intern. Med.* 72:875–882, 1970.

23. Ogilvie, R. I., Douglas, D. E., Lochead, J. R., Moscovich, M. D., and Kaye, M.   Ethchlorvynol (Placidyl) intoxication and its treatment by hemodialysis. *Can. Med. Assoc. J.* 95:954–956, 1966.

24. Erlanson, P., Fritz, H., Hagstam, K., Lilgenberg, B., Tryding, N., and Voight, G.   Severe methanol intoxication. *Acta Med. Scand.* 177:393–408, 1965.

25. Bennett, I. L., Cary, F. H., Mitchell, G. L., and Cooper, M. N.   Acute methyl alcohol poisoning: A review based on experiences in an outbreak of 323 cases. *Medicine* 32:431–463, 1952.

26. Kane, R. L., Talbert, W., Harlan, J., Sizemore, G., and Cataland, S.   A methanol poisoning outbreak in Kentucky. *Arch. Environ. Health* 17: 119–129, 1968.

27. Setter, J. G., Singh, R., Brachett, N. C., and Randall, R. E.   Studies on the dialysis of methanol. *Trans. Am. Soc. Artif. Intern. Organs* 13: 178–182, 1967.

28. Keyvan-harijarni, H., and Tannenberg, A. M.   Methanol intoxication: Comparison of peritoneal dialysis and hemodialysis treatment. *Arch. Intern. Med.* 134:293–296, 1974.

29. Schreiner, G. E., Maher, J. F., Marc-Aurele, J., Knowlton, D., and Alva, M.   Ethylene glycol: Two indications for hemodialysis. *Trans. Am. Soc. Artif. Intern. Organs.* 5:81–83, 1959.

30. Proudfoot, A. T., and Brown, S. S.   Acidemia and salicylate poisoning in adults. *Br. Med. J.* 2:547–550, 1969.

31. James, J. A., Kimball, L., and Read, W. T.   Experimental salicylate intoxication: 1. Comparison of exchange transfusion, intermittent peritoneal lavage, and hemodialysis as means of removing salicylate. *Pediatrics* 29:442–447, 1962.

32. Locket, S.   Hemodialysis in the treatment of acute poisoning. *Proc. R. Soc. Med.* 63:427–430, 1970.

33. Etteldorf, J. N., Dobbins, W. T., Summitt, R. L., Rainatis, W. T., and Fischer, R. L.   Intermittent peritoneal dialysis using 5% albumin in the treatment of salicylate intoxication in children. *J. Pediatr.* 58:226–236, 1961.

34. Hansen, A. R., Kennedy, K. A., Ambre, J. J., and Fischer, L. J.   Glutethimide poisoning: A metabolite contributes to morbidity and mortality. *N. Engl. J. Med.* 292:250–252, 1975.

35. Parry, M. F., and Wallach, R.   Ethylene glycol poisoning. *Am. J. Med.* 57:143–159, 1974.

36. Jeghers, H., and Murphy, R.   Practical aspects of oxalate metabolism. *N. Engl. J. Med.* 233:208–215, 238–246, 1945.

37. Berman, L. B., Schreiner, G. E., and Feys, J.   The nephrotoxic lesion of ethylene glycol. *Ann. Intern. Med.* 46:611, 1957.

38. Underwood, F., and Bennett, W. M.   Ethylene glycol intoxication:

Prevention of renal failure by aggressive management. *J.A.M.A.* 226: 1453–1454, 1973.

39. David, J. M., Bartlett, E., and Termini, B. P.   Overdosage of psychotropic drugs: A review. I. Major and minor tranquilizers. *Dis. Nerv. Syst.* 29:157–164, 1968.

40. Shader, R. I., and DiMascio, A.   *Psychotropic Drug Side Effects: Clinical and Theoretical Perspectives.* Chapter 22: Acute Poisoning with Psychotropic Drugs. Baltimore: Williams & Wilkins, 1970. Pp. 214–234.

41. Davis, J. M., Bartlett, E., and Termini, B. A.   Overdosage of psychotropic drugs: A review. II. Antidepressants and other psychotropic drugs. *Dis. Nerv. Syst.* 29:246–256, 1968.

NEUROLOGICAL EMERGENCIES

Martin A. Samuels

Metabolic
   Covered in other chapters
      Hypoglycemia and Hyperglycemia
      Hyponatremia and Hypernatremia
      Hypoxia and Hypercarbia
      Hypothyroidism and Hyperthyroidism
      Azotemia
      Hepatic Failure and Portosystemic Encephalopathy
      Hypertensive Encephalopathy
      Drug Overdose, Ingestion, and Withdrawal
   Wernicke's Encephalopathy
   Heat Stroke

EPILEPSY

Epileptic seizures only rarely require emergency treatment. Focal motor seizures, petit mal, and temporal lobe epilepsy are *never* emergencies and should not be treated as such. A great deal of harm can be done by attempting to control these types of seizures with aggressive anticonvulsant therapy. Generalized grand mal status epilepticus is the only type of epilepsy which requires deliberate, relatively rapid therapy on an emergency basis. Even in this situation, termination of the seizure within seconds or minutes is rarely required and should be sought only when the seizure activity has resulted in severe hypoxia or acidosis, which in turn threatens the patient's life. There is no evidence that seizures per se are of any harm to the individual experiencing them.

The diagnosis of grand mal status epilepticus is not a difficult one. The patient presents a picture of tonic and/or clonic movements of all limbs, usually associated with a conjugate deviation of the eyes (though the eyes may rove or show clonic movements in one direction at one moment and in the opposite direction in another). The direction of deviation of the eyes in grand mal status is usually not of lateralizing value in terms of the focus which precipitated the attack. The patient will fail to respond to either auditory or other sensory stimuli during the attack. The motor movements may be continuous, or they may stop intermittently. In the latter case, the patient may respond to stimuli or even follow simple commands, but before he regains total consciousness, another seizure intervenes. Thus, generalized grand mal status epilepticus includes both continuous seizures and seizures which are so frequent that each attack begins before the postictal period of the preceding one ends.

TREATMENT Therapy for grand mal status without life-threatening acidosis or hypoxia is as follows. The patient should be placed in the prone position, preferably with the head down to prevent aspiration of oral contents, until full consciousness is regained. Care should be taken to maintain an adequate airway. This usually can be accomplished with an oral airway, but rarely endotracheal intubation may be required. The patient should be placed in a safe environment with padded bed rails up but should not be restrained, for most intraictal injuries are due to restraint in abnormal postures. Initial blood serum samples should be taken to rule out hypoglycemia, hypocalcemia, and hyponatremia. Glucose, 25 to 50 gm, should be given in every case as an I.V. bolus. In cases secondary to hyponatremia (serum Na usually below 110 mg/100 ml), hypertonic (3%) NaCl should be given until seizure activity ceases. Such patients will usually be very resistant to conventional anticonvulsant therapy. In cases of hypocalcemia, one or two ampules (90 mg of elemental calcium per ampule) of calcium gluconate should be given very slowly intravenously over a 5 to 10 minute period. In cases of unknown etiology in which the suspicion of hypocalcemia is high (i.e., long Q-T interval on ECG or recent history of thyroid or parathyroid surgery), calcium should also be given.

Diphenylhydantoin (Dilantin) is the single most effective anticonvulsant drug, particularly in adults. In addition to having a higher therapeutic index than other anticonvulsants, it has the additional advantage of having very little effect upon the electroencephalogram, and it does not complicate the subsequent evaluation of the seizure disorder. Furthermore, diphenylhydantoin, even in large doses, has little or no effect on levels of consciousness, thus allowing full neurological evaluation once seizures have stopped. Despite earlier controversy, it now seems clear that levels of diphenylhydantoin sodium in the serum correlate with its clinical effectiveness [1]. With a large oral loading dose (1,000 mg), therapeutic levels (10 μg/ml to 15 μg/ml) can be reached in a few hours; and with intravenous administration, (1,000 mg at 50 mg/min), similar levels can be reached within a few minutes [2]. Thus, the initial therapy of grand mal status should be diphenylhydantoin sodium, 1,000 mg intravenously infused at a rate of 50 mg/min. This injection should preferably be given by a physician with monitoring of blood pressure, respiration rate, and electrocardiogram during the injection, for fatalities have occasionally been reported caused by hypotension, heart block, and respiratory depression during excessively rapid diphenylhydantoin injections (greater than 100 mg/min). The injection itself should require 20 minutes, after which the patient should be observed for 20 to 30 minutes, during which time most seizures will slow significantly or stop. If at this time no significant change is noted, phenobarbital should be administered. An initial dose of 90 to 120 mg I.M. may be administered followed by 30 to 60 mg every 15 minutes, to a maximum dose of 240 mg. Respiratory depression is common with barbiturates, and they should be given only when emergency endotracheal intubation is possible. In rare cases, the combination of diphenylhydantoin sodium and a barbiturate fails, requiring the use of a slow intravenous infusion of diazepam (Valium). In large enough doses, this therapy will stop virtually all seizures if only by the induction of coma. In very rare instances, neuromuscular blockade with d-tubocurarine or pancuronium (Pavulon) or general anesthesia has been required to control status epilepticus. An approach to therapy is summarized in Table 2-1.

When the course of grand mal status epilepticus is interrupted at any point by hypoxia or life-threatening acidosis, the seizure activity should be controlled as quickly as possible. The best method of accom-

TABLE 2-1 Treatment of Grand Mal Status Epilepticus

Step	Drug	Dose (mg)	Route	Rate
1	Thiamine	100	I.V.	Rapid (push)
	Glucose	50 gm	I.V.	Rapid (push)
2	Diphenylhydantoin	1,000	I.V.	50 mg/min
3	Phenobarbital	90–120	I.M.	—
4	Phenobarbital	30–60	I.M.	q. 15 min to total dose of 240 mg
5	Diazepam	Usually 5–10	I.V.	Over minutes
6	Pancuronium	4–5	I.V.	Rapid (push)

Note: If the course of treatment is interrupted at any point by life-threatening hypoxia or acidosis, one should proceed immediately to step 5 or 6. A reasonable amount of time should elapse between steps to assess drug action.

plishing this end is to administer diazepam by slow I.V. infusion until motor activity ceases (usually 5 to 10 mg is all that is required). This form of therapy, however, should be reserved for the relatively uncommon case which requires very rapid control of motor activity, because the patient so treated is likely to be comatose or stuporous for many hours afterward, making neurological examination difficult or impossible, an unfortunate situation, for many of these patients may have suffered head trauma and thus require careful sequential neurological evaluation once seizure activity has ceased.

NEUROMUSCULAR DISORDERS

Most diseases of peripheral nerves, neuromuscular junction, and muscle are chronic or subacute and are rarely seen as emergencies. There are only three reasonably common diseases in this category which are worthy of mention in the context of emergency treatment.

IDIOPATHIC POLYNEUROPATHY

Idiopathic polyneuropathy of the Landry-Guillain-Barré type is a treacherous disease primarily because of its insidious onset combined with its propensity to progress rapidly and to produce life-threatening respiratory depression within a very short time from its onset. It commonly occurs several days to three weeks after a viral illness. Its earliest symptoms are subtle, often producing mild subjective sensory changes in the lower legs and feet when the neurological examination is absolutely normal. Patients are often thought to be hysterical or malingering during this prodromal period and not uncommonly are referred to a psychiatrist. When weakness ensues, it can progress at a vicious rate, rapidly producing respiratory depression (within hours in some cases) caused by weakness of respiratory musculature. Although the classic type tends to ascend, affecting the longest nerves first, there are many other varieties of the same or similar process which begin in shorter nerves and may actually appear to descend. Probably most commonly, weakness appears in many areas at once, often progressing rapidly to total paralysis. Spinal fluid proteins are usually greatly elevated and almost invariably are elevated significantly at some point in the illness, but often a spinal fluid analysis early in treatment will reveal a normal protein level [3]. A *normal cerebrospinal fluid protein level should not, therefore, be taken as good evidence of the absence of serious polyneuropathy of the Landry-Guillain-Barré type.* A patient in whom this diagnosis is considered should be admitted for careful observation with frequent neurological examinations and measurements of vital capacity. In most cases, weakness does not proceed to respiratory paralysis, but there is no way to predict which patients will fall into the more severe group. Therefore, all such patients must be followed in the hospital at least until the weakness has peaked and is clearly improving for several days. With the advent of sophisticated respiratory and intensive care units, survival in the severe group has been greatly improved.

It is now clear that the vast majority of patients requiring tracheostomy for this illness will regain normal neurological function. The other 10% will virtually all regain nearly all function and return to essentially normal activity. The length of time for recovery is dependent on the rate of remyelination of the acutely demyelinated nerves, a process that can take as long as one year in severe cases. Trials of steroid therapy (prednisone, 45 to 60 mg daily) have shown inconsistent results, but a short trial in severe cases is probably warranted. The excellent prognosis of these patients with prompt diagnosis and therapy compared to their almost certain death without recognition places this disease in a rare category. That is, proper medical intervention can convert serious morbidity and significant mortality into total recovery and return to normal function. For this reason, this diagnosis should always be considered in the young patient complaining of vague dyasthesias or mild weakness, particularly when these follow a viral infection.

Myasthenia Gravis

Myasthenia gravis is a disease of the neuromuscular junction which can produce sudden, life-threatening weakness. It is presumably due to insufficient action of acetylcholine at the neuromuscular junction. Thus, muscle contraction will become progressively weaker with repeated contractions of that muscle. Rest will initially allow sufficient acetylcholine action to be reconstituted, but when the condition becomes severe, even rest will fail to restore normal muscle contractions on subsequent attempts. When this occurs the patient may become profoundly weak, be unable to breathe adequately, and require assisted ventilation. This predicament is known as *myasthenic crisis* and often can be diagnosed in the emergency room by a simple test. When a patient (usually a young woman or an older man) is first seen with severe weakness, an estimate of the relative strength of repeated contractions should be made. One useful way to assess this is to ask the patient to grasp and release repeatedly with one hand. If he becomes progressively weaker, myasthenic crisis is suggested. Often asking the myasthenic to maintain upward gaze will produce progressive weakness in the levator palpabrae muscle which may manifest itself by progressive ptosis or a twitching of the eyelid in an attempt to keep it open (myasthenic twitch). If this progressive weakness is relieved by allowing the patient to close his eyes for a few moments, myasthenic weakness is suggested.

The suspicion of myasthenia can be supported by performing the edrophonium (Tensilon) test, whereby a rapidly effective, short-acting anticholinesterase (edrophonium) is given and some objective measure of strength is made. Usually, the length of time that the patient can maintain upward gaze without ptosis is measured. The dose of edrophonium is 1 mg I.V. as a test dose followed by a 10-mg I.V. bolus. Another syringe should be filled with saline solution by a person who will not be doing the injection, and measurements of strength should be made with both the control (saline solution) and edrophonium injections by a person who does not know which syringe contains the edrophonium. This double blind procedure allows for unbiased interpretation of the test and rules out the placebo effect of the injection itself. Some physicians pretreat patients with 0.5 mg of atropine I.M. to prevent muscarinic side effects of the anticholinesterase. When clearly positive, the edrophonium test is pathognomonic for myasthenia gravis.

The patient should be admitted to the hospital and therapy should be started with a longer-acting anticholinesterase, usually pyridostigmine (Mestinon), 30 to 60 mg p.o. t.i.d. to start. The patient's strength should be rechecked frequently and vital capacities measured. Often such patients will require tracheostomy, but adequate control with anticholinesterases usually occurs before this becomes necessary. In patients with known myasthenia who are receiving anticholinesterase therapy and who are seen with weakness, an interesting differential diagnosis is presented. Is the patient receiving too little anticholinesterase? That is, is he in myasthenic crisis? Or has he been overdosed with anticholinesterase drugs, so that weakness has resulted (cholinergic crisis)?

Several points are of some use in making this distinction. If the patient has a history of muscarinic side effects of acetylcholine excess (that is, diarrhea, abdominal pain, etc.) this suggests cholinergic crisis. Often one can obtain a history of gradually increasing self-medication with anticholinesterases by the patient who, as he progressively felt weaker, mistakenly continued to raise his own dose, thereby overdosing himself. This is particularly common when intercurrent disease (particularly upper respiratory infection) causes the maintenance anticholinesterase requirement to rise slightly. The patient may overestimate the amount of increase in anticholinesterase that is required. When weakness increases, he may further raise his dose, thus bringing on cholinergic crisis. The edrophonium test is, of course, negative in cholinergic crisis, and may actually make the patient weaker. However, for unknown reasons, the absence of a positive edrophonium test in a treated myasthenic does not rule out myasthenic crisis. Thus, it is sometimes difficult or impossible to decide in the short run whether the weakness in a treated myasthenic is due to myasthenic or cholinergic crisis.

In this circumstance, as well as in clear cholinergic crisis, the treatment is hospitalization in an intensive or respiratory care facility with discontinuation of all medication and support of respiratory function as required. Again, frequent neurological examination and measurements of vital capacity are required. If the patient improves with no medication, the diagnosis is presumed to be cholinergic crisis, and when the patient is stable, anticholinesterase therapy is resumed at a slightly lower dose and the patient is reeducated in its use. If the patient does not improve, or worsens, the diagnosis is presumed to be myasthenic crisis, caused either by insufficient anticholinesterases or by resistance to adequate doses, but if a large dose is reached with no therapeutic benefit and severe muscarinic side effects, then anticholinesterases are discontinued and steroids begun, 25 mg of prednisone on alternate days, increasing gradually to 100 mg on alternate days [4]. The relatively recent discovery that steroids increase strength in this situation and perhaps even reestablish the patient's sensitivity to anticholinesterases has probably added significant numbers of years to the lives of some severely ill myasthenic patients. The mechanism for the relationship between anticholinesterase resistance and the steroid responsiveness is unknown.

It is important to remember in the emergency room that myasthenia commonly affects the extraocular musculature and levator palpabrae, but *never* affect the pupil size or reaction. Ocular myasthenia can imitate nearly any kind of neural eye movement disorder, especially partial third nerve palsies which may be erroneously attributed to diabetes or a vasculitis. All patients with disorders of extraocular movement should have an edrophonium test to rule out myasthenia gravis. Some forms of ocular myasthenia are benign in that they remain limited to the eye, but other forms are merely early signs of generalized myasthenia which can produce life-threatening weakness in a short time. When pupillary size is affected, myasthenia is ruled out (the differential diagnosis of anisocoria is discussed below in the section on increased intracranial pressure) and an edrophonium test need not be done.

Acute Rhabdomyolysis

Nearly all muscle diseases are chronic and are first seen as emergencies when weakness has progressed sufficiently to produce respiratory depression, aspiration of oral contents, or other mechanical difficulties. This is true of all types of muscular dystrophy, thyroid myopathy, alcoholic myopathy, and polymyositis. These diseases are characterized by progressive, primarily proximal muscle weakness (except for myotonic dystrophy, which is primarily distal) with nontender muscles, except for some cases of polymyositis, in which the muscles may be mildly tender. There is, however, one acute, dramatic disease of muscle which is a medical emergency—acute rhabdomyolysis with massive myoglobinuria and secondary acute tubular necrosis. This syndrome can be produced by massive trauma (primarily crush injuries), long periods of weight-bearing on muscular areas (particularly in patients found in coma in unusual postures), or by alcohol ingestion. It is characterized by acute severe proximal muscle weakness with very tender muscles and massive myoglobinuria [5]. The weakness itself is seldom life-threatening, but the myoglobin, being a relatively small molecule, is filtered completely by the kidneys and can produce acute tubular necrosis (ATN) and renal failure. Myoglobinuria can be easily diagnosed when the urine tests are positive for blood, with no red cells seen in the urine and a clear serum. If the serum is red, then the substance responsible for the positive result is hemoglobin, a larger molecule which is not completely cleared by the kidneys, accounting for the red serum. In the period before renal failure ensues, one should try to prevent concentration of the urine by administering large volumes of fluids. If urine output falls into the oliguric or anuric range with a urine sediment suggestive of acute tubular necrosis (i.e., renal tubular cells and "dirty brown" casts), high urine sodium levels, and low specific gravity, then the diagnosis of acute tubular necrosis secondary to myoglobinuria can be made and the patient treated for acute renal failure with fluid restriction to the amount of output plus insensible loss. If and when the patient enters the diuretic phase of ATN, fluid therapy is aimed at matching the massive outputs plus insensible losses. Most, but not all, such patients will recover from the ATN, whereas those who do not recover may require dialysis (see Chapter 9, Acute Renal Failure).

INFECTIOUS DISEASES

MENINGITIS

Meningitis may be bacterial, fungal, viral, or neoplastic in origin. The differential diagnosis among these four possibilities in a clinical case of meningitis is of vital importance, because bacterial meningitis is an unequivocal neurological emergency in which prompt appropriate therapy can spell the difference between life and death, whereas meningitis caused by fungi, viruses, and neoplastic infiltration rarely requires immediate therapy. History, physical examination, and spinal fluid examination can usually provide sufficient information to make this differential diagnosis reasonably certain within a matter of minutes.

Patients with bacterial meningitis are generally very ill systemically. They usually have high fevers, leukocytosis, tachycardia, and often evidence of underlying infections, most commonly pneumonia and/or endocarditis. Nuchal rigidity is variable, but will usually be impressive in a conscious adult with bacterial meningitis. Its absence, however, does not rule out meningitis, and it is not customarily seen in very young or very old patients or in patients who have slipped into deep coma. The level of consciousness varies, depending on the extent of disease. Early, patients may be perfectly alert, complaining of headache. Later, the level of consciousness deteriorates and any level can be seen, including deep coma. Focal neurological signs are unusual in uncomplicated bacterial meningitis, but seizures with Todd's paralysis and other focal signs such as Babinski signs, hemiplegias, etc., can be seen, probably on the basis of cortical vein thrombosis. The history in bacterial meningitis is generally not available, presumably because the onset of illness is so rapid that patients are often found critically ill by relatives or friends. When there is a history, bacterial infection, particularly purulent sputum production, is often associated.

The histories of viral, fungal, and neoplastic meningitis are rarely so catastrophic. Often the physical examinations are less dramatic, and generally there are fewer systemic symptoms and signs. Fevers are less impressive, and leukocytosis is usually absent. Tuberculous meningitis is the most widely variable type of meningitis. It may produce a subacute or acute illness and may in some fulminant cases be indistinguishable from other forms of bacterial meningitis. A rare case of cryptococcal meningitis may also be so fulminating as to mimic acute bacterial meningitis.

The spinal fluid should be examined in every case of possible meningitis. Even if intracranial pressure is suspected of being elevated, a lumbar puncture should be done, for the risk of herniation, even in the presence of known elevated intracranial pressure, is much less than the risk of missing a diagnosis of bacterial meningitis. In such situations the lumbar puncture may be done with mannitol immediately available and neurosurgical consultation near at hand to perform a ventricular tap if necessary. Every lumbar puncture should produce the following information: (1) opening pressure with the patient as relaxed as possible; (2) cell counts on tubes 1 and 3 (with differential count done if any white cells are present); (3) cultures of tube 2; (4) sugar and total protein on either tube 1 or 3 (a simultaneous blood sugar test should be done as well); (5) a Gram and Ziehl-Neelsen stain whenever *any* white cells are seen or whenever meningitis is suspected whether white cells are seen or not, and an India ink preparation if cryptococcal meningitis is suspected or in any immunocompromised host with signs of meningitis or white cells in the cerebrospinal fluid (CSF); (6) serological test for syphilis on either tube 1 or tube 3. If there is difficulty in obtaining cerebrospinal fluid, the most critical information is the cell count, culture, and CSF sugar, all of which can be done on as little as 1 ml of CSF if necessary. The results often provide strong evidence for one of four types of meningitis (Table 2-2).

Obviously there may be a great deal of overlap, but usually the history, physical examination, and CSF formula together produce a fairly strong case for one or another type of meningitis. Generally, when there is a reasonable possibility of bacterial meningitis on the basis of the above results, even when organisms are not seen on Gram and Ziehl-Neelsen stains, it is best to treat the patient empirically until culture results are available. Evidence of basilar meningitis, such as cranial nerve palsies, may be a clue to tuberculous meningitis, and in these patients, along with individuals with known pulmonary tuberculosis, treatment should be empirical for tuberculous meningitis until culture results are available.

Treatment of acute bacterial meningitis depends upon the organism. If an organism is unequivocally seen on Gram or Ziehl-Neelsen stains or if it can be demonstrated rapidly by other means, such as counterimmunoelectrophoresis [6] or Limulus lysate test [7], then the therapy can be specific, but if the organism cannot be demonstrated despite an otherwise strong case for bacterial meningitis, then the therapy largely depends on one's knowledge of the most likely causative organisms, which depend to a large extent on the age of the patient (Table 2-3). A ra-

TABLE 2-2 Common Spinal Fluid Findings in Meningitis

Constituent or Test	Bacteria	Fungi	Viruses	Neoplasms
Cells (per mm³)	>500	>500	<500	Variable
Differential count	Polymorphonuclear leukocytes	Polymorphonuclear leukocytes early, lymphocytes later	Polymorphonuclear leukocytes early, lymphocytes later	Lymphocytes Tumor cells (rarely)
CSF-glucose	<15% blood glucose	<50% blood sugar	60–90% blood sugar	<50% blood sugar
Protein	Normal or elevated	Usually very high	Normal	Usually high
Organisms (stain)	+	±	0	0
Organisms (culture)	+	+	0	0
Cell types (cytology)	0	0	0	Tumor cells

TABLE 2-3 Common Causes of Bacterial Meningitis

Patient's Age	Organisms in Order of Frequency
<2 months	*Escherichia coli; Aerobacter; Proteus; Staphylococcus; Streptococcus*
2 mo–6 yr	*Hemophilus influenzae; Neisseria meningitides; Diplococcus pneumoniae*
6 yr–15 yr	*N. meningitides; D. pneumoniae; H. influenzae*
Over 15 yr	*D. pneumoniae; N. meningitides; H. influenzae; Staphylococcus aureus;* Group A streptococci; coliforms; *Pseudomonas* (usually secondary to LP spinal anesthesia or shunting procedures); *Salmonella; Shigella; Clostridium; Neisseria gonorrhoeae; Listeria monocytogenes; Mima polymorpha; Amoeba*

tional antibiotic choice can then be made with some knowledge of the likely sensitivities for the major organisms (Table 2-4).

The intrathecal and intraventricular use of antibiotics in bacterial meningitis is still debatable. It has now been well shown that bacteriocidal concentrations of antibiotic can better be maintained in the meninges when combined intrathecal and parenteral gentamicin are used [8]. Thus, intrathecal antibiotic should be administered in fungal and gram-negative meningitides (Table 2-3).

The utility of steroids in meningitis (particularly tuberculous) is an equally unsolved question. At present, one should probably use steroids only when the basilar meningitis (usually tuberculous) is causing impending subarachnoid block or cerebral edema [9].

ABSCESSES

Abscesses in the central nervous system primarily occur in three places: in the brain, in the subdural space (subdural empyema), and epidurally. Antibiotics alone are not curative in any of these abscesses but must always be combined with surgical drainage. These abscesses become emergencies only when they act as masses and produce either transtentorial herniation or spinal block. These syndromes are discussed below in the section on neoplasms, but are mentioned again here to emphasize the point that surgical intervention is required to treat abscesses in the central nervous system and that antibiotics alone, even if of the appropriate spectrum, are insufficient therapy.

TRAUMA

CONCUSSION

Concussion is defined as the loss of consciousness caused by head trauma. No matter how brief the period of unconsciousness, all patients with concussion should be hospitalized and observed for at least 12 hours. During the period of observation, the patient should be awakened at

TABLE 2-4 Antibiotic Choices in Various Forms of Meningitis Before Sensitivities

Suspected Organism	Antibiotic and Dose in Order of Preference
Diplococcus pneumoniae	Penicillin, 2–3 million units q4h I.V. Chloramphenicol, 1 gm q4h I.V. Erythromycin, 1 gm q6h I.V.
Neisseria meningitides	Penicillin, 2–3 million units q4h I.V. Chloramphenicol, 1 gm q4h I.V.
Hemophilus influenzae	Ampicillin, 2 gm q4h I.V. Chloramphenicol, 1 gm q4h I.V.
Coliforms	Gentamicin, 5 mg/kg/day in divided doses I.V., plus gentamicin, 4–5 mg q.d. intrathecally
Pseudomonas	Gentamicin, 5 mg/kg/day in divided doses I.V., plus gentamicin, 4–5 mg q.d. intrathecally
Staphylococcus aureus	Nafcillin or oxacillin, 2 gm q4h I.V. Chloramphenicol, 1 gm q4h I.V. Erythromycin, 1 gm q6h I.V.
Mycobacterum tuberculosis	Isoniazid, 300 mg p.o. q.d., streptomycin, 1 gm I.M. q.d., and ethambutol, 25 mg/kg p.o. q.d.
Fungi (*Coccidioides immitis* and *Cryptococcus neoformans*)	Amphotericin B, 1 mg I.V. q.d. increasing as rapidly as tolerated to 75 mg I.V. q.o.d. to total of 3 gm, plus amphotericin B, 0.5 mg q.o.d. intrathecally

least hourly and neurological vital signs tested (i.e., pulse, blood pressure, respiratory rate, temperature, pupillary size and reaction to light, and estimate of strength). Skull x-rays should be made of all such patients, with special reference made to pineal location, if visible, and the presence or absence of fractures. Patients suffering skull fractures have a much higher incidence of serious sequelae than patients without fractures. There is no need to do a lumbar puncture on patients with concussion, because a high percentage show red cells in the CSF and do not go on to develop serious complications. Furthermore, the absence of red cells does not rule out the presence of serious sequelae of head trauma.

ACUTE SUBDURAL HEMATOMA AND EPIDURAL HEMATOMA

Acute subdural hematoma and epidural hematoma are usually not difficult diagnoses to make. These patients have nearly always suffered massive head trauma, with the mechanism of the hematoma in the epidural form being a fracture through the middle meningeal artery. The exception to this rule is that children may develop epidural hematomas with minor head trauma. It is said that such patients have a "lucid interval" between the occurrence of head trauma and the onset of neurological symptoms. This is certainly true in some cases, but equally often neurological abnormality begins coincident with the injury. These patients are first seen in coma, often with a severe hemiparesis, probably caused by a brain contusion in association with the subdural or epidural hematoma. The only therapy is rapid evacuation of the hematoma, removal of destroyed brain tissue, and control of bleeding from the bisected middle meningeal artery. Patients should be treated with hypertonic agents (e.g., mannitol) and dexamethasone until an operation can be performed. Even when these patients are diagnosed early and reach the operating room rapidly, the mortality rate from this disease is about 80%, with nearly all the survivors suffering major sequelae.

Chronic Subdural Hematoma

Chronic subdural hematoma is another matter entirely. Head trauma responsible for this lesion may be trivial or even nonexistent. The onset of symptoms may occur anywhere from a few minutes to many weeks or even months after the presumed insult. Its manifestations are protean. In some patients the lesion acts like a tumor, producing gradually increasing hemiparesis. In others it produces no lateralizing or focal signs but merely a change in mental status, with memory loss, inattention, dementia, or lethargy. Some patients have only headache. The most typical situation, however, is increasing apathy, lethargy, and inattention, with a dearth of lateralizing or focal signs. The spinal fluid is rarely of help in making the diagnosis; in the majority of cases it is abnormal in some nonspecific way (i.e., increased protein, xanthochromia, or a few red blood cells), but a perfectly normal cerebrospinal fluid analysis is compatible with a potentially fatal subdural hematoma. Skull x-rays are sometimes of help because of a shifted pineal body, but the pineal is all too often not calcified and even when in the midline does not rule out the relatively frequent occurrence of bilateral subdural hematomas.

The same criticism can be leveled against the echoencephalogram, which is useful only when abnormal and even then is not specific for subdural hematoma. The presence of a visual field defect in a hemiparetic patient is of some use in making subdural hematoma less likely, because an intracerebral lesion should be required to interfere with the optic radiations as they course from the lateral geniculate bodies toward the occipital cortex. However, defects in the patient's attention may interfere with one's ability to make an accurate assessment of visual fields, making this distinction of more academic than practical interest. Another area of some help is that of speech. When an aphasia is produced by a subdural hematoma, it is usually an anomic type (i.e., a fluent aphasia with good repetition and comprehension). Other aphasias (i.e., Wernicke's, Broca's, conduction, etc.) are only rarely caused by subdural hematomas, but rather by intracerebral lesions (i.e., strokes, tumors, etc.).

Despite all of these clinical clues, one can definitively rule out a subdural hematoma only by arteriography. Unless there is an unequivocal lateralizing sign such as a large unreactive pupil on one side, a nondominant carotid arteriogram should be done (usually a right carotid study). Three questions should be answerable in this way: (1) Are the middle cerebral vessels seen to reach the inner table of bone or is there a visible subdural collection? (2) Is the anterior cerebral in the midline? and

(3) Are the ventricles of normal size? If possible, the carotid study should be done by means of a femoral catheterization, not only because of the technical superiority of such a study but also because the opposite carotid can be studied immediately if necessary, without the unnecessary hazard of bilateral direct carotid punctures. Furthermore, if hydrocephalus is observed, a vertebral study can easily be done. Computerized transaxial tomography (CTT), if available, may demonstrate a subdural hematoma, thereby avoiding an arteriogram. However, when the CTT is negative in a patient in whom the diagnosis of chronic subdural hematoma is considered likely, an arteriogram should still be done.

Recently there has been some debate about the necessity for operation in chronic subdural hematomas. Certainly, many small hematomas, if allowed to follow their own natural history, will resolve spontaneously. In patients with no focal or lateralizing signs, who will return for follow-up, it may be reasonable to treat small subdural hematomas medically. However, for the majority of patients the therapy remains surgical removal, because the patient either has debilitating symptoms or is unreliable for careful follow-up. The greatest danger of subdural hematoma is that the lesion may act like a tumor, gradually increasing in size and suddenly resulting in transtentorial herniation and death. It is difficult to know at any given time where a patient fits on this spectrum, so it is probably safer in most situations to remove the hematoma when it is discovered.

INTRACEREBRAL HEMORRHAGE

Serious head trauma can produce intracerebral hemorrhages nearly everywhere in the brain, but there are two locations where the hemorrhages are eminently treatable. The first is in the lateral temporal lobes, which may produce transtentorial herniation if the mass of blood increases in size rapidly, and the second is in the cerebellum, which can cause death by tonsillar herniation, direct dissection into the brain stem, or the production of acute hydrocephalus by blockade of the fourth ventricle. In both cases the patient may be awake and alert early in the course but may have strong focal signs, such as a severe hemiplegia, aphasia, or ataxia, depending on the location of the lesion.

At present this diagnosis can be best made by computerized transaxial tomography (CTT) of the brain. Of all the lesions seen by this new technique, results are most dramatic in intracerebral hemorrhage. In 15 minutes, without invasive procedures, the exact location of such a hemorrhage can be ascertained and the patient can be operated upon without the risk of an arteriogram. If CTT is not available, arteriography is the next best study. The only therapy is prompt evacuation of the hematoma and control of hemorrhage. Depending on the location of the lesion, the patient may make an excellent recovery. Cerebellar lesions have the best prognosis, but nondominant temporal lobe hemorrhages are also worth looking for and removing, if present. Dominant temporal lobe lesions are, of course, equally accessible, but serious aphasic sequelae are common when extensive bleeding has occurred.

Brain Contusion

Brain contusion is diagnosed by exclusion. If intracerebral and subdural masses are excluded in a patient who has suffered head trauma and who has focal or lateralizing signs, the probable cause is contusion of the brain. Treatment is symptomatic and supportive and should include glycerol and dexamethasone (Decadron) to attempt to control cerebral edema. Occasionally, when massive edema ensues, a large bifrontal decompression craniotomy is done, but the outlook for such patients is very poor.

VASCULAR DISORDERS

Subarachnoid Hemorrhage

Subarachnoid hemorrhage refers to hemorrhage directly into the subarachnoid space. The vast majority of such hemorrhages are caused by rupture of intracranial aneurysms and bleeding from arteriovenous malformations. In younger patients the latter is the more frequent, whereas the reverse is true in older patients. Many patients who suffer subarachnoid hemorrhage die before they reach the hospital, but those who do reach the hospital and are able to give a history relate a fairly typical story. The event usually occurs during strenuous exercise, very suddenly, and is heralded by the onset of excruciating headache. Most patients say it is the worst headache they have ever had but find it difficult to localize. Some note that the pain is behind one eye. Some lose consciousness for varying periods of time and may arrive in the emergency room in deep coma. Others are able to recall that their legs became weak without loss of consciousness (presumably because of rupture of an anterior communicating artery aneurysm), but generally there is a dearth of focal or lateralizing symptoms or signs. There may be nuchal rigidity, but, as in meningitis, this is a highly variable finding and may be absent in older patients or persons in deep coma. Subhyaloid hemorrhages may be seen in the fundus, presumably caused by rupture of retinal vessels with the sudden rise in subarachnoid pressure.

The spinal fluid is under increased pressure and is grossly bloody (nearly always more than 100,000 red cells [RBC]/mm^3 and usually in excess of 1,000,000 RBC/mm^3). The location of the ruptured aneurysm is difficult to ascertain clinically, but there are two rare focal signs which when present are of localizing value. If frontal lobe signs are prominent, such as weakness in the legs, prominent sucking and rooting, and an abulic (unconcerned) affect, then the lesion may be in the anterior communicating artery, either with bleeding directly into the frontal lobes or with compromise of flow in one or both anterior cerebral arteries. If one pupil is widely dilated with poor or absent direct and consensual light reflex in a conscious patient, then the aneurysm may be in the posterior communicating artery, with pressure being exerted on the third cranial (oculomotor) nerve. Because the oculomotor nerve is laminated with the parasympathetic pupillary constrictor fibers on the outside and the extraocular movement fibers on the inside, the eye movements are preserved in such a lesion. The same would be true, of course, in transtentorial herniation, but in the latter situation, the patient would always be stuporous or in coma by the time the pupil has dilated.

In the absence of focal signs, an arteriogram is the only method by which the etiology of the hemorrhage can be determined. A three-vessel arteriogram by the femoral approach should always be done, because multiple aneurysms are relatively common, and study of only one vessel may fail to demonstrate the aneurysm which caused the current episode of bleeding. If two angiograms are done, about two weeks apart, a cause can be found for about 80% of subarachnoid hemorrhages. The remaining 20% have a better prognosis with respect to bleeding again, presumably because many of these aneurysms or small arteriovenous (AV) malformations were destroyed in the process of bleeding. Thus, the angiograms should be done both to identify operable causes of subarachnoid hemorrhage and to identify a group which is at low risk for additional bleeding without operation.

There are several modalities available for treatment of subarachnoid hemorrhage, some standard and some controversial. Almost everyone would agree that patients with recent subarachnoid hemorrhage should not be operated on immediately. These patients should be treated with antihypertensive agents in order to maintain their blood pressure in the mildly hypotensive range (i.e., about 90 systolic). Some utilize propranalol in an attempt to decrease the rate of pressure development (dP/dT) as well as the pressure itself. Other agents such as methyldopa, reserpine, and diuretics should also be utilized as necessary to control the blood pressure. Potent vasodilators such as diazoxide and hydralazine are relatively contraindicated because of their adverse effect on dP/dT. Initially, blood pressures may be in the malignant range (i.e. >250/150 mHg), in which case nitroprusside and trimethaphan would be the agents of choice.

It is also generally agreed that patients should be sedated and kept at bed rest in a dark room during the acute period (about two weeks). Spasm generally ensues about the second or third day and may become a life-threatening problem. There is great controversy as to whether anything can be done to control or prevent spasm, and studies are in progress to assess the use of isoproterenol (beta stimulation), reserpine (catecholamine depletion), and oral kanamycin (sterilization of the colon of organisms which produce serotonin and other vasoactive amines) to control spasm. At present none of these agents is used routinely.

The other serious concern after subarachnoid hemorrhage is another episode of bleeding. About 10% will bleed again during the first week, and 5% more during the next week after the initial event. There is good evidence that use of antifibrinolytic agents (e.g., epsilon-aminocaproic acid and related drugs) can decrease significantly the incidence of repeated bleeding [10]; but again, this method of therapy is relatively controversial. If, however, one intends to use either the antispasm or the antifibrinolytic regimen, it is obviously necessary to document that aneurysmal rupture was the cause of the subarachnoid hemorrhage, for neither form of therapy has been tested in hemorrhages from AV malformations.

The only definitive therapy of intracranial aneurysms or AV malformations is surgical removal when possible. Posterior communicating aneurysms have long been approachable, and with recent advances in microneurosurgical techniques, anterior communicating aneurysms are also treatable by direct removal; success in treating aneurysms in other locations and AV malformations depends entirely upon their location. Some unreachable AV malformations can be decreased significantly in size by directed embolization.

HYPERTENSIVE INTRACEREBRAL HEMORRHAGE

Hypertensive intracerebral hemorrhages arise primarily from five locations: putamen (50%), thalamus (20%), pons (10%), cerebellum (10%), and other locations (10%) [11]. The importance of recognizing this syndrome is that one of the hemorrhages (cerebellar) is eminently treatable, one is possibly treatable (putaminal), and two are untreatable (pontine and thalamic). Whether hemorrhages located in other areas are surgically treatable depends on their location. Nearly all such patients are hypertensive when the event occurs. The history, when available, is usually that of the rapid onset of headache and paralysis over the period of a few minutes, often occurring during exertion. The onset is rarely as dramatic as that of a subarachnoid hemorrhage, and the headache is usually not as severe. Depending on the location and extent of the lesion the patient will become gradually more lethargic and slip into coma over minutes or hours. In patients who survive, progression has usually stopped before the person reaches the hospital. Deepening coma or increasing paralysis in the hospital is a bad prognostic sign. The spinal fluid is nearly always bloody at some time during the course, but may be absolutely clear early, presumably because intracerebral blood has not yet dissected to the subarachnoid space or into the ventricles. Even when the fluid is bloody, the red cell count is significantly lower than that seen in subarachnoid hemorrhage (Table 2-5).

It has been noted that the eyes often give a clue to the location of the hemorrhage. In putaminal hemorrhage, there is a hemiparesis and the eyes are conjugately deviated to the opposite side. In thalamic hemorrhage, there is usually a hemiparesis and the eyes are deviated downward as if looking at the tip of the nose. Vertical eye movements are impaired, and the pupils are usually small and fixed. In pontine hemorrhage the eyes are in the central position and the pupils are very small (pinpoint),

TABLE 2-5 Common Spinal Fluid Cell Counts in Stroke (Lumbar Puncture within 72 Hours of Onset)

Blood Cells/ mm³	Subarachnoid Hemorrhage	Intracerebral Hemorrhage	Embolus	Thrombosis
Red	>100,000 (usually >10⁶)	500–100,000	0–500	0
White	100–1,000	1–100	0–1	0

but reactive. The eyes may bob in the vertical plain but horizontal movements are absent even on ice water stimulation (calorics). In cerebellar hemorrhage there is a forced conjugate lateral deviation or a sixth nerve palsy without paralysis of the limbs. The pupils are of average size and reactive [11].

Cerebellar hemorrhage is the most treatable but most treacherous and difficult to diagnose. There is very little interval between little or no signs and death because of dissection of the hemorrhage into the brain stem. The typical history is that of moderate headache and severe vertigo, with nausea, vomiting, and inability to stand. One may find unilateral cerebellar ataxia as shown by finger-nose and heel-knee-shin testing, but this is not always present. Inability to walk is nearly always seen and is not generally noted in other forms of acute vertigo. Whenever a hypertensive patient is seen who had sudden inability to stand or walk, cerebellar hemorrhage should be seriously considered. Two-thirds of the patients show some abnormality in the spinal fluid when first seen (xanthochromia or a few RBC), but a normal CSF should not dissuade one from studying a patient with a compatible history and physical examination. If CTT is available, it is the study of choice, and, if a hemorrhage is demonstrated, it should be surgically removed. If CTT is not available, arteriography can be done to search for evidence of hydrocephalus on a carotid study, and if there is hydrocephalus to follow with a vertebral angiogram. Angiography is more difficult to interpret in intracerebral hemorrhage than is CTT, however. Putaminal hemorrhages are theoretically relatively accessible but probably should be operated upon only when the patient appears to be deteriorating rapidly despite medical supportive management. Such medical management should include rapid control of blood pressure and correction of any abnormalities in blood coagulation. Treatment for cerebral edema with glycerol, mannitol, and dexamethasone has been relatively unsuccessful in patients with intracerebral hemorrhages.

CEREBRAL INFARCTION

Cerebral infarction caused by thrombosis or embolus may or may not be a neurological emergency, depending on one's point of view. In general, thrombosis occurs in large vessels, the major one in the head and neck being the carotid, most commonly the internal carotid just at the bifurcation of the common carotid. Cerebral infarction caused by internal carotid thrombosis is probably the most common of all strokes. It may or may not be preceded by transient ischemic attacks (TIA) characterized by transient hemiplegias, transient aphasias, or transient monocular blindness (amaurosis fugax). A given patient may have anywhere from none to literally hundreds of such attacks before having a cerebral infarction. On the other hand, patients have had multiple TIA and never have a stroke. In some cases the TIA actually cease and never terminate in stroke. The major question is whether a patient suffering his first such attack or a patient suffering accelerated numbers or lengths of attacks should undergo carotid angiography to determine the extent of his carotid stenosis, and if the stenosis is extensive, whether he should undergo carotid endarterectomy in an effort to prevent a stroke. In short, this question is presently unanswered. In some centers, such patients will be advised to undergo endarterectomy, and those who cannot be operated on for medical reasons are placed on anticoagulation therapy. In other centers, no such effort is made. It is now fairly clear that anticoagulation decreases the incidence of transient ischemic attacks, but there is no evidence at present to suggest that anticoagulation influences the progression to stroke [12].

In the vertibrobasilar circulation, the situation is somewhat different. Surgery for most sorts of vascular disease in this distribution is not possible, but the debate rages as to the utility of anticoagulation in TIA of the brain stem (i.e., transient diplopia, dysarthria, quadriparesis, dysphagia, etc.) and whether such anticoagulation protects in any way against brain stem infarction caused by basilar artery thrombosis. There is some evidence that aspirin in a low dose (300 to 600 mg/day) may decrease the frequency of the attacks, and perhaps even influence the development of stroke [13].

Cerebral embolus accounts for most of the cerebral infarctions caused by occlusion of the anterior, middle, or posterior cerebral arteries themselves or their smaller branches. In about half of these cases, a possible source for the embolus can be found in the form of atrial fibrillation, cardiomyopathy, recent myocardial infarction, or bacterial endocarditis; but in the remainder of the cases the source remains obscure. Again, debate rages as to the utility of anticoagulation after an occlusion of one of these smaller arteries. Some feel that if the spinal fluid is clear, anticoagulation therapy should be begun immediately. Others feel that this should be deferred for 24 to 48 hours to ensure that the infarction was not hemorrhagic (a repeat spinal tap in 24 to 48 hours as the criterion) before beginning anticoagulation. Others believe that anticoagulation is not of any use regardless of when it is used during the course of an embolic infarction. There are presently no hard data to support any of these points of view. It is known, however, that the incidence of systemic emboli is greatly increased in atrial fibrillation with mitral valve disease and somewhat increased in atrial fibrillation without mitral valve disease. Thus, from a neurological point of view, all patients with mitral valve disease and atrial fibrillation should have anticoagulant therapy. If a patient has a cerebral infarction caused by demonstrated occlusion of a small cerebral vessel and has a possible source of emboli (e.g., atrial fibrillation), he should probably have anticoagulants once it is clear that the infarction is not primarily hemorrhagic. Two lumbar punctures (one on admission and one 24 to 48 hours later) should satisfy this criterion, if both specimens are absolutely free of red blood cells. All patients admitted with infarction caused by probable cerebral emboli should have blood cultures taken and, if bacterial endocarditis is demonstrated, should *not* have anticoagulants. At the present state of our knowledge, if no possible source for systemic embolization can be found, anticoagulants should probably not be used. If red blood cells are found in the CSF either on admission or 24 hours later, anticoagulants should not be used, because there is some evidence that they can increase the size of hemorrhagic cerebral infarction and perhaps produce significant intracerebral hemorrhage.

NEOPLASTIC DISORDERS

Tumors are rarely first seen as emergencies, but occasionally the results of an expanding mass within the nervous system require prompt emergency therapy. Obviously, similar syndromes can be caused by masses other than tumors, such as edema, hematomas, or abscesses, but these are less common causes of the following emergency situations.

SPINAL CORD COMPRESSION

Spinal cord compression is usually the result of tumors involving the spinal cord, most frequently metastatic, but they can also be seen secondary to trauma, abscesses, or vertebral collapse. It is vitally important to recognize the syndrome for what it is, because failure to relieve the compression promptly may spell the difference between complete recovery and severe, even life-threatening, paralysis. The patient will usually complain of rapidly progressive weakness, stiffness, or numbness. There may be symptoms of urinary or fecal incontinence or failure to sense a full bladder or rectum. Weakness, spasticity, and Babinski signs may be noted below the level of the block, and sometimes flaccid weakness with hyporeflexia and fasciculations can be seen in a radicular distribution at the level of the lesion. The hallmark of spinal block is a spinal level below which sensation is impaired (sensory level). This may be obvious and present for all modalities of sensation or may be subtle in the early stages, with defects in hot-cold discrimination, but intact pinprick, light touch, joint position sense, and vibration. Whenever spinal compression is suspected, an emergency myelogram should be performed, and if a block is found it should be relieved surgically as soon as possible.

INCREASED INTRACRANIAL PRESSURE

Increased intracranial pressure is a problem which has many causes, but it is included in this section because tumors produce the most ominous form of increased pressure and are most likely to result in serious complications with diagnostic procedures. The symptoms of increased intracranial pressure are headache, lethargy, nausea, and vomiting (sometimes but not invariably projectile). On physical examination, there may be remarkably little to see, especially if the onset has been acute. Papilledema may be present, but this often takes as long as 12 hours to develop. The lethargy and inattention are nonspecific and the skull x-ray may be normal, because erosion of the clinoid processes occurs only in chronic increases in intracranial pressure. Thus, a lumbar puncture may be done, with the physician surprised and dismayed to find a very high CSF pressure. If the patient deteriorates neurologically as the lumbar puncture is being done, the needle should *not* be removed, but rather the valve should be closed and an intravenous line begun with immediate infusion of 20% mannitol as rapidly as possible. Simultaneously, a neurosurgical consultation should be obtained in the event that a ventricular tap is required. Usually, however, even in this rather unusual circumstance, the pressure can be lowered with the use of hypertonic agents to a safe level and the spinal needle removed. This circumstance is usually precipitated in cases of posterior fossa tumors in which cerebellar tonsillar herniation occurs when pressure in the lumbar subarachnoid space is lowered by a lumbar puncture (L.P.). It should be strongly emphasized, however, that this is an *extremely rare* situation, and it is certainly true that many more errors are made by failing to do lumbar punctures than by doing inappropriate ones.

Nonetheless, if papilledema is noted, there are probably some situations in which an arteriogram should precede a lumbar puncture. A short discussion of the principles of herniation is required in order to recognize such situations.

In general, there is a risk of herniation only when there is a focal mass in the brain. For example, in benign intracranial hypertension (pseudotumor cerebri), where there is a generalized increase in fluid within the brain, there is no risk of herniation with lumbar puncture. In fact, reduction of pressure by means of lumbar puncture often produces relief of symptoms and is one of the accepted forms of therapy of pseudotumor. On the other hand, brain tumors, particularly in the posterior fossa, which produce increased intracranial pressure, do have a small but finite chance of producing herniation. Thus, in situations in which a strong suspicion of tumor is present in a patient with papilledema, the first study should probably be a three-vessel arteriogram. If a definite tumor is demonstrated, a ventricular tap may be required to reduce the pressure and to examine the CSF. Although massive cerebral infarction, intracerebral hemorrhage, and subdural hematomas can certainly produce herniation, the process is rarely, if ever, precipitated by a lumbar puncture. Thus, lumbar puncture is permissible and, in fact, strongly indicated as an early diagnostic procedure when stroke is likely in the differential diagnosis. If there are no signs of increased intracranial pressure, even when brain tumor is suspected, a lumbar puncture is a safe procedure.

The herniation syndrome, when it occurs, is important to recognize and treat promptly. There are three major types of herniation: transtentorial uncal (temporal), subfalcial, and cerebellar tonsillar. The latter is rarely preceded by a prodrome and is treacherous for its sudden onset and lack of orderly deterioration of neurological function. It often presents with sudden dilation of the pupils and respiratory arrest. Subfalcial herniation, in which a mass in one cerebral hemisphere causes herniation of brain under the falx cerebri, has no clinical significance. Transtentorial herniation is the most common and is due generally to a supratentorial mass lesion, which as it increases in size forces the temporal lobe over the rigid tentorium, proceeding to destroy the brain stem in an orderly rostral to caudal manner [14]. In fact, one generally does not see all of the classic signs of this event, since the torque on the brain stem during herniation produces hemorrhages (Duret hemorrhages), which obscure the neurological picture. Two important points are worth making, however. One is that the most reliable sign of laterality for the mass causing uncal herniation is a dilated, fixed pupil on the side of the mass (Hutchinson's pupil), as the oculomotor nerve is trapped between the tentorium and the herniating temporal lobe. A dilated, fixed pupil caused by transtentorial herniation is *never* seen in a fully conscious individual, so anisocoria in an alert patient should never be interpreted as a sign of herniation. The second point is that the side of a hemiparesis is of no value in lateralizing the mass, because in many cases the herniating mass causes compression of the opposite cerebral peduncle, producing an ipsilateral hemiparesis, which is a falsely localizing sign (i.e., Kernohan's notch).

When the transtentorial herniation syndrome is observed, an immediate neurosurgical consultation should be obtained and mannitol, 20% solution I.V., should be initiated as quickly as possible. Dexamethasone, 10 mg I.V., may be given but cannot be expected to abort the acute episode, because it will not begin to be effective for several hours. The prognosis for such patients depends upon the nature of the underlying lesion and the stage at which herniation was observed and treated. Tumors often respond dramatically to hypertonic agents, and prominent neurological deficit can often be prevented. Benign tumors with a significant degree of edema associated with them are just as capable of producing herniation as malignant tumors or strokes, so the long-term prognosis cannot be ascertained when the patient is first seen.

Sudden or Rapid Loss of Vision

Sudden or rapid loss of vision is a neurological emergency. When bilateral, it often represents tumor involving the optic chiasm. Immediate pneumoencephalography is indicated and an early decompressive operation recommended if an operable lesion can be found. Sudden or rapid unilateral blindness may be vascular in origin, but an early effort should be made to rule out lesions of the optic nerve, because vision, once lost, rarely returns, even if successful decompression of the optic nerve is accomplished. Very rapid or even sudden visual loss (usually unilateral) can be caused by cranial arteritis with or without polymyalgia rheumatica. Though most patients show gradual visual impairment along with headache, tender temporal arteries, generalized malaise, arthralgias, and myalgias, some cases of cranial arteritis may be first seen as sudden or rapid loss of vision. Most patients are elderly and have very high Westergren erythrocyte sedimentation rates (usually over 75 mm/hr and often greater than 100 mm/hr). When the diagnosis is suspected, the patient should be immediately given corticosteroids in high doses (i.e., methylprednisolone, 40 to 60 mg p.o. q.d.). Temporal artery biopsy may be done for definitive diagnosis, but therapy should not be delayed for this procedure.

METABOLIC ENCEPHALOPATHY

Metabolic encephalopathy is probably the most common neurological syndrome seen in a general hospital. In general, a metabolic abnormality should be considered likely when there is an acute disturbance of consciousness without localizing or lateralizing signs and normal cerebrospinal fluid. Metabolic encephalopathies may include all disturbances of consciousness from mild inattention to confusion to delirium to stupor to coma. The nature and extent of the insult superimposed on the baseline neurological function of the patient will produce the particular syndrome seen in an individual case. The problem is made increasingly complex when an old, even resolved, neurological deficit is exacerbated by a superimposed metabolic abnormality; for example, patients who have recovered completely from strokes may have a dramatic exacerbation of their old symptoms, including aphasias, hemiplegias, etc.

Most of the common metabolic derangements which can produce neurological disturbance are covered elsewhere. They include hypo- and hyperglycemia, hypo- and hypercalcemia, and hypo- and hypernatremia; hypoxia and hypercarbia, hypothyroidism, azotemia, hypertensive encephalopathy, hepatic coma, and portosystemic encephalopathy; drug overdose, ingestion, and withdrawal; and delirium tremens. All of these must be systematically ruled out when a metabolic encephalopathy is suspected.

WERNICKE'S ENCEPHALOPATHY

In addition, there are two specific syndromes which are worthy of further mention here. Wernicke's encephalopathy is a neurological emergency. It is caused by thiamine deficiency and characterized by mental disturbance, paralysis of eye movements, and ataxic gait. The abnormalities are caused by symmetrically located lesions in the thalamus, hypothalamus, mammillary bodies, periaqueductal region, floor of the fourth ventricle, and anterior lobe of the cerebellum. It is potentially fatal and must be treated promptly. The most common eye movement abnormalities are bilateral sixth nerve palsies, horizontal and vertical nystagmus, and gaze palsies. Internuclear ophthalmoplegias and downward gaze palsy are occasionally seen. Some patients are so severely affected that no eye movements whatsover can be seen. Others merely show nystagmus or have diplopia on lateral gaze. Most patients are alcoholics, but the disease can be seen in any poorly nourished person [15]. The treatment is immediate thiamine parenterally (100 mg I.V. if severe or I.M. if mild), hospitalization in every case, and thiamine daily, 100 mg I.M. for 5 days or until a normal diet is resumed. One should avoid administering glucose to patients with possible thiamine deficiency before thiamine is given, because this can precipitate an acute attack of Wernicke's encephalopathy. Although many such patients also have Korsakoff's psychosis, the two diseases are not always seen together. It should be remembered that the memory disturbance (Korsakoff's), when seen alone, is not an emergency and is caused by many things other than alcoholism and vitamin B_1 deficiency, the most common being head trauma.

HEAT STROKE

Heat stroke is extreme hyperpyrexia in which the central mechanism for heat dissipation fails. Although most often caused by extensive exposure to the sun, this exposure is not necessary, and heat stroke can be seen in persons who have been in hot environments out of the sun. It is most common in elderly patients with underlying diseases such as alcoholism, arteriosclerosis, and diabetes mellitus, or who are receiving phenothiazine-related drugs. Sweating ceases and internal temperature rises to above 106°F (41.1°C). Death is usually caused by vascular collapse. Treatment is aimed at artificially dissipating heat until the intrinsic temperature control mechanism regains competence. This may be done by placing the patient in a cool place and using tepid water or alcohol baths. Fluids are given intravenously with careful monitoring of the central venous pressure. Mortality in true heat stroke is high despite aggressive appropriate therapy [16].

REFERENCES

1. Kutt, H., and McDowell, F.   Management of epilepsy with diphenylhydantoin sodium. *J.A.M.A.* 203:167–170, 1968.
2. Wallis, W., Kutt, H., and McDowell, F.   Intravenous diphenylhydantoin in treatment of acute repetitive seizures. *Neurology* 18:513–525, 1968.
3. Asbury, A., Arnason, B. G., and Adams, R. D.   The inflammatory lesion in idiopathic polyneuritis. *Medicine* 48:173–215, 1969.
4. Seybold, M. E., and Drachman, D. B.   Gradually increasing doses of prednisone in myasthenia gravis. *N. Engl. J. Med.* 290:81–84, 1974.
5. Adams, R. D.   Principles of myology and myopathology. *Johns Hopkins Med. J.* 131:45–63, 1972.
6. Coonrod, J. D., and Rytel, M. W.   Determination of the aetiology of bacterial meningitis by counter-immunoelectrophoresis. *Lancet* 1:1154–1157, 1972.
7. Nachum, R., Lipsey, A., and Siegel, S. E.   Rapid detection of gram negative bacterial meningitis by the Limulus lysate test. *N. Engl. J. Med.* 289:931–934, 1973.
8. Rahal, J. J., Phineas, J. H., Simberkoff, M. S., and Rubinstein, E.   Combined intrathecal and intramuscular gentamicin for gram negative meningitis. *N. Engl. J. Med.* 290:1394–1398, 1974.
9. Stead, W. W.   Tuberculosis. In Wintrobe, M. M. (Ed.), *Harrison's Principles of Internal Medicine.* 7th ed. New York: McGraw-Hill, 1974. P. 156.
10. Tovi, D.   The use of antifibrinolytic drugs to prevent early recurrent aneurysmal subarachnoid hemorrhage. *Acta Neurol. Scand.* 49:163–175, 1973.
11. Fisher, C. M.   Some neuro-ophthalmological observations. *J. Neurol. Neurosurg. Psychiatry* 30:383–392, 1967.
12. Millikan, C. H.   Reassessment of anticoagulant therapy in various types of occlusive vascular disease. *Stroke* 2:201–207, 1971.
13. Dyken, M. L., Kolar, D. J., and Jones, F. H.   Differences in the occurrence of carotid transient ischemic attacks associated with antiplatelet aggregation therapy. *Stroke* 4:732–756, 1973.
14. Plum, F., and Posner, J. B.   *The Diagnosis of Stupor and Coma.* 2d ed. Philadelphia: Davis, 1972.
15. Victor, M., Adams, R. D., and Collins, G. H.   *The Wernicke-Korsakoff Syndrome.* Philadelphia: Davis, 1971.

16. O'Donnell, T. F., Jr., and Clowes, G. H. A., Jr. The circulatory abnormalities of heat stroke. *N. Engl. J. Med.* 287:734–737, 1972.

SELECTED READINGS

Brewer, N. S., MacCarty, C. S., and Wellman, W. C. Brain abscess: A review of recent clinical experience. *Ann. Intern. Med.* 82:571–576, 1975.

Browne, J. R., and Poskanzer, D. C. Treatment of strokes. *N. Engl. J. Med.* 281:594–600, 650–656, 1969.

Carpenter, R. R., and Petersdorf, R. G. The clinical spectrum of bacterial meningitis. *Am. J. Med.* 33:262–275, 1962.

Flacke, W. Treatment of myasthenia gravis. *N. Engl. J. Med.* 288:27–31, 1973.

Millichap, J. G. Drug treatment of convulsive disorders. *N. Engl. J. Med.* 286:464–468, 1972.

New, P. F. J., et al. Computerized axial tomography with the EMI scanner. *Radiology* 110:109–123, 1974.

Nishioka, H. Report of the cooperative study of intracranial aneurysms and subarachnoid hemorrhage. *J. Neurosurg.* section V, part 2. 25:321–704, 1966.

Perkoff, G. T., Dioso, M. D., Bleisch, V., and Klinkerfuss, G. A spectrum of a myopathy associated with alcoholism. Part 1: Clinical and laboratory features. *Ann. Intern. Med.* 67:481–510, 1967.

Perlo, V. P., Poskanzer, D. C., Schwab, R. S., et al. Myasthenia gravis: Evaluation of treatment in 1,355 patients. *Neurology* 16:431–439, 1966.

Rowbotham, G. F. *Acute Injuries of the Head.* 4th ed. Baltimore: Williams & Wilkins, 1964.

Schwartz, M. N., and Dodge, P. R. Bacterial meningitis—A review of selected aspects. *N. Engl. J. Med.* 272:725–731, 779–787, 842–848, 898–902, 954–960, 1003–1010, 1965.

Scott, W. R., New, P. F. J., Davis, K. R., and Schnur, J. A. Computerized tomography of intracerebral and intraventricular hemorrhage. *Radiology* 112:73–80, 1974.

3 CARDIOPULMONARY RESUSCITATION

WILLIAM B. HOOD, JR.

CARDIAC ARREST and respiratory arrest, occurring alone or in combination, constitute the ultimate medical emergency and demand both immediate recognition and prompt institution of a well-rehearsed sequence of resuscitative efforts. Certain basic principles apply in all cardiopulmonary resuscitations, and these include establishment of a patent airway and of proper ventilation, and restoration of cardiac pumping action. The precise sequence of events will depend upon the underlying cause of the arrest and the setting in which resuscitation occurs.

GENERAL APPROACH

Regardless of the setting, the initial approach to cardiopulmonary resuscitation will usually be directed toward establishment of a patent airway and of ventilation, and restoration of cardiac pumping action if this is absent. This will be followed by definitive therapy of the underlying cause of the cardiopulmonary arrest. The initial process has been labeled the ABCs of cardiopulmonary resuscitation. Initially, patency of the *airway* is established by hyperextending the neck, pulling the mandible forward to displace the tongue from the back of the throat, and inserting an oropharyngeal airway if available. Foreign bodies must be removed from the mouth and throat. If this does not restore respiration, *breathing* must be initiated either by mouth-to-mouth or mouth-to-nose ventilation, or by face mask with bag ventilation if this is available. A ventilatory rate of 12/min is recommended. Subsequently, an esophageal airway or an endotracheal tube may be inserted for more precise control of ventilation. This, however, should await adequate oxygenation and the availability of experienced personnel.

If the presenting problem is respiratory arrest, this treatment may be adequate; however, once ventilation is restored, the operator must quickly palpate the pulses and ascertain whether cardiac pumping action is evident. If not, *circulation* must be restored by closed-chest cardiac massage. This is accomplished by cyclical depression of the lower precordial sternum, with a displacement of approximately 5 cm, using the flat of the hand. If one operator is present, a rate of 80/min should be employed, with two rapid insufflations of the lung interjected every 15 strokes. If two operators are present, a rate of 60/min should be employed, with one insufflation of the lungs for every fifth stroke (without interrupting precordial compression). Under no circumstances should external compression be stopped for more than 5 seconds until an effective circulation is restored. Clues to proper conduct of the resuscitation include palpation of peripheral pulses during chest massage and, more important, maintenance of constricted pupils.

SETTINGS FOR CARDIOPULMONARY RESUSCITATION

The exact approach to cardiopulmonary resuscitation may well depend upon the setting in which the arrest occurs and also upon the etiology. Arrest occurring outside the hospital can be treated by applying the ABCs of resuscitation, but definitive therapy may well await arrival at the hospital. When the arrest occurs in the emergency room (accident floor), attention can more readily be directed to the cause of the arrest. Definitive treatment of cardiopulmonary arrest may depend upon special techniques such as cardiac defibrillation or pacing, injection of drugs, or insertion of endotracheal tubes with use of artificial ventilators. Vigilance must be maintained toward reversal of potentially treatable complications, such as pneumothorax or intravascular volume depletion from blood loss.

In the patient who is already in the hospital and being carefully monitored in a coronary or intensive care unit, cardiopulmonary arrest may often be anticipated and treated the instant it occurs. In certain situations it may be desirable to alter the usual protocol; for example, ventricular fibrillation may be treated within a few seconds after its occurrence by defibrillation, without initiating the ABCs of resuscitation.

ETIOLOGY

Arrests occur not infrequently in patients with complex medical and surgical diseases. In such cases, the immediate cause of the arrest may not always be obvious and the physician may find himself faced with the necessity of dealing with the specific complications, i.e., apnea, ventricular fibrillation, cardiac standstill, without knowing the exact causes. Quite frequently, however, a specific diagnosis and a specific mechanism resulting from the disease process are responsible for cardiopulmonary arrest (Table 3-1), and a demonstrably effective plan of action can be undertaken. In acute myocardial infarction, ventricular fibrillation and standstill, as well as other arrhythmias, pulmonary edema, and cardiogenic shock are all mechanisms which may be responsible for arrest. In pulmonary embolization, massive obstruction of the pulmonary ves-

TABLE 3-1 Some Causes of Cardiopulmonary Arrest

Disease State	Mechanisms
Acute myocardial infarction	Ventricular fibrillation, standstill, or other arrhythmias; shock and/or pulmonary edema
Pulmonary embolism	Pulmonary vascular obstruction
Dissecting aneurysm	Intravascular volume loss
Hypoxia, acidosis	Advanced pulmonary or cardiac failure Prolonged seizures Drowning, aspiration, tracheal obstruction, pneumothorax, drug overdose, CNS lesions
Renal failure	Hyperkalemia

sels with an ensuing drop in cardiac output is responsible, but resuscitation should be carried out nonetheless because of the possibility that clots may be broken up with chest massage and circulatory competence restored. In dissecting aneurysm, intravascular volume depletion from blood loss should be sought and corrected, with further consideration of immediate surgical intervention. Other forms of intravascular volume loss from gastrointestinal bleeding, pancreatitis, dehydration, diabetic ketoacidosis, and adrenal insufficiency should also be kept in mind. Hypoxia and acidosis, though they result from cardiopulmonary arrest, may also be a cause of it, and may result from prolonged seizure activity, drowning, advanced pulmonary or cardiac failure, aspiration, pneumothorax, drug overdosage, or expanding central nervous system lesions with respiratory depression. Advanced renal failure may result in hyperkalemia with cardiac arrest. Other causes of arrest may include smoke or carbon monoxide inhalation, electrocution, and anaphylaxis.

PROCEDURE

The treatment of respiratory arrest is relatively straightforward, and establishment of artificial ventilation can maintain the patient for an indefinite period of time even if spontaneous respirations do not return. The treatment of cardiac arrest is more complicated, and it is essential that cardiac pumping action be restored if the patient is to survive. With this in mind, a detailed presentation of the approach to cardiac arrest, based on the occurrence of ventricular fibrillation or standstill, is given.

Successful resuscitation from cardiac arrest depends upon organized team effort and smooth execution of a well-rehearsed and standardized procedure. Promptness of action is the chief factor determining likelihood of success, which also depends upon immediate recognition of arrest and the presence of adequate personnel and equipment in the immediate vicinity of the patient.

Many patients may be prevented from having cardiac arrest by prompt recognition and treatment of predisposing arrhythmias such as ventricular tachycardia and heart block. In others, cardiac arrest develops as the terminal event in the sequence of progressive and unremitting cardiac failure. Presently available methods of treatment will not save such patients, and indeed, a decision may be made in advance that resuscitation is not in order if arrest occurs. The patients of concern here are those in whom cardiac arrest develops suddenly with little or no warning, and in whom there is a reasonable chance of resuscitation with prompt action.

Cardiac arrest is defined as ventricular fibrillation or standstill resulting in absent cardiac pumping. Certain arrhythmias such as rapid ventricular tachycardia or idioventricular rhythm may result in virtually ineffective cardiac pumping action and are tantamount to cardiac arrest.

The resuscitation procedure may be divided into four phases on the basis of elapsed time, status of the patient, number of personnel available at the bedside, and progress of treatment (Table 3-2): Phase 1, initial treatment, begins with alarm and ends with first defibrillator shock (for ventricular fibrillation) or first attempt to restart the heart by pounding on chest (for standstill). Requires one physician and ideally should require only a few seconds. Phase 2, initiation of cardiopulmonary support, begins with initiation of continuous cardiac massage and pulmonary ventilation and ends with arrival of the full resuscitation team. It requires one or two persons. Ideally it should require one minute or less. Phase 3, sustained resuscitative effort, begins with arrival of adequate personnel to allow initiation of drug therapy and decision regarding further electrical therapy including electroshock or pacing. It lasts until resuscitation is successful or until a decision to discontinue resuscitative attempts is made. It requires at least five persons, two of whom are physicians, and it may last up to one hour. Phase 4, postresuscitation care is instituted.

Phase 1

The alarm sounds and is answered by a nurse or physician, who quickly determines whether the alarm is real. If cardiac arrest is discovered, the mechanism is ascertained and is treated as follows. For ventricular fibrillation, an initial sharp blow to the lower precordium should be applied ("thump version"); if this is unsuccessful, one should quickly grease electrode paddles and apply 400 watt-sec shock. Unless there has been excessive delay this is done without initiating artificial ventilation or closed chest massage. A second shock of 400 watt-sec can be given if the first is unsuccessful. For cardiac standstill, a sharp blow is delivered to the precordium. If results are inadequate (ventricular fibrillation, persistent asystole, or slow rhythm with feeble or absent pulses, patient remaining or becoming unconscious) one should proceed directly to phase 2 treatment.

Under certain circumstances, a modified approach should be used. When cardiopulmonary arrest has lasted for a minute or more prior to phase 1 treatment, three quick inflations of the lung should be employed initially (mouth-to-mouth, face mask) to ensure adequate oxygenation prior to electrical treatment. When an electrocardiographic diagnosis is not available initially, "blind" defibrillation is permissible.

TABLE 3-2 Resuscitation Procedure

Phase	Title	Number of Personnel	Duration	Arrhythmia	Treatment
1	Initial treatment	1	<10 sec	Ventricular fibrillation (VF) Ventricular standstill	Chest thump; electrical defibrillation Chest thump
2	Cardiopulmonary support	1 or 2	<1 min	Ventricular fibrillation Ventricular standstill	Chest massage and ventilation
3	Sustained resuscitative effort	5 or 6	<1 hr	Ventricular fibrillation	Repeat defibrillation; in addition, for "large-amplitude" VF: antiarrhythmics (lidocaine, procainamide); for "small-amplitude" VF: epinephrine, CaCl$_2$ NaHCO$_3$ adjusted according to pH
				Ventricular standstill	Isoproterenol-atropine External, transthoracic, or transvenous pacing, if indicated
4	Postresuscitation care	CCU or ICU staff	Hours to days		Proper ventilation, vital signs, arterial, central venous, or pulmonary arterial pressure monitoring (if indicated); check for complications (aspiration, pneumothorax, fractures, rupture of viscus); antiarrhythmic drugs (if indicated); treatment of heart failure (if required); special care for comatose patients

PHASE 2

Failure of phase 1 treatment calls for initiation of closed chest massage and artificial ventilation. It is often possible to sustain the patient's life for many minutes or even to effect a successful resuscitation by these maneuvers alone. The patient should be flat in bed with a bed board behind his back. Ventilation with self-inflating bag supplied with 100% oxygen and face mask should be carried out. Vomitus is suctioned.

PHASE 3

With arrival of additional personnel, a second effort at resuscitation is made. The ideal team includes:

1. One physician who directs the entire operation, and who remains unencumbered by technical operations
2. One physician giving closed chest massage
3. One physician giving ventilatory support (who should insert an endotracheal tube if face mask ventilation is inadequate. Intubation should be attempted only by experienced personnel in a well-oxygenated patient, unless other means of ventilation are impossible)
4. One physician giving drugs intravenously, inserting intravenous line if none is present
5, 6. Two nurses, one to prepare intravenous or intracardiac drugs, and one to assist, to procure equipment, and to keep records

At least five persons are needed; the physician-in-charge may if necessary fill one of the other positions. However, a team of more than six persons is undesirable and cumbersome.

TREATMENT OF PERSISTENT VENTRICULAR FIBRILLATION   Treatment is as follows:

1. Initially give 1 mEq/kg of $NaHCO_3$; this may be repeated once after 10 minutes. When pH determination is available, adjust the dosage accordingly. However, if pH measurements are not immediately available, give one-half the initial dose every 10 minutes thereafter until acid-base status can be ascertained.
2. If ventricular fibrillation is of the "large amplitude" type, or if each defibrillation results in transient reversion followed by ventricular tachycardia degenerating into ventricular fibrillation, give 100 mg of lidocaine I.V. or intracardiac and repeat shock; if this is unsuccessful give 100 mg of procainamide and repeat shock. The intracardiac route poses dangers, such as tamponade, accidental intramyocardial injection of drugs, and necessity for stopping chest massage. The intravenous route should be used if a centrally placed venous line is in position.
3. If the above measures are unsuccessful, or if tracing degenerates into "low amplitude" ventricular fibrillation, give 0.5 ml of epinephrine 1 : 1000 (0.5 mg) and repeat shock. If this is unsuccessful give 5 ml of $CaCl_2$ (500 mg) and repeat shock.

4. Arterial P_{O_2}, P_{CO_2}, and pH should be determined every 15 minutes. Note: Shocks should all be 400 watt-sec.

TREATMENT OF VENTRICULAR STANDSTILL   Treatment is as follows:

1. Give $NaHCO_3$ as (1) above.
2. Infuse isoproterenol, 1.0 mg in 500 ml of 5% D/W I.V., giving up to 4.0 ml/min (8 μ/min). Atropine (1.0 mg) may also be injected, but it is less effective than isoproterenol.
3. If electrical activity is not restored, give 0.5 ml of epinephrine 1 : 1000 as (3) above, then 5 ml $CaCl_2$ as (3) above.
4. If electrical activity is not restored, an attempt at external or trans-thoracic pacing may be made. These may be employed much earlier if they do not hamper the efforts at ventilation and chest massage. However, if at any point the patient's condition stabilizes, plans should be made for insertion of a transvenous pacemaker.
5. Determine blood gases and pH every 15 minutes, as (4) above.

TREATMENT OF SUPERIMPOSED POWER FAILURE   Restoration of normal or near-normal cardiac excitation after either ventricular fibrillation or cardiac standstill is often accompanied by ineffectual cardiac contraction despite normal activation, resulting in weak or absent peripheral pulses and low or unobtainable blood pressure. This is identical to the shock syndrome, and should be treated with norepinephrine, 8 mg in 500 ml 5% D/W, infused at rates up to 2.0 ml/min (32 μ/min).

TREATMENT OF OTHER ARRHYTHMIAS   Rapid ventricular tachycardia (rates greater than 200) and slow idioventricular rhythm are often accompanied by ineffectual cardiac pumping, and in such cases should be considered the equivalent of cardiac arrest. Rapid ventricular tachycardia is treated with lidocaine, 100 mg I.V., with a second dose approximately one minute later if required. If reversion does not occur, apply precordial shock starting with 50 watt-sec, and working up to 400 watt-sec. Idioventricular rhythm should be treated as standstill, except that the situation is sometimes stable enough to allow elective transvenous pacemaker insertion.

During resuscitation a variety of arrhythmias may be observed. A characteristic recurrent "cycle" may be noted, for example, ventricular fibrillation—precordial shock—standstill—idioventricular rhythm—ventricular tachycardia—ventricular fibrillation. Initial standstill may be converted into this cycle by administration of catecholamines or calcium. No method for interrupting the cycle exists which uniformly succeeds, and treatment must be directed to the arrhythmia of the moment. However, restoration of effective ventilation and cardiac output using closed chest massage, and adjustment of pH using $NaHCO_3$ infusions, are essential.

PHASE 4

If initial resuscitation is successful, attention should be directed to the following points:

1. Take care of endotracheal tube and ventilator.
2. Monitor frequently vital signs, intake and output, and, in presence of shock or pulmonary edema, arterial, central venous, or pulmonary arterial pressure.
3. Check for aspiration, pneumothorax, fractured ribs, ruptured viscera; determine hematocrit frequently.
4. Use lidocaine drip or procainamide as prophylaxis against further ventricular arrhythmia.
5. Insert transvenous pacemaker as prophylaxis against recurrent ventricular standstill.
6. Use continuous catechol infusions, digitalis, or manipulation of blood volume to treat shock or pulmonary edema.

TABLE 3-3 Contents of Emergency Carts at Boston City Hospital

---

Syringes and needles
Face mask and tubing to oxygen tank
Self-inflating bag and mask (Ambu) with tubing to oxygen tank
Oropharyngeal tube
Endotracheal tubes sizes 28F, 32F, 38F, and metal stylet
Laryngoscope set and handle with extra bulbs
Backboard
Suction tubing
Blood pump
Intracardiac needles
Intracaths
Arm boards
Sterile goods: gloves, cutdown kits, sponges, etc.
Extension cord and outlet box
Drugs and fluids
   aminophylline ampules (250 mg)
   atropine ampules (1.0 mg)
   digoxin ampules (0.5 mg)
   diphenhydramine hydrochloride (Benadryl) ampules (50 mg)
   epinephrine (Adrenalin) ampules (1 mg = 1 : 1,000)
   heparin vials (5,000 U/ml)
   isoproterenol (Isuprel) ampules (1.0 mg)
   lidocaine ampules (1,000 mg)
   metaraminol bitartrate (Aramine) ampules (100 mg)
   methyl prednisolone vials (1.0 gm) and H_2O
   norepinephrine bitartrate (Levophed) ampules (8.0 mg)
   potassium chloride vials (40 mEq)
   procainamide hydrochloride (Pronestyl) vials (1.0 gm)
   sterile water and saline solution for injection
   succinylcholine vials (200 mg)
   calcium chloride prefilled syringes (1.0 gm)
   epinephrine prefilled syringes (1.0 mg)
   lidocaine prefilled syringes (100 mg)
   sodium bicarbonate prefilled syringes (44.6 mEq)
   lactated Ringer's solution (1,000 ml)
   physiologic saline solution (1,000 ml)
   5% D/W (1,000 ml)
   5% sodium bicarbonate solution (500 ml)

---

7. If patient is comatose, turn frequently, and use indwelling urinary catheter, ophthalmic ointment, etc.

EMERGENCY CART

In order to be prepared for a cardiopulmonary resuscitation, the house officer should become intimately acquainted with the contents of the emergency carts which are available to him. He should examine all of the drugs and equipment and should rehearse in his own mind and in actual practice sessions the sequence of actions that he would pursue in the event of a real cardiopulmonary resuscitation. A list of the contents of the emergency carts at the Boston City Hospital is given in Table 3-3.

CARDIOPULMONARY RESUSCITATION AT BOSTON CITY HOSPITAL

Cardiopulmonary arrest is a frequent event at Boston City Hospital, occurring in about 3% of admissions and being encountered, on the average, about once daily on the medical and surgical wards alone. Many other episodes occur in the emergency room or in the coronary and intensive care units. In recent years, 37% of cardiopulmonary resuscitation attempts have been initially successful, with 9% of patients surviving to leave the hospital, despite the advanced age of the patient population (average age, 63).

Though the majority of patients do not survive cardiopulmonary resuscitation, because of serious underlying cardiac or pulmonary pathology, the number of patients who can be salvaged is considerable. This calls for an expectant approach to, and vigorous therapy of, patients who develop cardiopulmonary arrest.

SELECTED READINGS

Cardiopulmonary resuscitation. Statement by the Ad Hoc Committee on Cardiopulmonary Resuscitation of the Division of Medical Sciences, National Academy of Sciences–National Research Council. *J.A.M.A.* 198: 374–379, 1966.

Goldberg, A. H. Cardiopulmonary arrest. *N. Engl. J. Med.* 290:381–385, 1974.

Goldberg, A. H., Ramirez, A., and Ransil, B. J. Cardiopulmonary resuscitation (CPR) on medical and surgical wards. In *Abstracts of Scientific Papers, American Society of Anesthesiology.* Pp. 347–348, 1974.

Standards for cardiopulmonary resuscitation (CPR) and emergency cardiac care (ECC). *J.A.M.A.* 227(suppl.):833–868, 1974.

CARDIAC ARRHYTHMIAS
Enobong A. Ekong

Lidocaine
Propranolol Hydrochloride (Inderal)
Diphenylhydantoin Sodium (Dilantin)

AMONG THE EMERGENCIES encountered in daily medical practice, few appear to be as anxiety-provoking, both to the patient and to the physician, as cardiac emergencies. The increased public awareness of coronary risk factors and the syndrome of sudden death heighten this anxiety. It is no surprise then that when a patient is first seen with chest pain, "skipped beats," or any of the other myriad manifestations of cardiovascular impairment, great attention is paid by the physician (and rightly so) to prompt evaluation and treatment.

Part of the complex of cardiac emergencies is the sudden or chronic disruption of normal cardiac rhythm with potential or attendant hemodynamic impairment. Experience has shown that immediate and prompt correction of potentially fatal cardiac arrhythmias not only saves but also prolongs life. It is beyond the scope and intent of this chapter to discuss all the cardiac arrhythmias that may be encountered. Emphasis will be given instead to the arrhythmias most commonly observed and treated at Boston City Hospital, and to ways of diagnosing and treating them.

GENERAL MANAGEMENT OF ARRHYTHMIAS

The patient should be made comfortable. All diagnostic and therapeutic maneuvers should be carried out with a functioning intravenous line in place and within easy access to emergency resuscitation equipment. The procedures should preferably be carried out under continuous electrocardiographic monitoring and by someone with competence in the interpretation of electrocardiograms. A careful and thorough physical examination should be performed, with special emphasis on the cardiovascular system. Several valuable diagnostic clues may be obtained by the presence or absence of such signs as jugular venous A waves, heart murmurs, clicks, and gallops, and by the varying intensity and splitting of the heart sounds. It is important to determine whether the patient has been taking other drugs which might interfere with, potentiate, or contraindicate the form of treatment chosen, e.g., digitalis preparations. The type of treatment and the route of administration of drugs will depend very much on the patient's clinical state and the nature of the arrhythmia. A thorough knowledge of the pharmacokinetics of the various antiarrhythmic agents is invaluable in selecting which drugs to use and when to employ them.

INTERPRETATION OF ARRHYTHMIAS

Arrhythmias should always be interpreted within the context of the total clinical state of the patient, rather than as an isolated electrocardiographic finding. For instance, the approach to a young patient with a run of paroxysmal atrial tachycardia, but whose hemodynamic status is stable, would be totally different from that employed in an elderly patient with similar electrocardiographic findings, but with chest pain and congestive heart failure (CHF). One should always search for P waves and their relationship to QRS complexes. It is unwise to "eyeball" tracings, because subtle, crucial changes in rate and interval may be missed; hence, it is helpful to invest in a good pair of calipers. The least harmful diagnostic maneuver should always be performed for identification and clarification of any uncertain rhythm prior to treatment. Sometimes these diagnostic maneuvers can be therapeutic.

GENERAL MEASURES AND HEMODYNAMIC CONSEQUENCES OF ARRHYTHMIAS

The ultimate effects of any arrhythmia depend on many variables such as underlying coronary artery disease, other coexistent disease states, the rapidity of the rate and duration of the arrhythmia, the effects upon cardiac output and ventricular function, prior drug therapy, and absence or presence of increased sympathetic tone. In general, young patients without underlying coronary artery disease tolerate extremes of heart rate better than older patients with coronary artery disease (CAD), in whom more severe hemodynamic alterations are frequently observed. These alterations include diminution of cardiac output, coronary hypoperfusion with attendant ischemic pain, and reduction of blood flow to the kidneys, brain, and mesenteric circulation. Patients with arrhythmia are often seen with associated signs and symptoms suggesting dysfunction in these various organ systems, and frequently these signs and symptoms persist for some time after correction of the arrhythmia. It is therefore prudent to have a high index of suspicion for underlying arrhythmias in patients who are first seen with sudden unexplained CHF, syncope, transient neurological symptoms, renal impairment, mesenteric ischemia with abdominal pain, diarrhea or gastrointestinal bleeding, and sometimes even cyanosis or gangrene of the extremities.

As a general rule, hypotension caused by an arrhythmia can be corrected with appropriate treatment of the arrhythmia. Elevation of blood pressure by vasopressor agents may also terminate an arrhythmia and at the same time correct hypotension by improved coronary perfusion. Some arrhythmias may be related to underlying electrolyte disorders and hypoxia, which may require correction before antiarrhythmic therapy can be successful.

SUPRAVENTRICULAR TACHYARRHYTHMIAS

PAROXYSMAL SUPRAVENTRICULAR TACHYCARDIA

Paroxysmal supraventricular tachycardia (SVT) is an inclusive term for paroxysmal atrial tachycardia (PAT) in which the P waves are abnormal, but not of retrograde configuration, and have a constant relationship to the QRS complex; for paroxysmal junctional tachycardia (P waves retrograde, or with no P waves); and for an undefined group of arrhythmias in which the ectopic focus cannot definitely be determined. The majority are due to atrioventricular (AV) node or sinoatrial node reentry. SVT may be seen in young healthy persons, in patients without heart disease, in Wolff-Parkinson-White (WPW) syndrome, in rheumatic heart disease, in myocardial infarction (MI), with chronic obstructive pulmonary disease (COPD), or with the "sick-sinus" syndrome. The rhythm is precisely regular and is marked by abrupt onset (usually following a premature beat) and by abrupt termination, either spontaneously or during vagotonic maneuvers. The rate is usually 150 to 220, with a range of 140 to 250/min. P waves may be absent or present at identical rate but with abnormal contour. The QRS complex may be normal, or sometimes wide when aberrancy or conduction disturbances are present. Carotid sinus massage (CSM) either stops the arrhythmia abruptly or has no effect. The lack of this response cannot be used as a foolproof method for diagnosis, especially if wide QRS complexes are present. The differential diagnosis includes sinus tachycardia, atrial flutter with 2 : 1 conduction, paroxysmal atrial tachycardia with block, atrial fibrillation with rapid ventricular response, and paroxysmal ventricular tachycardia.

The diagnostic features of common, untreated tachyarrhythmias are as noted in Table 4-1.

TREATMENT AND PREVENTION An order of priority should be established, from the simplest, least dangerous and uncomfortable to more complicated regimens.

1. Sedation and reassurance. In many instances these measures might be the only modalities required to terminate the tachyarrhythmia.

2. Simple physiologic maneuvers. Vagal tone may be increased by CSM, the Valsalva maneuver, eyeball pressure, and induced vomiting or gagging. The best and most productive procedures are CSM and the Valsalva maneuver. The patient should be under continuous ECG monitoring in the recumbent position. Check both carotid pulses to be certain that they are present. Absence of the carotid pulse on one side is a contraindication to massage of the carotid sinuses. Both carotid pulses should never be massaged simultaneously, because a fatal outcome could ensue (cerebrovascular accident or cardiac standstill). The right carotid sinus should be identified and massaged first in brisk, rotating fashion for no more than 10 seconds. If there is no effect, the maneuver should be repeated on the left side. The Valsalva maneuver may potentiate the CSM. Although occasionally useful, eyeball pressure should be applied with caution, if at all, in patients with glaucoma, contact lenses, and possible retinal detachment. Induction of vomiting or gagging should be avoided in patients with acute MI.

3. Parasympathomimetic agents. The preferred drug is edrophonium chloride (Tensilon), after testing for hypersensitivity with an initial 1-mg I.V. injection, followed by administration of 9 mg (total 10 mg). The drug should be given slowly, and blood pressure and ECG should be continuously monitored. If no immediate effect is noted, the CSM should be repeated within one minute. An effect from the Tensilon should be observed within 1 to 2 minutes and dissipated within 10 to 15 minutes. Should this not occur, the dose can be repeated one more time. Side effects include nausea and vomiting, and the drug should be used with caution in patients with possible digitalis toxicity.

TABLE 4-1 Features of Common Untreated Tachyarrhythmias

| Rhythm | Rate (beats/min) | | Regularity | | Atrial Complexes | Ventricular Complexes | AV Conduction | Carotid Sinus Massage |
	Atrial	Ventricular	Atrial	Ventricular				
Supraventricular tachycardia (SVT)	140–250	140–250	Regular, "like clockwork"	Regular, "like clockwork"	Often not identifiable	Usually of normal duration (may be abnormal)*	1 : 1	No effect or rhythm is terminated
Atrial fibrillation	350–600	100–160	Irregular	Irregular	Irregular F waves	Usually of normal duration (may be abnormal)*	Variable block	Transient slowing of ventricular rate
Atrial flutter	240–350	120–175	Regular	Regular or irregular	Sawtooth pattern in II, III, AVF, V1	Usually of normal duration (may be abnormal)*	May be variable but usually fixed 2 : 1 or 4 : 1	Transient, stepwise slowing of ventricular rate
Paroxysmal atrial tachycardia (PAT) with block	150–250	150–250 or less	Regular	Regular or irregular	Small "spiked" P waves with isoelectric intervals	Usually of normal duration (may be abnormal)*	Fixed 2 : 1 or variable	Transient, stepwise slowing of ventricular rate
Ventricular tachycardia (VT)	Usually slower than the ventricular rate	120–250	Regular	Regular or irregular	Normal but usually not identifiable	Wide, bizarre complexes	1 : 1 with retrograde conduction; or no relationship of P to QRS if AV dissociation present	No effect on ventricular rate; atrial rate may be slowed

* With bundle branch block or aberration.

4. Pressor amines. These agents act to initiate a reflex increase in vagal tone and prolong conduction in the AV node by stimulating the carotid and aortic baroceptors. They should be used with extreme caution in hypertensive patients and in elderly patients, because they may precipitate a cerebrovascular accident. In such patients, other modalities of treatment are preferable. The blood pressure level at which reflex vagal bradycardia occurs is variable, but a rough rule of thumb is to aim for a systolic pressure between 140 and 180 and a diastolic pressure of 90 to 110 mHg.

a. Metaraminol bitartrate (Aramine), 250 mg diluted in 500 ml D_5W, may be used to titrate the blood pressure upward. The drug may also be given in a dose of 0.5 to 2.0 mg intravenously over 2 to 5 minutes. However, regulation of blood pressure level by the latter method is not reliable.

b. Phenylephrine (Neo-Synephrine), 0.5 to 1.0 mg, may also be injected intravenously over 2 to 5 minutes.

5. Alternatives. If there has been no response to the therapeutic maneuvers discussed above, there are several alternatives.

a. Rapid digitalization is still a most effective way of reverting an episode of SVT. Digitalization should preferably be carried out by the intravenous route. Useful digitalis preparations in this regard are (1) ouabain, which may be given in an initial dose of 0.2 to 0.5 mg I.V., followed by 0.1 mg every half hour until a digitalizing dose of 0.5 to 1.0 mg has been reached or the arrhythmia has been terminated; (2) digoxin, 0.75 to 1.0 mg I.V. initially, followed by 0.25 to 0.50 mg every 60 to 90 minutes, for a total of 1.0 to 2.0 mg in 24 hours; (3) lanatoside-C (Cedilanid), 0.4 to 0.8 mg I.V. followed by 0.4 mg every 60 to 90 minutes, for a total of 1.2 to 2.0 mg in 24 hours. CSM will potentiate the effect of any of these preparations in terminating the arrhythmia. The ECG should be monitored continuously.

b. Intravenous propranolol, procainamide, or intramuscular quinidine may also be useful in terminating refractory SVT. Care should be taken in the administration of propranolol to patients who have developed congestive heart failure (CHF) as a manifestation of their arrhythmia, and in those patients in whom CHF is likely to be provoked by its negative inotropic effect, for example, patients with enlarged hearts or a history of CHF. The doses for these drugs are shown in Table 4-2.

c. Electrical cardioversion is very useful for rapid restoration of sinus rhythm, especially in the patient who has developed chest pain, in the setting of acute myocardial infarction, and with development of hypotension or CHF (see section on cardioversion).

6. Electrical pacing of the right atrium. This technique is especially valuable if the patient has been fully digitalized; in this case, high energy shock may lead to worsening of arrhythmias. It is also useful for defining the atrial mechanism during insertion of the atrial wire. Generally, the pacing rates for overdriving are in the range of 100 to 400/min, with increasing stimulus strengths between 4 and 15 ma until conversion occurs. Sometimes, this procedure may convert the SVT to atrial fibrillation, which can then be more easily controlled with digitalis.

7. Prevention of recurrent attacks. The patient should be advised to avoid tobacco, tea, high-caffeine beverages, and excessive fatigue. Mild

TABLE 4-2 Antiarrhythmic Drugs

Drug	ECG Effect	t½ (hr)	Dosage Schedules	Route	Adverse Effects	Therapeutic Serum Levels
Digitalis—See Table 4-4 and section on CHF						
Quinidine	Prolongs QT, QRS, and PR (±)	6	200–600 mg q 6 h	P.O. or I.M.	Nausea, diarrhea, rash, thrombocytopenia, syncope, cinchonism, hypotension, heart block, VT, VF	2.5–6.0 mg/L
Procainamide hydrochloride (Pronestyl)	Prolongs QT, QRS, and PR (±)	3–4	500 mg–1 gm loading dose; then 250–500 mg q 3–4 h 250–500 mg q 3–4 h 100–200 mg q 5 min until 1 gm; then 1–3 mg/min drip for maintenance	P.O. I.M. I.V.	Rashes, arthralgias, lupus-type syndrome with +ANA, +LE prep on long-term therapy; hypotension, VT, VF, heart block	4–8 mg/L
Lidocaine (Xylocaine)	Shortens QT, shortens PR (±), QRS–no effect	1.5–2	50–100 mg; then 2–4 mg/min	I.V.	Lethargy, confusion, somnolence, seizure, disorientation, coma, paresthesias, hypotension, heart block	2–5 mg/L
Propranolol hydrochloride (Inderal)	Shortens QT, prolongs PR (±), QRS–no effect	2–4 2	10–40 mg q 6 h 1–3 mg by slow push in 1-mg increments	P.O. I.V.	Hypotension, heart block, CHF, asthma	50–100 ng/ml
Diphenylhydantoin sodium (Dilantin)	Shortens QT, shortens PR (±), QRS–no effect	24–36 4–6	1 gm loading in divided doses over 12–24 hr; followed by 300–400 mg/day 100–200 mg q 5–10 min until 1 gm; then 300–400 mg/day	P.O. I.V.	Tremors, diplopia, ataxia, nystagmus, coma, blood dyscrasias, megaloblastic anemia, skin rash, gingival hyperplasia, hypotension	10–18 mg/L

sedatives are helpful. For recurrent attacks, combinations of digitalis preparations with quinidine, procainamide, propranolol, or diphenylhydantoin sodium (Dilantin) may be helpful. Chronic symptomatic SVT may require further therapy such as interruption of cardiac sympathetics, induction of hypothyroidism by radioactive iodine, permanent ventricular pacing after surgical interruption of the AV node, or electrical pacing of the carotid sinus nerve.

ATRIAL FIBRILLATION

Atrial fibrillation is characterized by atrial rates above 350/min with a varying ventricular response, which is usually in the range of 100 to 160/min. Sometimes the ventricular response may be relatively slow, and this should alert one to the possibility of coexistent AV node disease or to concurrent therapy with digitalis. The ventricular response is determined by the degree of AV junctional conduction, refractory period, and degree of concealed conduction. On physical examination, patients in atrial fibrillation have a varying intensity of the first sound, a pulse deficit with an irregular pulse rate, and absent jugular A waves. As with SVT, patients with atrial fibrillation may conduct with widened QRS complexes caused by aberration or preexistent conduction defects, and this pattern sometimes raises the differential diagnosis of ventricular tachycardia. Another irregular rhythm to be differentiated from atrial fibrillation is atrial flutter with varying conduction.

Atrial fibrillation may occur in clinical situations such as rheumatic heart disease, hypertension, pulmonary embolism, coronary artery disease, atherosclerotic heart disease, thyrotoxicosis, pericarditis, alcohol or heroin intoxication, congestive heart failure, pneumonia, acute myocardial infarction, chronic obstructive pulmonary disease, cardiomyopathy, or after thoracotomy. It may also occur in paroxysmal fashion ("lone atrial fibrillation") in normal persons. This rhythm predisposes to peripheral and pulmonary embolism, especially in susceptible patients (e.g., with valvular heart disease, severe congestive heart failure). It also deprives the heart of the contribution to the cardiac output of the "atrial kick," which usually amounts to 20 to 25%. Restoration of this reserve may sometimes make the difference in the myocardial performance of a hemodynamically compromised patient.

Various forms of atrial fibrillation have been described, depending on the appearance on the surface electrocardiogram. "Coarse" fibrillation is seen more commonly in rheumatic heart disease and left atrial enlargement and is thought to be more responsive to cardioversion. The "straight line" form is seen in ischemia and hypertension and is less responsive to cardioversion. It is important to note that atrial fibrillation is rarely a digitoxic arrhythmia.

TREATMENT The procedure for atrial fibrillation is as follows:

1. Control of ventricular rate. The initial emphasis in the treatment of atrial fibrillation is directed at controlling the ventricular response. Digitalis is the drug of choice. It can usually reduce the ventricular rate to

less than 90/min. Larger doses of digitalis may be required to slow down the ventricular response in patients with thyrotoxicosis, anemia, fever, or other high-output states. The drug may be given orally or intravenously, depending on the patient's clinical status—orally if the patient is stable, intravenously if the patient is acutely ill with a very rapid heart rate. The aim is to slow down the ventricular rate to around 70 to 80/min, with a narrowing of the pulse deficit after mild exercise to less than 20 to 30 beats/min. The patient should be completely digitalized and placed on maintenance doses after successful control of the heart rate. In some situations, ectopic ventricular beats may develop prior to adequate digitalization and control of the heart rate. Propranolol p.o. in the dosage of 10 to 40 mg t.i.d. is usually an effective adjunctive therapy. Digitalis toxicity in the presence of atrial fibrillation can sometimes be recognized by the development of nonparoxysmal junctional tachycardia with "regularization" of the ventricular response or by the appearance of bidirectional tachycardia or ventricular premature beats (VPBs).

In the patient (usually elderly) who manifests a slow ventricular response to atrial fibrillation (rate less than 60/min), there should be no urgency to use digitalis preparations unless he has intractable congestive heart failure when first seen, for which digitalis or reversion to normal sinus rhythm (NSR) would normally be employed. In such patients, there may be a high incidence of AV nodal disease, and it may be wise to withhold digitalis therapy or an attempt at cardioversion until after placement of a ventricular pacing wire, to guard against a high degree of AV block.

Following the slowing down of ventricular response with digitalization, one of two things can occur: the rhythm may convert spontaneously to normal sinus rhythm or atrial fibrillation may persist. The choice of further therapy for the atrial fibrillation depends on many variables, such as the duration of atrial fibrillation, the size of the left atrium, the prior history of the patient in maintaining sinus rhythm after cardioversion, and history of embolic episodes (see section on cardioversion below for further discussion). Should it be decided that the rhythm needs to be converted to a sinus mechanism, there are two choices available: electrical cardioversion or drug-induced reversion.

2. Electrical cardioversion. The procedure of choice, this method is successful in 77 to 92% of patients. It is the simplest, safest, and fastest way of achieving the desired result. Should a cardioverter not be available, should the patient not consent to its use, or should the heart fail to convert to sinus rhythm after an adequate attempt at cardioversion, then the next modality is reversion using pharmacologic agents.

3. Reversion using drug agents. This should be attempted only after the patient has been fully digitalized and has a slow ventricular response between 80 and 90/min. The success rate is 50 to 90%. The patient should be hospitalized. The drug of choice is quinidine sulfate. A test dose of 200 mg is given initially p.o. to check for idiosyncratic reactions or hypersensitivity (rash, hypotension). With the Levine method, quinidine sulfate is given in 3 divided doses each day, starting with 200 mg, and with an increment of 200 mg with each subsequent dose, until either

conversion occurs or a maximum dose of 3.0 gm/day has been achieved. With the Sokolow method, 5 divided doses of 200 to 300 mg of quinidine sulfate are given at 2-hr intervals, followed by a daily increase of each individual dose by 100 mg until conversion or toxicity occurs.

Reversion of atrial fibrillation by drug agents is rarely employed in contemporary medical practice, with the advent of cardioversion. However, in situations as indicated above, further administration of the drug should be stopped should serum quinidine levels exceed the therapeutic range of 6 mg/liter or should evidence of toxicity develop with signs such as severe vomiting, diarrhea, widening of the QRS complex greater than 50% of the initial value (25% if conduction defect is present originally), and multiple premature ventricular contractions (PVCs). After successful conversion, the patient can be maintained on both digitalis and quinidine (usually 200 to 300 mg q.i.d.).

ATRIAL FLUTTER

Atrial flutter is usually seen with an atrial rate between 240 and 350/min and with a varying ventricular response. In the untreated patient, the most common type is flutter with 2 : 1 conduction, which may give the appearance of sinus tachycardia or PAT with a rate of 150. Atrial flutter may sometimes be seen with 1 : 1 conduction with a ventricular response over 250 (WPW syndrome; atrial flutter improperly treated with quinidine). The circulatory system cannot usually tolerate such a rapid rate, and these cases should always be treated as acute emergencies. Occasionally, flutter rhythm with varying AV conduction may resemble atrial fibrillation, but diagnostic maneuvers usually bring out the typical flutter waves. Flutter rhythm with a 4 : 1 ventricular response (sometimes seen after digitalis administration) may also superficially resemble normal sinus rhythm at a regular rate of approximately 75/min.

The diagnosis is usually easy to make if the typical flutter waves with "sawtooth" pattern and undulating baseline are seen in ECG leads II, III, and AVF. In the right precordial leads the flutter waves are often also clearly visible. This is an important differential point between flutter waves and the P waves seen in paroxysmal atrial tachycardia with block, which usually have an isoelectric baseline in both limb leads and precordial leads. Should the diagnosis not be immediately apparent, the flutter waves can be made manifest by carotid sinus massage, which increases the degree of AV block transiently by a stepwise reduction in rate (e.g., 150 to 100 or 75) as the block is increased. On careful physical examination, the diagnosis of a flutter mechanism can sometimes be made by observing the neck veins for rapidly occurring A waves, in "fluttering" fashion. Atrial flutter is rare in normal persons but may occur during acute illness, in ischemic heart disease, and acute myocardial infarction.

TREATMENT   The options for atrial flutter are:
1. Ventricular response. As in atrial fibrillation, the ventricular response may be slowed by digitalis preparations. The rhythm may revert to normal sinus or to atrial fibrillation following digitalization. In the

latter instance, quinidine or cardioversion may then be employed to revert the atrial fibrillation to sinus rhythm.

2. Electrical cardioversion. This is currently the treatment of choice. It is effective in 90% of patients. Low energy settings of less than 50 watt-sec are often effective. At even lower energy settings (1 to 10 watt-sec) the rhythm can often be converted to the more stable and more manageable atrial fibrillation in patients who are unable to maintain sinus rhythm.

Multifocal Atrial Tachycardia

The atrial rate is at least 100/min. There should be at least three types of P-wave morphology visible in any particular ECG lead. The P-P and R-R intervals are irregular, and there are varying P-R intervals. The rhythm is usually associated with underlying conditions such as chronic obstructive pulmonary disease, intercurrent illnesses, and diabetes mellitus. It may sometimes resemble atrial fibrillation, and the differentiation occasionally has to be made by intra-atrial electrograms. Multifocal atrial tachycardia responds poorly to drugs, digitalization, or cardioversion. Treatment should be directed toward correction of the underlying conditions. The arrhythmia is often paroxysmal and self limited.

Ventricular Preexcitation

1. Wolff-Parkinson-White syndrome. This syndrome is characterized by the onset of a tachyarrhythmia, usually supraventricular, in a patient whose resting electrocardiogram shows the typical WPW morphology: a short P-R interval of less than 0.10 sec and a delta wave which is typically noted on the ECG as widening of the QRS with slurring at the onset of the QRS (best seen in the precordial leads). The two classic types described are type A, with the anteriorly directed delta wave vector (RBBB configuration in V_1), and type B, with the leftward directed delta wave vector (LBBB configuration in V_1). Intermediate types are also possible. Tachyarrhythmia results from a macro-reentry circuit between the normal conduction pathway and the anomalous AV connections (Kent's bundle, James fiber, Mahaim fibers, AV connection of Ohnell). Several types of arrhythmias have been reported with WPW attacks—atrial tachycardia, atrial fibrillation, atrial flutter, and SVT. Ventricular tachyarrhythmias are rare, although during an attack, the wide aberrant complexes may resemble ventricular tachycardia. The condition is not usually lethal, although recurrent attacks can be uncomfortable and incapacitating. Death has, however, been reported during an attack. Therapy is directed toward reducing the frequency of tachyarrhythmias. The most useful drugs are quinidine or procainamide (increased block in the anomalous pathway) and propranolol (exerts effect on both normal and anomalous pathways). Atrial or ventricular pacing and electrical countershock have also been found to be useful in terminating an attack. Although digitalis may not be absolutely contraindicated, it should be used with caution in these patients, because it may

shorten the refractory period of the anomalous pathway while at the same time delaying normal AV conduction. It could thus lead paradoxically to an increased ventricular response. In troublesome refractory cases, surgical ablation of the anomalous pathway (especially in type B) has been successful.

2. Lown-Ganong-Levine syndrome. This syndrome is seen with ECG evidence of short P-R interval (less than 0.12 sec) and normal QRS duration. Frequent atrial ectopic beats are present, and the syndrome is defined by the onset of a supraventricular tachyarrhythmia. Treatment is the same as that employed in SVT.

Paroxysmal Atrial Tachycardia with Block

Paroxysmal atrial tachycardia (PAT) with block is diagnosed when a rapid atrial rate between 150 and 250 is observed with regular or varying ventricular response at a slow rate. The rhythm may be confused with atrial flutter, sinus tachycardia, or SVT, especially when the "buried" P waves (in the QRS complex) are not visible. When compared with atrial flutter, the P waves are noted to be upright in leads II, III, and AVF, with an isoelectric baseline, and upright, discrete, and of spiking nature in V_1. Carotid sinus massage, if effective, transiently slows the ventricular rate by decreasing AV conduction, without any change in the atrial rate. PAT with block may occur spontaneously in the elderly patient in the absence of digitalis therapy; or, as frequently observed (in 50 to 60% of cases), it may occur together with PVCs during digitalis therapy; in this instance, the diagnosis of digitalis excess should be strongly entertained and the drug withheld. This rhythm should be thoroughly delineated from atrial flutter or SVT by the use of intra-atrial leads if necessary, because treatment regimens are quite dissimilar.

TREATMENT If arrhythmia is associated with concurrent digitalis excess:
1. Discontinue digitalis.
2. Give potassium chloride by mouth, 2 to 4 gm initially followed by 1 to 2 gm every 3 to 4 hours as needed. It is, however, preferable to give KCl by the intravenous route in a slow infusion of about 10 to 15 mEq/hr (40 mEq in 500 ml of 5% D/W). Better control of the potassium level can then be achieved. The electrocardiogram should be monitored continuously for evidence of possible hyperkalemia (tall, symmetrically peaked T waves in the precordial leads). Note that hyperkalemia can sometimes occur as a concomitant of digitalis toxicity as a result of its effect on the myocardial membrane Na-K ATPase. Therefore, potassium should be given with careful monitoring of both the ECG and the electrolyte levels.
3. Diphenylhydantoin has been found effective in reversing this toxic arrhythmia caused by digitalis. It may be given in doses of 100 to 200 mg I.V. slowly over a 4- to 5-minute period. This dose may be repeated in 5 to 10 minutes, up to a total dose of 1.0 gm in 24 hours.

If the arrhythmia is clearly not due to digitalis, digitalis preparations should be used to treat the arrhythmia. Electrical cardioversion can also be employed.

SINUS TACHYCARDIA

In sinus tachycardia the rate usually varies between 100 and 180/min. In infants tachycardia is usually diagnosed when the rate exceeds 130 to 140/min. Adults with severe underlying disease or hypermetabolic states may be seen with rates in excess of 160/min. This rhythm is considered here because it can entail a troublesome differential diagnosis with other supraventricular rhythms such as PAT, SVT, atrial flutter with 2 : 1 conduction, and sometimes rapid atrial fibrillation when the variation in R-R intervals is not immediately apparent. CSM usually has no effect in terminating the tachycardia but may cause a slight, gradual, and simultaneous slowing of both atrial and ventricular response such that the P-R interval stays the same. The rate usually increases again in gradual fashion after massage is terminated. Sinus tachycardia can be a physiologic response as seen in exercise, excitement, infancy, or early childhood. Several pharmacologic agents may also induce the rhythm, the most commonly used ones being caffeine, atropine, isoproterenol, ephedrine, nicotine, amylnitrate, and epinephrine. Sinus tachycardia can also be a manifestation of underlying disease states such as hypotension, infection, fever, hyperthyroidism, congestive heart failure, beriberi, and pulmonary embolism.

TREATMENT Treatment is directed at the underlying cause of sinus tachycardia. Electrical cardioversion is not indicated, although it may erroneously be attempted if the rhythm has been misdiagnosed as SVT (intra-atrial leads are helpful). In troublesome cases, the rate may be slowed by the administration of propranolol, 10 to 40 mg t.i.d. orally, or 1 mg, given slowly by the I.V. route. This modality is obviously contraindicated in situations in which negative inotropy would be deleterious. Several diagnostic aids that may be useful in defining atrial mechanisms are listed below:

1. Carotid sinus massage, eyeball pressure, Valsalva maneuver, gagging
2. Lewis leads, V$_3$R leads
3. Edrophonium chloride (Tensilon), parasympathomimetic drugs
4. Esophageal leads
5. Right intra-atrial leads
6. His bundle recording

EXTRASYSTOLIC RHYTHMS

Extrasystolic rhythms originate frequently on the basis of the reentry phenomenon; however, other mechanisms, such as increased automaticity of pacemaker foci, may also be operative.

ATRIAL PREMATURE BEATS

Atrial premature beats (APBs) are generally innocuous beats which require no specific treatment except when they occur with increasing frequency or multifocality with symptoms, or as premonitory signs of documented tachyarrhythmias, e.g., reciprocating tachycardia. Atrial premature beats may or may not be conducted to the ventricles, depending on their site of origin and degree of prematurity. If they are non-conducted, they may be seen commonly as a cause of a "pause" which may be mistakenly diagnosed as AV block. Atrial premature beats may occur in normal persons, with alcohol ingestion, with atrial distension or ischemia, or with fatigue. Treatment, if deemed necessary, is usually with quinidine sulfate, 200 to 400 mg orally every 4 to 6 hours. Other effective drugs are procainamide, propranolol, or, when congestive heart failure resulting in atrial distension is present, digitalis.

Ventricular Premature Beats

Ventricular premature beats (VPBs) represent probably the commonest form of rhythm disturbance. They may have a compensatory pause, retrograde conduction, or be interpolated. They occur in normal persons, in acute MI, with hypoxemia, infections, exercise, coronary artery disease, ventricular aneurysms, congestive heart failure, anesthesia (especially with cyclopropane), digitalis toxicity (especially with associated hypokalemia), and with other drugs such as amphetamines, isoproterenol, epinephrine, and caffeine. The decision to treat or not to treat VPBs depends on other associated diseases (e.g., MI) and on their arrhythmogenic potential (multifocal nature, coupling closeness to the T-wave vulnerable period, and frequency greater than 5 to 10/min). When VPBs are not a reflection of underlying coronary artery disease, they may be treated by having the patient abstain from the precipitating cause such as drugs and caffeine, and by mild sedation. For life-threatening arrhythmogenic VPBs, especially in the setting of acute MI or severe underlying heart disease, the irritable focus can be treated with (1) intravenous boluses of lidocaine, 50 to 100 mg followed by an I.V. infusion of lidocaine at 2 to 4 mg/min (1 gm lidocaine in 1,000 ml 5% D/W), or (2) procainamide boluses, 100 mg every 10 minutes, up to a total dose of 800 to 1,000 mg, or (3) intravenous diphenylhydantoin (Dilantin) in doses of 100 to 200 mg slowly over a 4- to 5-minute period, and repeated in 5 to 10 minutes, up to a total dose of 1.0 gm in 24 hours. For less urgent situations, oral therapy can be initiated with procainamide, 250 to 500 mg every 3 hours, depending on the patient's body weight, quinidine sulfate, 200 to 400 mg t.i.d.–q.i.d. or diphenylhydantoin, 250 mg t.i.d.–q.i.d. In some cases, combinations of several of these drugs may be found to be effective. The ECG should be monitored constantly during the administration of these potent drugs, and potential side effects should be carefully watched for (see Table 4-2). In intractable cases, overdrive pacing with the use of a temporary pacing wire may be effective.

When ectopic activity is present, a common problem is differentiation of VPBs from supraventricular ectopic beats with aberrant conduction. Table 4-3 may prove helpful in this task.

TABLE 4-3 Differentiation of Aberrantly Conducted Beats from
Ventricular Ectopic Beats

Criterion	Aberration	Ectopy
Right bundle branch block configuration		
RSR in V_1	++++	—
R or qR in V_1	+	++
Left bundle branch block configuration	+	++
Fixed coupling	+	++
"Compensatory" pause	+	++
Identical initial vector to normally conducted QRS	++++	—
Identical slope of initial vector	++++	—
Long-short cycle sequence in AF (Ashman beats)	++	+
Short-long cycle sequence in AF	—	+++
Fusion beats	—	+++
Preceding atrial activity	++	+
Like known aberrancy	++++	—
Dressler or capture beats	—	+++

Note: VPBs originating from the left ventricle may be seen with RSR configuration
in V_1; similarly those from the right ventricle may show left bundle branch block
configuration.

VENTRICULAR TACHYARRHYTHMIAS AND VENTRICULAR FIBRILLATION

VENTRICULAR TACHYCARDIA

Two types of ventricular tachycardia (VT) have been identified: a
rapid, paroxysmal form, and slow VT or accelerated idioventricular
rhythm. VT is defined as the occurrence of three or more repetitive
premature ventricular contractions. It may be sporadic or sustained. The
highest incidence is during acute MI and in the setting of severe coronary, arteriosclerotic, or hypertensive heart disease. It may occur as a
result of iatrogenic causes such as irritation of the ventricle by a pacing
wire or central venous pressure line; from drugs (isoproterenol, digitalis,
atropine); or from other underlying conditions like malignancies, sarcoidosis, myxedema, cardiomyopathy. The ECG shows a ventricular rate
between 120 and 250, with a slight beat-to-beat variation of less than 0.33
sec. The rhythm is seldom grossly irregular (to be distinguished from
atrial fibrillation with aberrancy and slow ventricular tachycardia). The
four ECG diagnostic features are (1) wide QRS complexes of 0.12 sec
or greater duration, (2) AV dissociation with atrial rate slower than the
ventricular rate (not always present), (3) VPBs at times when sinus
rhythm is present and of morphology similar to those seen during the
paroxysm, and (4) fusion or capture beats, which if present, may sub-
stantiate the diagnosis of a ventricular ectopic focus (to be sometimes
differentiated from an aberrantly conducted SVT). On physical examination, there may be a wide splitting of the first and second sounds

caused by asynchrony of ventricular contraction. Gallop sounds may be present. The first heart sound may vary in intensity because of AV dissociation and a varying P-R interval. Cannon A waves may be observed in the jugular venous pulse as a consequence of AV dissociation. The blood pressure may be low. CSM may slow the atrial rate (if AV dissociation is present) without affecting the ventricular rate.

The slow type of VT is generally a benign rhythm disturbance recognized with increasing frequency following acute MI, especially inferior MI. It occurs most frequently in the presence of bradycardia or during the slow phase of sinus arrhythmia. It begins as an escape rhythm; however, unlike idioventricular escape rhythms, the discharge rate is faster than that of the underlying sinus mechanism. The rate is usually between 60 and 120/min. It does not adversely affect prognosis and generally does not require treatment. Sometimes, when associated with VPBs, it may degenerate into rapid ventricular tachycardia, requiring treatment by acceleration of the slow sinus rate with atropine or pacing.

TREATMENT Treatment of rapid VT is directed not only at the arrhythmia per se but also at correction of some of the associated hemodynamic derangements. Hypotension should be corrected with vasopressors if restoration of normal rhythm does not correct it. Hypoxemia and acid-base disturbances should be corrected. A functioning airway should be maintained.

The preferred treatment of ventricular tachycardia is lidocaine given in an I.V. bolus of 100 mg. It is effective in 80% of cases. If sustained VT is not abolished, a second bolus may be given. Should this again fail, cardioversion at 25 watt-sec should be carried out directly, provided that the arrhythmia is not thought to be a manifestation of digitalis toxicity. It is effective in 97% of cases. Intravenous procainamide in boluses of 100 mg every 5 minutes, up to a total of 1.0 gm, may also be used if no response has been obtained with lidocaine, if the patient manifests CNS symptoms from lidocaine, or if a cardioverter is not available. The ECG and blood pressure should be monitored constantly. The drug is effective in about 78% of cases. Should hypotension develop, the blood pressure must be maintained with vasopressors. Widening of the QRS beyond 50% of control is an indication to stop the drug immediately. After successful termination of the arrhythmia oral therapy may be begun with procainamide, 250 to 500 mg every 3 hours to guard against further recurrence.

Another agent of secondary choice in the treatment of premonitory VPBs or VT is diphenylhydantoin. This is often quite effective in the treatment of digitalis-induced arrhythmias. The dosage schedule is discussed under VPBs. Propranolol (Inderal) may also be used as a second-line drug with doses of 1 mg injected slowly I.V. and repeated at 5-minute intervals to a maximum of 3 mg.

When VT occurs because of possible digitalis overdosage, procainamide or lidocaine should be tried as described under the treatment of VPBs. If these agents prove unsuccessful, diphenylhydantoin and propranolol may be used as discussed above. When pharmacologic measures prove unsuccessful, "overdrive" of ventricular tachycardia may be attempted with transvenous pacing.

As discussed in the section on VPBs, a combination of the various drugs will sometimes be found effective. However, such combinations should be undertaken with caution because of possible added drug toxicity. Parenteral quinidine gluconate is rarely indicated because of its marked side effects. In intractable cases, quinidine may be given I.M. in doses of 0.4 gm initially and every 2 hours until toxicity or reversion occurs. Surgical techniques such as aneurysmectomy, stellate ganglionectomy, coronary artery bypass, and sympathectomy have also been employed in refractory cases.

Ventricular Fibrillation

The incidence of this uniformly fatal arrhythmia can be appreciably diminished in the hospital by the aggressive treatment of the foregoing premonitory arrhythmias (VPBs, VT). However, when it occurs in any setting, prompt treatment must be instituted. The only definitive therapy of this arrhythmia is rapid defibrillation (not synchronized countershock). Defibrillation should be carried out within 15 to 45 *seconds*, with maximum energy levels of the machine (i.e., 400 watt/sec). If prompt defibrillation attempts are made, a high success rate in reversion to sinus rhythm may be expected. Precious time should not initially be expended in other resuscitative maneuvers.

If efforts at defibrillation are not immediately successful, cardiopulmonary resuscitation must be carried out (see Chapter 3, Cardiopulmonary Resuscitation).

CARDIOVERSION

Synchronized precordial electrical shock, or cardioversion, is employed for the elective reversion of certain arrhythmias to normal sinus rhythm (NSR).

Indications

1. Atrial fibrillation. The success rate is about 90%, but with "lone" atrial fibrillation only about 79% of patients will revert to NSR following cardioversion. Cardioversion for atrial fibrillation should be used for the following reasons: (a) fast, symptomatic, or uncontrollable ventricular response; (b) occurrence of systemic or pulmonary emboli; and (c) atrial fibrillation of less than one year's duration. Chances of reversion to and maintenance of sinus rhythm are increased in the patient with a normal-sized left atrium. For patients with atrial fibrillation of about 5 years' duration the success rate is about 50%. Despite administration of digitalis and/or antiarrhythmic drugs after conversion to sinus rhythm, less than two-thirds of patients remain in NSR at the end of one year.

There is currently no uniformity of opinion regarding the use of anti-coagulant therapy prior to cardioversion. Some observers advocate routine anticoagulation in all patients before cardioversion. In general, high-risk patients with prosthetic valves, mitral stenosis, or history of systemic or pulmonary emboli should be anticoagulated for 4 to 6 weeks prior to cardioversion.

2. Atrial flutter. Easy to convert at low energy settings, the success rate is 90%.

3. SVT. Cardioversion is successful in 80% of patients. Start with low energy settings if digitalis toxicity is suspected.

4. Ventricular tachycardia. Initial therapy should be with lidocaine as discussed previously, followed by cardioversion for sustained, symptomatic VT. A success rate of 97% has been reported for treatment of this rhythm by cardioversion.

CONTRAINDICATIONS

Patients with digitalis-induced arrhythmias usually should not be cardioverted except in extreme circumstances, because most of the complications of cardioversion have occurred in this group. Treatment for these arrhythmias should be by withdrawing the drug, improving electrolyte, renal, and metabolic status, and by administration of potassium and antiarrhythmic drugs. Cardioversion should not be used in sinus tachycardia or in patients with unstable or recurrent arrhythmias (for instance, the patient who goes in and out of PAT, atrial fibrillation, or flutter). Elderly patients with a slow ventricular response to atrial fibrillation do not require cardioversion if they are asymptomatic. Patients with multifocal atrial tachycardia (MAT) as a manifestation of underlying disease such as chronic obstructive pulmonary disease (COPD) should not be cardioverted. In similar fashion, hyperthyroid patients who have atrial fibrillation should be treated medically with propranolol or digitalis and the hyperthyroidism corrected before cardioversion is attempted.

MECHANICS

When the procedure is entirely elective, ordinarily digitalis preparations are discontinued 24 hours in advance of the procedure, and quinidine, 0.3 gm q.i.d. is given p.o. (for atrial fibrillation or flutter). The patient is given nothing by mouth the morning of the procedure. When the procedure is not elective, the above measures may be dispensed with, provided that proper precautions are taken to avoid provocation of digitalis-induced arrhythmias at the time that cardioversion is carried out (see below). For purely elective procedures, high-risk groups such as patients with chronic CHF, prior embolization, prosthetic heart valves, and long-standing mitral disease should be anticoagulated for 4 to 6 weeks prior to cardioversion. Before the cardioversion procedure, an explanation is given to the patient, and a permit is signed if time and the patient's condition permit.

For the cardioversion procedure, an intravenous line, preferably an Intracath, is inserted. The patient is placed supine and gown removed from the arms and upper torso. A full 12-lead ECG is made, and the presence of the arrhythmia which is being treated is confirmed. The cardioversion machine is tested by choosing an artifact-free lead with ample positive R-wave deflection and by setting the gain so that the synchronizing circuit is just being triggered. Synchronization should be upon the R-wave, not beyond (in those machines in which such an adjustment can be made). These two maneuvers are of utmost importance to avoid delivering an electrical shock at an improper phase of the cardiac cycle, thereby possibly inducing ectopic arrhythmias or possibly even ventricular fibrillation. A permanent record is made of this synchronization pattern.

Lidocaine and atropine should be drawn up in syringes and ready for use. Other drugs which should be immediately on hand include isoproterenol, procainamide, diphenylhydantoin, quinidine, propranolol, epinephrine, calcium chloride or gluconate, and sodium bicarbonate. On occasion it may be useful to have some of these other drugs already prepared in syringes or dripsets as well; for example, isoproterenol in cases of slow atrial fibrillation, when bradyarrhythmias not infrequently ensue upon reversion.

The electrode paddles are liberally greased over their entire surface (to avoid burns). The patient normally will be rendered amnestic for the event by giving intravenous diazepam (Valium), starting with 3 to 5 mg, and increasing the dose as necessary to 15 mg or sometimes even more. If the patient becomes stuporous, and if respirations are feeble, he may be temporarily assisted with an Ambu bag and face mask, with delivery of 100% O_2. Repeated measurement of blood pressure by cuff is begun. An anesthetist should preferably be in attendance.

When the effect of the diazepam is apparent, the patient is lifted up, and the posterior paddle is placed behind his back, with care taken to clear the paddle from gowns and bedclothes. The machine is charged to an appropriate joule setting (see below), and, with one hand, an operator places the anterior paddle squarely on the precordium just to the left of the sternum. The ECG recorder is started, all personnel stand away from the patient, and the machine is discharged. Immediately thereafter, the ECG is inspected, and, if there is doubt about the rhythm, lead V_1 is taken (especially helpful in cases of atrial fibrillation and flutter). If reversion has not taken place, higher joule settings are employed in sequence (see below), with additional doses of diazepam as required. If reversion occurs, the patient's vital signs are closely observed for at least 15 minutes; in some cases reversion to junctional rhythm or other bradyarrhythmias may require longer periods of observation, or even administration of isoproterenol or atropine, especially if hypotension is present. Induction of ventricular irritability, especially if possibly caused by digitalis, requires intravenous administration of lidocaine, in one or more boluses of 50 mg. Generally it is safe to proceed with higher energies after such therapy. On occasion diphenylhydantoin (Dilantin) may also be required to control such arrhythmias. Intravenous procainamide and propranolol represent additional useful therapeutic agents but are rarely needed. Occurrence of severe ventricular arrhythmias requiring such drugs will generally discourage further attempts at cardioversion.

Starting joule settings appropriate for various arrhythmias are as follows:

Atrial fibrillation	50 joules
Atrial flutter	25 joules
Ventricular tachycardia	25 joules
PAT and junctional tachycardia	50 joules

The sequence of energy titration should be 25, 50, 100, 200, and 400 joules. On occasion when digitalis status is suspect, it is appropriate to give "test doses" of energy at settings as low as 5 or 10 joules. If ventricular irritability is induced, lidocaine therapy should be employed prior to giving more energetic shocks.

When atrial fibrillation or flutter, or ventricular tachycardia, is reverted as an emergency procedure, quinidine, 0.3 gm p.o., should be given immediately after cardioversion for the former, and a lidocaine drip started for the latter. Unless digitalis toxicity is present, digitalis therapy may be resumed after cardioversion.

COMPLICATIONS

The overall incidence of complications is about 14%.

1. Burns and chest wall soreness. These conditions tend to occur especially in the emergency setting when not enough electrode paste has been applied to the paddles. Care should be taken not to apply too much electrode paste, however, because this may dissipate the energy delivered.
2. Hypotension. Usually this complication occurs at high energy settings and as a result of the sedative or anesthesia used.
3. Increased serum enzymes. Concentrations of SGOT, LDH, and CPK may be found elevated in the skeletal muscle fractions. Should acute myocardial infarction be in the differential diagnosis, appropriate serum samples should be drawn prior to cardioversion or enzymes should be fractionated.
4. Rhythm disturbances. Few serious arrhythmias occur after cardioversion. Most of the arrhythmias are limited to transient VPBs, APBs, and sinus bradycardia, thought to be due to release of acetylcholine and catecholamines.
5. Pulmonary and systemic emboli. Emboli may be seen in about 1.5% of cases.
6. Pulmonary edema. This complication occurs only rarely.

BRADYARRHYTHMIAS

SINUS BRADYCARDIA

Sinus bradycardia is defined as a heart rate of less than 60/min. It may be associated with acute myocardial infarction (especially inferior wall), with the "sick-sinus" syndrome, or may occur as a manifestation of a sensitive carotid sinus. A slow heart rate may predispose to ventricular ectopy by temporal dispersion of refractoriness. It may lead to syncopal attacks, or to congestive heart failure. Sinus bradycardia can be seen with several pathologic states such as myxedema, hypothermia, increased cerebrospinal fluid pressure, or typhoid fever. It may be physiologic (in athletes, with sleep, with carotid sinus massage). Several drugs can also induce sinus bradycardia, including digitalis, propranolol, morphine, and reserpine.

Treatment is directed at the underlying condition. However, for symtomatic slow rates usually $\leq$ 40/min, treatment may be initiated with atropine, 0.5 to 1.0 mg I.V. or I.M. and repeated every 3 to 4 hours. An intravenous isoproterenol drip (1 amp in 500 5% D/W) may also be used to increase the rate. This treatment may not be the modality of choice in the setting of an acute myocardial infarction. For chronic, recurrent symptomatic cases, ventricular pacing has been successfully employed.

"Sick-Sinus" Syndrome

The "sick-sinus" syndrome is characterized by multiple arrhythmias resulting in both slow and fast heart rates, and often with dizzy spells, syncopal attacks, or CHF. It tends to occur in the elderly patient, although it has been reported in all age groups. The ECG may show sinus bradycardia, sinus node exit block unrelated to drug therapy, or periods of prolonged sinus arrest with or without sinus or junctional escape rhythm. Should such escape rhythms occur, they may be seen at a rapid rate as paroxysmal atrial tachycardia, junctional tachycardia, atrial fibrillation, or supraventricular tachyarrhythmia. Patients with associated AV nodal disease may show atrial fibrillation with a slow ventricular response.

There are many associated causes for this syndrome. It has been described with infiltrative diseases such as amyloid, sarcoid, and hemachromatosis, with collagen disease, surgical injury, cardiomyopathies, pericarditis, acute myocardial infarctions (especially inferior), and as a concomitant of sclerotic or ischemic coronary disease. The clinical manifestations are usually due to inadequate organ perfusion.

Diagnosis is facilitated by having a high index of suspicion, especially in elderly patients with sinus bradycardia or unexplained slow atrial fibrillation or SVT. The patients usually have an inappropriately slow heart rate response to exercise or atropine. For instance, atropine in 1 to 2 mg doses I.V. may not speed up the sinus rate to over 90/min as would be expected. Long-term ECG monitoring may reveal periods of sinus arrest or exit block. The patients may demonstrate an exaggerated slowing of the sinus node recovery time as measured by overdrive suppression of the SA node by atrial pacing (pauses in excess of 1,200–1,400 msec are characteristic). A false negative test may occur with atrial pacing as a consequence of entrance block.

The treatment of choice is permanent ventricular pacing (not atrial pacing, because associated AV conduction disturbances may coexist), a procedure which prevents bradycardia and also permits safe administration of antiarrhythmic agents if tachyrrahythmias persist. To permit digitalization for CHF or tachyarrhythmias, or prior to cardioversion for tachyarrhythmias, standby pacing should also be employed. Temporary measures include use of atropine, isoproterenol, or oral ephedrine.

HEART BLOCK

First-Degree AV Block

First-degree AV block is defined as a P-R interval of 0.21 sec or greater. It may be seen with drug therapy with digitalis, quinidine, or procainamide, with disease states such as myocarditis, hypoxia, inferior myocardial infarction, or as a consequence of increased vagotonic influences. Usually no treatment is indicated, but atropine or isoproterenol may be used if needed.

Second-Degree AV Block

Second-degree AV block is defined as such when both conducted and dropped beats are present. Two types may be observed.

1. Mobitz type I (Wenckebach phenomenon). Although this condition is seen in digitalis excess most commonly it may occur also without digitalis. It may also be observed in the setting of an acute MI. It is defined as progressive P-R prolongation leading to dropped beats, with progressive R-R shortening until the dropped beat occurs. The R-R interval encompassing the dropped beat is usually shorter than the sum of the preceding two R-R intervals. The usual ratios are 2 : 1, 3 : 2, 4 : 3, and 5 : 4. If the phenomenon is seen with digitalis excess, the drug must be discontinued.

2. Mobitz type II. Dropped beats occur in type II also, but the P-R interval of the conducted beats stays constant. Type II block usually denotes serious conduction disturbance below the AV junction and may be a premonitory sign prior to development of complete AV block. The most common type is 2 : 1 AV block. It is commonly seen in acute myocardial infarction.

Third-Degree (Complete) AV Block

In third-degree heart block the ECG shows independent atrial and ventricular activity, with the P waves bearing no relationship to the QRS complex. The atrial rate is faster than the ventricular rate, and the P-R intervals vary. If the ventricular pacemaker is below the bifurcation of the bundle of His, the QRS complex may have a wide duration, and this configuration is associated with more severe symptoms and poorer prognosis. The ventricular rates vary depending on the site of the ventricular focus.

Junctional pacemaker	40–60/min
His bundle pacemaker	40–50/min
Idioventricular rhythm	15–40/min
Congenital complete heart block	60/min
Surgical complete heart block	40–50/min

TREATMENT

Complete heart block may be seen in various clinical states: infiltrative cardiomyopathy, Chagasic cardiomyopathy, acute myocardial infarction, diphtheria, digitalis or potassium excess, congenital heart lesions, and myxedema. The treatment of choice is ventricular pacing.

CARDIAC PACEMAKING

INDICATIONS

The indications for emergency use of temporary transvenous pacing are as follows.

1. Acute myocardial infarction complicated by
   (a) complete heart block
   (b) Mobitz type II block
   (c) advanced Mobitz type I AV block unresponsive to atropine, or when atropine is contraindicated
   (d) certain cases of junctional or sinus bradycardia
   (e) first-degree AV block superimposed on new or preexisting LBBB, or RBBB with left anterior or left posterior hemiblock
2. Overdrive suppression of arrhythmias as discussed in the section on arrhythmias, such as intractable ventricular premature beats, ventricular tachycardia, and supraventricular tachyarrhythmias, including refractory digitalis-induced arrhythmias
3. Therapy of Stokes-Adams attacks prior to permanent pacing
4. Improving the clinical status prior to long-term pacing in patients with carotid sinus syncope, "sick-sinus" syndrome, symtomatic refractory CHF, or angina pectoris associated with sinus bradycardia or complete AV block
5. Coronary angiography or cardiac surgery (ventricular or atrial pacing)
6. Cardiac arrest with ventricular asystole
7. Permanent pacemaker failure

TECHNIQUE

An adequate intravenous pathway is inserted. A solution of 2 mg of isoproterenol in 500 ml of 5% D/W is readied for infusion with a microdrip. A portable monitor should be attached to the patient, and a defibrillator should be on hand. Lidocaine and atropine should be drawn up in labeled syringes.

  1. Inserting the pacemaker under fluoroscopic control. Sterile surgical techniques should always be employed. Select the right or left brachial (median basilic), left external jugular, or left subclavian vein, but do not use the right jugular nor the right subclavian vein, because insertion of a permanent transvenous pacemaker is usually performed by way of the right jugular or cephalic vein. If a percutaneous method is used, introduce the catheter through a plastic sleeve. (A metal Intracath needle may shear off the catheter insulation.) Monitor fluoroscopically as well as electrocardiographically, because VPBs are frequently noted when the

catheter touches the right ventricular endocardial wall, especially the outflow tract.

2. Inserting the pacemaker under ECG control. After the pacing catheter has been introduced into the vein, it should be attached by means of a sterile alligator cable to the V lead of a grounded ECG machine. Large P waves are recorded from the right atrium (negative, biphasic, or positive, depending on high, mid, or low atrial position). The P wave diminishes in size when the right ventricle is entered, and a characteristic right ventricular complex appears: small R, deep S, and inverted T wave. An endocardial current of injury will also be noted by the appearance of markedly elevated S-T segments.

The pacing threshold should not exceed 1.5 ma if the catheter is at the right ventricular apex. The pacing current should be set at 2 to 3 times the threshold for ventricular capture. In all instances it is preferable to utilize the pacemaker on the "demand" mode.

After placement, the catheter should be sutured to the skin 1 to 2 inches from the insertion site. If the brachial (median basilic) vein is used, the arm should be slung or held to the chest, as arm abduction or elevation may displace the catheter tip. Topical antibiotic ointment should be applied over the skin entrance sites; dressings must be changed every 24 hours and ointment reapplied each time. Immediately after placement of the pacemaker an overpenetrated portable chest film should be obtained for baseline reference as to the position of the catheter tip. A 12-lead ECG should be taken.

Failure to pace is not uncommon and is usually due to (1) displacement of the electrode from the endocardial surface, or (2) perforation of the right ventricular wall. In these two instances a pacing artifact without ventricular capture will be noted in the electrocardiograph when the pacemaker is operated in the "fixed" mode. Failure to visualize the pacing artifact indicates (1) poor connection of pacing catheter to the pacer, (2) displacement of the ground needle in cases of unipolar electrodes, or (3) battery failure.

Cautionary Measures

Although most of the cases of heart block following acute myocardial infarction are transient and normal sinus rhythm is restored within 7 days, AV conduction may be delayed in some cases for weeks or may even become permanent. In patients who revert to sinus rhythm, heart block may later reappear; therefore, the pacemaker should be left in place for at least 5 days after return of normal sinus rhythm. Patients who have progressed to complete heart block following Mobitz II block may eventually require permament pacer insertion, whether or not return to NSR occurs; however this is seldom true for transient complete heart block which develops following Mobitz I block.

In all instances the following precautions should be observed.

1. The temporary pacer should be a battery-powered unit. Only in extreme circumstances when a battery-powered unit is not available should wall outlets be used.

2. Any electric bed of a patient with a temporary pacemaker should have 3-pronged grounding and should be disconnected from the wall power source when not in use. When a change in position is desired, no part of the patient should be in contact with metal while the bed is in operation.
3. All electrical equipment coming into even remote contact with the patient (x-ray equipment) must be plugged into a 3-pronged grounded electrical outlet.
4. Electric razors for patients with temporary pacemakers are not permitted.

ANTIARRHYTHMIC DRUGS

DIGITALIS

The various antiarrhythmic preparations are summarized in Table 4-2. Table 4-4 outlines the dosages for digitalization. Higher doses of digitalis are sometimes required for the treatment of arrhythmias than are necessary for CHF. Dosages and pharmacokinetics have been extensively discussed in recent publications. Patients receiving digitalis preparations should be carefully watched for clinical and ECG signs of toxicity.

QUINIDINE

Quinidine exerts its effect by slowing conduction velocity, prolonging the effective refractory period, and depressing the rate of atrial and ventricular pacemaker discharge. It is thus useful for treating APBs and VPBs. It is less useful for treating SVT. An oral dose of quinidine sulfate is almost completely absorbed. It peaks in 1 to 3 hours and lasts for 6 to 8 hours. Therapeutic levels are in the range of 2.5 to 6.0 mg/liter. It may be given I.M. as the gluconate form, and it tends to peak earlier. Serum levels are helpful as therapeutic guides. The drug prolongs the action potential duration (Q-T), the P-R interval, and may cause a widening of the QRS complex in the therapeutic range. It is metabolized in the liver and is also excreted unchanged in urine. It should be discontinued if the QRS complex is widened to greater than 50% of the control. The most common side effects are nausea, vomiting, and diarrhea. Toxic reactions may include hypotension, cinchonism, thrombocytopenia, and "quinidine syncope." The dosages are as discussed under treatment of specific arrhythmias and in Table 4-2. Preparations include quinidine sulfate, 0.2 gm in tablet or capsule form; quinidine gluconate (Quinaglute), 0.33-gm tablets in sustained release form (0.2-gm base), and quinidine polygalacturonate (Cardioquin) in tablets containing the equivalent of quinidine sulfate 0.2 gm.

PROCAINAMIDE

Procainamide is similar in its mode of action to quinidine. It is most commonly used to treat VPBs and VT. Occasionally supraventricular tachyarrhythmias may also respond to it. Procainamide may also be use-

TABLE 4-4 Properties of Digitalizing Drugs

Preparation	GI Absorption (%)	Onset of Action (min)	Peak (hr)	t½	Excretion Route	Oral Dose (mg) Average	Oral Dose (mg) Range	I.V. or I.M. Dose (mg) Average	I.V. or I.M. Dose (mg) Range
Ouabain	–	5–10	0.5–2	22 hr	Renal	–	–	0.3–0.5	0.3–1.0
Cedilanid	10	10–30	1–3	36 hr	Renal	6.0	5.0–10.0	1.6	1.2–2.0
Digoxin	55–75	15–30	1.5–5	36 hr	Renal	1.25–1.5	1.0–4.0	0.75–1.0	0.75–2.0
Digitoxin	90–100	25–120	4–12	4–6 days	Hepatic	0.7–1.2	0.7–2.0	1.0	1.0–2.0

ful in patients who are sensitive to quinidine. It may be given p.o., I.M., or I.V. For I.V. use, 100- to 200-mg boluses may be given every 5 minutes until the arrhythmia is abolished or until 1 gm has been administered. To maintain normal rhythm, an infusion rate can be maintained at about 1 to 3 mg/min. Sixty percent of the drug is excreted unchanged in the kidney. Therapeutic serum levels are 4 to 8 mg/liter. Oral doses are usually given in 250- to 500-mg tablets every 3 hours, depending on the patient's body weight: <125 lb (250 mg); 125 to 175 lb (375 mg); >175 lb (500 mg). Sixty percent of patients on long-term therapy may require discontinuation of the drug because of severe side effects such as fever, rash, lupus-type syndrome, or arthralgias. The antinuclear antibody (ANA) levels should be monitored closely with long-term therapy. The lupus syndrome usually disappears when the drug is discontinued. Like quinidine, procainamide may cause ventricular arrhythmias and heart block at toxic levels. QRS complex widening and Q-T prolongation also occur as with quinidine, and the drug should be stopped when the QRS complex is prolonged beyond 50% of control.

LIDOCAINE

Lidocaine is a water soluble, synthetic local anesthetic which has been found extremely useful in the treatment of ventricular arrhythmias, especially those associated with acute myocardial infarction or digitalis intoxication. It is usually administered by the intravenous route in boluses of 50 to 100 mg followed by an I.V. drip at 2 to 4 mg/min to maintain a serum therapeutic range of 2 to 5 mg/liter. The drug is not usually effective for supraventricular arrhythmias. It should be used at reduced dosages in patients with liver failure, shock, and reduced hepatic blood flow due to CHF, because it is metabolized by the liver. Lidocaine shortens the action potential duration and refractoriness of the Purkinje fibers while at the same time exerting no effect on the arterial blood pressure, left ventricular (LV) end diastolic pressure, or ventricular contractile force. Its toxic side effects are usually seen at levels exceeding 5 mg/liter, at which point CNS symptoms predominate: lethargy, confusion, somnolence, and seizures. At very high levels (exceeding 9 to 10 mg/liter), cardiovascular impairment may be seen. Hypotension, heart block, and arrhythmias have also been reported.

PROPRANOLOL HYDROCHLORIDE (INDERAL)

This is a beta adrenergic-blocking drug with quinidine-like properties which has been found effective for atrial arrhythmias and supraventricular tachyarrhythmias (especially if caused by digitalis or if unresponsive to digitalis). The drug is not very effective and is not recommended for controlling acute ventricular arrhythmias, although its combination with other antiarrhythmic drugs may be found useful. It may be used for controlling the fast symptomatic ventricular response from sinus tachycardia of diverse causes until the underlying factors can be defined and corrected (e.g., thyrotoxicosis, pheochromocytoma). Propranolol may precipitate congestive heart failure because of its negative inotropic effect, even in doses as low as 1 mg intravenously, or after many days of oral therapy. It is contraindicated in patients with severe bronchospasm or those with a history of allergic manifestations (asthma, allergic rhinitis). The drug may mask the expected tachycardia from hypoglycemia in a diabetic patient on hypoglycemic agents. Propranolol effect may persist for hours to days after discontinuation of the drug. Its half-life is prolonged in liver disease. The dosage schedules are as recorded in Table 4-2.

DIPHENYLHYDANTOIN SODIUM (DILANTIN)

The exact mechanism of action of diphenylhydantoin is poorly understood, but the drug appears to suppress ectopic pacemaker activity by reducing the rate of spontaneous diastolic depolarization. Its effect on the ECG is usually limited to slight shortening of the P-R and Q-T intervals. The therapeutic range is 10 to 18 mg/liter (the same as for antiepileptic therapy). It is useful for treating both ventricular and supraventricular arrhythmias, especially in the setting of digitalis toxicity. It may be given orally or intravenously. The onset of action after an I.V. dose is almost immediate; the duration of action is variable. Intramuscular administration leads to erratic absorption and may cause tissue necrosis. The drug is almost completely hydroxylated in the liver and excreted in the urine. Toxic effects are primarily neurological but include hypotension (especially if it is given too rapidly by I.V. injection), tremors, ataxia, nystagmus, coma, and blood dyscrasias. Megaloblastic anemia, skin rash, and gingival hyperplasia have also been reported. The dosage schedules are as shown in Table 4-2.

REFERENCES

1. Bellet, S.   Diagnostic features and management of supraventricular arrhythmias. *Prog. Cardiovasc. Dis.* 8:483, 1966.
2. Ticzon, A., and Whalen, R.   Refractory supraventricular tachycardias. *Circulation* 47:642–653, 1973.
3. Moss, A. J., and Davis, R. J.   Brady-tachy syndrome. *Prog. Cardiovasc. Dis.* 16:439–454, 1974.
4. Pick, A., and Langendorf, G.   Differentiation of supraventricular and ventricular tachycardias. *Prog. Cardiovasc. Dis.* 2:391, 1959.
5. Chung, K. Y., Walsh, T. J., and Massie, E.   Wolff-Parkinson-White syndrome. *Am. Heart J.* 69:116, 1965.
6. Lown, B., Ganong, W., and Levine, S.   The syndrome of short P-R interval, normal QRS complex and paroxysmal rapid heart action. *Circulation* 5:693–704, 1952.
7. Shine, K., Kastor, J., and Yurchak, P.   Multifocal atrial tachycardia. *N. Engl. J. Med.* 279:344, 1968.
8. Lown, B., Temte, J., and Arter, W.   Ventricular tachyarrhythmias—Clinical aspects. *Circulation* 47:1364–1381, 1973.
9. Kastor, J. A.   Atrioventricular block. *N. Engl. J. Med.* 292:572, 1975.
10. Hecht, H. H., Kossman, C. E., et al.   Atrioventricular and intraventricular conduction—Revised nomenclature and concepts. *Am. J. Cardiol.* 31:232–244, 1973.

11. Resnekov, L.   Present status of electroversion in the management of cardiac dysrhythmias. *Circulation* 47:1356–1363, 1973.
12. Javier, R., Maramba, L., Hildner, F., et al.   Temporary cardiac pacing: Technique and indications. *Chest* 59:498, 1971.
13. Lown, B., Kleiger, R., and Wolff, G.   The technique of cardioversion. *Am. Heart J.* 67:282, 1964.
14. Lown, B., and Kosowsky, B.   Artificial pacemakers (3 part series). *N. Engl. J. Med.* 283:907–916, 971–977, 1023–1031, 1970.
15. Smith, T., and Haber, E.   Digitalis (4 part series). *N. Engl. J. Med.* 289:945–952, 1010–1016, 1063–1072, 1125–1128, 1973.
16. Mason, D. T.   Digitalis pharmacology and therapeutics: Recent advances. *Ann. Intern. Med.* 80:520–530, 1974.
17. Surawicz, B., and Lasseter, K. C.   Effect of drugs on the electrocardiogram. *Prog. Cardiovasc. Dis.* 13:26–54, 1970.
18. Gianelly, R. E., and Harrison, D. C.   Drugs used in the treatment of cardiac arrhythmias. *D.M.* Jan., 1969. Pp. 1–53.
19. Koch-Weser, J.   Serum drug concentrations as therapeutic guides. *N. Engl. J. Med.* 287:227–231, 1972.
20. Treatment of cardiac arrhythmias. *Med. Lett. Drugs Ther.* 16:101–108, 1974.

ACUTE CARDIAC FAILURE

PANTEL S. VOKONAS

ACUTE CARDIAC FAILURE, i.e., acute pulmonary edema secondary to cardiac disease, is a common life-threatening medical emergency that requires prompt identification and decisive treatment.

PRIMARY THERAPEUTIC GOALS

In the initial treatment phase of acute cardiac decompensation two primary therapeutic goals must be kept in mind: (1) the improvement and maintenance of adequate tissue oxygenation, and (2) the diminution of the work load of the heart, i.e., reduction of circulatory demands by measures to decrease venous return. Eight specific measures used in the management of acute cardiac failure frequently effective in achieving the two primary goals of treatment are as follows.

UPRIGHT POSITION

In the absence of significant hypotension, the patient should be rapidly placed in a sitting position either in bed or in a chair. Proper positioning of the patient in this manner increases lung volume and vital capacity while simultaneously decreasing venous return and the work of breathing. Occasionally, this simple maneuver alone will markedly improve the overall degree of acute respiratory distress.

MORPHINE SULFATE

In the presence of acute pulmonary edema, the majority of patients will tolerate 5 to 10 mg of morphine sulfate intravenously. This drug can also be given subcutaneously, 10 to 15 mg, but in the presence of reduced peripheral tissue perfusion the intravenous route is mandatory. Although the beneficial effects of morphine are not completely understood they are derived from multiple factors, i.e., (1) its sedative effect; (2) a decrease in musculoskeletal and respiratory activity; (3) venodilation resulting in reduction of venous return with a decrease in pulmonary arterial pressure and pulmonary vascular resistance (producing what is in effect a pharmacologic or "internal" phlebotomy); and (4) possibly inhibition of autonomic reflexes mediated by the central nervous system, which may contribute to the development of pulmonary edema [1, 2, 3].

The use of morphine sulfate requires close and continuous observation for evidence of respiratory depression and the immediate availability of morphine antagonists such as nalorphine hydrochloride (Nalline) or naloxone hydrochloride (Narcan). Because of its depressive effect on the respiration, the use of morphine sulfate should always be accompanied by the concomitant administration of oxygen and should be used only with extreme caution or not at all in patients with severe chronic obstructive lung disease.

Oxygen

Oxygen is administered to patients in acute cardiac failure to elevate alveolar oxygen tension and enhance alveolar-capillary diffusion of oxygen. This must be done whether or not detectable cyanosis is present. The best technique for administering humidified oxygen is by means of a well-fitted face mask. The frequently used nasal catheter system usually cannot deliver high concentrations of oxygen and is relatively ineffective in elevating inspired air oxygen tension.

Intermittent Positive Pressure Breathing (IPPB)

Oxygen administered under intermittent positive pressure is the most effective technique for supplementing inspired oxygen under conditions of severe cardiac decompensation. IPPB used in this manner aids in regulating the patient's respiration; provides more uniform pulmonary ventilation; increases intra-alveolar pressure, thus reducing capillary to alveolar transudation of fluid; and decreases venous return to the lungs, further resulting in a decrease in pulmonary artery pressure. By partially diminishing the increased lung stiffness already present, this technique reduces the overall work of breathing.

IPPB, however, must be used with careful regulation of oxygen flow rates, inspiratory pressure levels, and timing, since the resultant reduction in venous return can sometimes be dramatic and result in markedly diminished cardiac output and systemic hypotension. Oxygen should always be administered with humidification in order to avoid drying of the mucous membranes of the tracheobronchial tree and inspissation of bronchial secretions. In the presence of large amounts of frothy sputum, some clinicians recommend that oxygen be bubbled through antifoaming agents such as 20 to 50% ethyl alcohol or propylene glycol. This is in an effort to decrease the partial respiratory obstruction related to the mechanical presence of edema fluid in the tracheobronchial tree.

In the absence of hypotension, the two additional measures to decrease venous return which follow will enhance the effect of the measures described above.

ROTATING TOURNIQUETS

Application of tourniquets to three extremities at a pressure greater than venous but lower than arterial diastolic pressure should be performed at once. Tourniquets are rotated every 20 minutes and removed sequentially when no longer needed. Equipment is now available which will automatically inflate and deflate pneumatic cuffs applied to the extremities in a sequential fashion every 20 minutes. In this context, tourniquets reduce venous return, lower central blood volume, and decrease preload (i.e., ventricular filling pressures), thereby reducing overall cardiac work. Presumably the concomitant reduction in pulmonary capillary pressure also reduces the gradient for capillary to alveolar transudation of fluid.

PHLEBOTOMY

If reduction of venous return by tourniquets is inadequate, as is often the case in the presence of massive peripheral edema and/or marked venous distension, phlebotomy, with removal of 300 to 500 ml of blood, should be performed. This is best done with the use of a sterile donor collection bag in order to permit retransfusion of the patient's red blood cells. In selected patients with severe anemia and acute cardiac decompensation such a course of sequential plasmaphoresis may prove extremely effective. Phlebotomy must be performed with great caution in acute pulmonary edema following acute myocardial infarction, especially in a patient with a normal heart size and blood volume, because significant hypotension may rapidly ensue. Under these circumstances, continuous monitoring of the blood pressure and urinary output is essential to prevent this complication.

DIURETIC THERAPY

Parenteral administration of rapidly acting diuretic agents such as furosemide (Lasix), 20 to 40 mg, or ethacrynic acid (Edecrin), 25 to 50 mg I.V., is an important additional measure that may promote relief of pulmonary congestion. This effect, however, is not necessarily related to the diuretic effect of these agents [4, 5]. Recent studies with furosemide in patients with acute cardiac failure following acute myocardial infarction have demonstrated that critical relief of the symptoms of acute pulmonary congestion frequently precedes apparent diuresis. The mechanisms involved may be related to an increase in peripheral venous capacitance and to an early rise in renal plasma flow [5]. Both agents must be used judiciously, because the prompt and profound diuresis which is soon initiated may occasionally result in a severe reduction of intravascular volume, producing a significant decrease in cardiac output and systemic hypotension.

Aminophylline

In patients with significant bronchospasm, aminophylline, 250 to 500 mg, may be given intravenously. Aminophylline decreases bronchoconstriction and in addition has a direct vasodilating effect, promotes diuresis, and may improve cardiac contractility. The intravenous administration of aminophylline must be carried out slowly over a period of 15 minutes, since side effects include hypotension and cardiac arrhythmias in the presence of hypoxia as well as metabolic or respiratory acidosis [1].

When a patient critically ill with acute pulmonary edema fails to respond to the above measures and when arterial blood gas determinations suggest rapidly progressive deterioration, endotracheal intubation should be performed and continuous positive pressure ventilation applied (see Chapter 7, Acute Respiratory Failure). Under conditions of controlled assisted respiration, further use of larger incremental doses of intravenous morphine sulfate is permitted and is frequently effective in reversing even the severest forms of acute pulmonary edema.

SECONDARY THERAPEUTIC GOALS

Secondary therapeutic goals which must be pursued immediately after the initial phase of treatment are designed: (1) to improve cardiac contractility, (2) to identify precipitating or aggravating factors leading to the development of acute cardiac failure, and (3) to investigate the underlying nature of the specific heart disease involved [1, 2].

Digitalization

Digitalis augments cardiac contractility, which in turn tends to increase cardiac output, promote diuresis, and reduce filling pressures in both ventricles, thereby promoting relief of pulmonary congestion. Thus, digitalization may be of potential benefit in the majority of patients with cardiac failure regardless of underlying cause. In the treatment of acute cardiac failure, however, digitalis must be considered a secondary or ancillary measure in comparison with the rapid effectiveness of the measures outlined above. If the patient has not received prior digitalis therapy, Digoxin, 0.5 to 1.0 mg I.V., may be given followed by additional 0.25-mg increments every 2 to 4 hours as indicated. The peak effect is usually reached between 1½ and 6 hours. Alternatively, oubain, 0.2 mg I.V., may be given followed by 0.1- to 0.2-mg increments every 1 to 2 hours, to an average digitalizing dose of 0.8 mg. The onset of action is approximately 5 minutes, with a peak effect usually in 30 to 60 minutes. It is imperative that the physician have an adequate working knowledge of the mode of action, metabolism, dosage schedule, toxic side effects, and conditions under which toxicity is likely to occur for whichever cardiac glycoside is used [6, 7, 8]. Electrocardiographic monitoring as well as consideration of each patient's electrolyte balance, renal function, and arterial blood gas status is essential to avoid digitalis toxicity.

Digitalis provides little or no benefit in patients with constrictive pericarditis, cardiac tamponade, untreated hyperthyroidism, mitral stenosis in normal sinus rhythm without right ventricular failure, the circulatory overload state of acute glomerulonephritis, and acute pulmonary edema related to noncardiac causes. It should be used only with great caution in patients with myocarditis, hypothyroidism, and acute cor pulmonale secondary to chronic obstructive lung disease.

RECOGNITION AND TREATMENT OF CARDIAC ARRHYTHMIAS

Prompt recognition and treatment of cardiac arrhythmias are imperative in the management of acute cardiac failure (see Chapter 4, Cardiac Arrhythmias). In the presence of adequate blood pressure and tissue perfusion, supraventricular tachycardia, atrial flutter, and fibrillation with moderately rapid ventricular rates frequently respond to rapid digitalization. In patients with ventricular tachycardia, unresponsive to the usual antiarrhythmic therapy, or with supraventricular tachyarrhythmias (not related to digitalis toxicity) associated with extremely rapid ventricular rates or significant hypotension, immediate cardioversion by direct current countershock should be performed. Acute cardiac failure associated with severe bradycardia should be treated with atropine, 1 mg I.V., or by transvenous insertion of a cardiac pacemaker.

In some patients, cautious mechanical removal of fluid from large accumulations in pericardial, pleural, or peritoneal spaces may occasionally result in marked symptomatic improvement.

Severe hypertension associated with acute pulmonary edema requires prompt treatment (see Chapter 7). Recently, sodium nitroprusside, phentolamine, and nitroglycerin, agents which decrease both afterload and venous return, have been used in selected patients with acute cardiac failure following myocardial infarction characterized by low cardiac output and high peripheral vascular resistance.

Prompt identification and treatment, whenever possible, of precipitating or aggravating factors related to acute cardiac failure may be of critical importance in the continuing management of each patient. Following is a list of these factors.

Hypertension	Hyperthyroidism
Arrhythmias	Fever
Acute myocardial infarction	Anemia
Pulmonary emboli	Infection
Bacterial endocarditis	Excessive intake of salt
Myocarditis	Discontinuation of cardiac medications
Pericarditis	

The nature of the specific heart disease involved is frequently suggested by the clinical history and physical findings aided by standard laboratory studies, including chest roentgenogram and electrocardiogram. Noninvasive studies, such as cardiac series, phonocardiography, and echocardiography, may be done at a later time and, if indicated, followed by cardiac catheterization and angiographic studies to assess the specific cardiac disease involved.

During the early phase of patient evaluation and treatment, however, the physician must maintain a high level of awareness for those specific cardiac lesions, initially seen as acute cardiac failure, which may require immediate study and surgical intervention. Three examples of such lesions are (1) massive mitral regurgitation related to ruptured chordae tendiniae manifested by the presence of a new early systolic or pansystolic murmur over the apex or precordium in a patient with normal sinus rhythm; (2) massive aortic regurgitation secondary to bacterial endocarditis indicated either by the presence of a new decrescendo diastolic murmur over the aortic area and left sternal border or by marked increase in intensity of a similar preexisting murmur; (3) perforation of the interventricular septum or (partial) papillary muscle rupture manifested by the development of new systolic murmurs or thrills in a patient with acute myocardial infarction. In many instances, prompt identification and appropriate surgical therapy of such lesions may be life-saving.

REFERENCES

1. Ramirez, A., and Abelmann, W. H.   Cardiac decompensation: Current concepts. N. Engl. J. Med. 290:499–501, 1974.
2. Hurst, J. W., and Spann, J. F.   Treatment of Heart Failure. In Hurst, J. W., Logue, R. B., Schlant, R. C., and Wenger, N. K. (Eds.), The Heart. 3d ed. New York: McGraw-Hill, 1974.
3. Robin, E. D., Cross, C. E., and Zelis, R. M.   Pulmonary edema. N. Engl. J. Med. 288:239–304, 1973.
4. Lesch, M., Carnasos, G. J., Mulholland, M. D., and the Osler Medical House Staff.   Controlled study comparing ethacrynic acid to mercaptomerin in the treatment of acute pulmonary edema. N. Engl. J. Med. 279:115–122, 1968.
5. Dikshit, K., Vyden, J. K., Forrester, J. S., Chatterjee, K., Prakash, R., and Swan, H. J. C.   Renal and extrarenal hemodynamic effects of furosemide in congestive heart failure after acute myocardial infarction. N. Engl. J. Med. 288:1087–1091, 1973.
6. Beller, G. A., Smith, T. W., Abelmann, W. H., Haber, E., and Hood, W. B., Jr.   Digitalis intoxication: A prospective clinical study with serum level correlations. N. Engl. J. Med. 284:989–997, 1971.
7. Doherty, J. D.   Digitalis glycosides: Pharmacokinetics and their clinical implications. Ann. Intern. Med. 79:229–238, 1973.
8. Smith, T. W.   Digitalis glycosides. N. Engl. J. Med. 288:719–722, 942–946, 1973.

Aram V. Chobanian

THE HYPERTENSIVE CRISIS is a life-threatening condition which requires immediate therapy and prompt reduction of blood pressure. Any form of hypertension may be associated with this critical state, the major determinant being the degree of elevation of blood pressure rather than the etiologic basis for the hypertension. The blood pressure level required to precipitate hypertensive crisis will vary from patient to patient and will depend to some extent on the rate of rise and the prior level as well as the absolute height of blood pressure. A child with acute glomerulonephritis or a young woman with eclampsia may be in hypertensive crisis with blood pressures as low as 170/110 mHg. On the other hand, adults with chronic hypertension may show no evidence of hypertensive crisis even with blood pressure levels as high as 280/170 mHg.

The different clinical conditions which may be considered as hypertensive emergencies are summarized below.

RAPID LOWERING OF BLOOD PRESSURE MANDATORY

Hypertensive Encephalopathy

The classic form is hypertensive encephalopathy, which is characterized by marked elevation of blood pressure in association with severe headache, agitation, convulsions, coma, or other neurological signs. Cerebral edema and increased intracranial pressure are common and may contribute to the elevation in blood pressure by stimulating reflex responses which tend to increase systemic blood pressure. Cerebral vasospasm and decreased cerebral perfusion have been considered as important factors in the pathogenesis of hypertensive encephalopathy [1], although recent studies suggest that the cause of the encephalopathy is a failure of autoregulation of cerebral blood flow with hyperperfusion rather than hypoperfusion and resultant development of cerebral edema [2]. In the vast majority of patients, rapid lowering of blood pressure produces marked

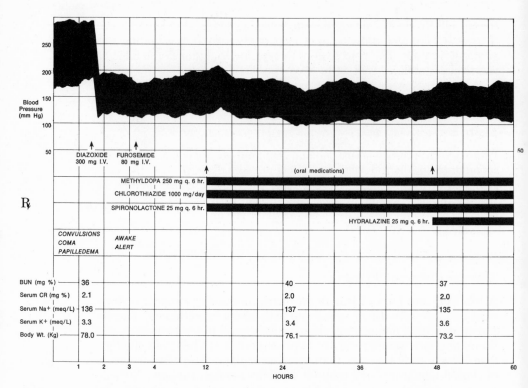

FIGURE 6-1   Clinical course of a 39-year-old man with acute hypertensive encephalopathy treated with antihypertensive drugs.

improvement in symptoms within a matter of minutes. When such improvement is not readily apparent, the diagnosis of hypertensive encephalopathy should be questioned and other diagnoses such as cerebral hemorrhage or other space-occupying lesions should be considered. The clinical course of a typical patient with hypertensive encephalopathy is depicted in Figure 6-1.

Eclampsia

Eclampsia is another form of hypertensive emergency in which immediate lowering of blood pressure is required. The symptoms associated with eclampsia are comparable to those in hypertensive encephalopathy. A prior history of toxemia is generally present, and the eclampsia develops in the latter half of pregnancy.

Dissecting Aortic Aneurysms

Acute antihypertensive therapy is also beneficial for patients with dissecting aortic aneurysms. The current evidence indicates that many patients with this disorder, particularly those with uncomplicated dissections originating beyond the origin of the left subclavian artery, may be treated effectively by blood pressure lowering alone. Antihypertensive therapy is warranted initially, even in patients ultimately requiring surgical intervention. The objectives of therapy are to diminish the force of ventricular systole as well as to keep the blood pressure at the lowest level consistent with the maintenance of adequate perfusion to vital organs [3].

ACUTE PULMONARY EDEMA WITH SEVERE HYPERTENSION

Patients with severe hypertension and acute pulmonary edema usually respond dramatically to lowering of blood pressure. Reduction of the pressure load on the left ventricle is usually the most effective method of treating the heart failure in these persons, and patients will generally recover even without administration of digitalis glycosides.

RAPID LOWERING OF BLOOD PRESSURE BENEFICIAL

TRANSIENT ISCHEMIC EPISODES

A relatively rare form of hypertensive crisis is the development of transient ischemic episodes in association with severe hypertension. The appearance of focal neurological signs can be related to cerebral vasospasm developing in response to severe hypertension. It is likely that such patients have significant preexistent cerebrovascular disease which becomes of clinical significance as a result of the reflex vasoconstriction.

SEVERE BLEEDING AND SURGICAL TREATMENT

Hypertensive patients who have severe bleeding from any cause may benefit from immediate treatment of the hypertension. In addition, patients with severe hypertension who are to undergo angiographic studies, biopsies, or other surgical treatments should have their blood pressure reduced prior to the procedure to minimize bleeding problems.

CEREBRAL HEMORRHAGE

The presence of severe hypertension in patients with cerebral hemorrhage is generally considered to be an indication for parenteral antihypertensive drugs, although the benefits of such aggressive therapy have not been demonstrated clearly. The blood pressure usually increases with the cerebrovascular accident, presumably as a result of increased intracranial pressure. In contrast to hypertensive encephalopathy, blood pressure lowering in such patients will not produce rapid improvement in the clinical picture. The objective of therapy is to reduce the pressure to a level which will decrease the possibility of rebleeding without inducing critical reductions in organ perfusion. However, this optimum level of blood pressure has not been clearly delineated. Because in patients with cerebral thrombosis the area of infarction may be extended following marked blood pressure lowering, it is important to try to exclude the diagnosis of cerebrovascular occlusion before embarking on a program involving marked reduction of blood pressure.

Myocardial Infarction or Coronary Insufficiency

A new approach to the treatment of patients with myocardial infarction or coronary insufficiency involves the rapid lowering of blood pressure to diminish cardiac work. The available evidence strongly supports the use of rapidly acting antihypertensive drugs in patients with moderate or severe hypertension and myocardial ischemia. In addition, experimental data suggest that rapid blood pressure lowering may have a beneficial effect even in some normotensive or mildly hypertensive patients with myocardial ischemia.

Renal Failure

Patients with severe hypertension and renal failure may also be candidates for acute antihypertensive therapy even though renal function can deteriorate further with lowering of blood pressure and anuria can be induced. Fortunately, the decrease in renal function is usually transient, although, in rare instances, the patients will need dialysis until renal function improves.

DRUGS IN THE TREATMENT OF HYPERTENSIVE CRISIS

A summary of the individual drugs, the dosage information, onset and duration of action, and toxicity is given in Table 6-1. The hemodynamic effects of the agents are described in Table 6-2.

Quick-Acting Drugs

Diazoxide This drug appears to be the most valuable agent except in patients with significant ischemic heart disease. It acts almost instantaneously and in contrast to the other compounds in this group (e.g., nitroprusside and trimethaphan), its duration of action is prolonged. It produces a marked peripheral vasodilation and a reflex compensatory increase in cardiac output, and increase in renal and cerebral blood flow may occur. Because of its marked binding to serum albumin, it should be administered very rapidly as an intravenous bolus [3]. The solution containing the drug is very alkaline (pH approximately 12), and therefore it is highly irritating if not injected directly into the vein. A hypotensive response to the drug may occur, particularly if the patient is receiving propranolol or some other beta-blocking drug. The dose used in the presence of beta-blocking treatment should be only ⅓ to ½ that of the usual recommended dosage. Any hypotension should be treated with norepinephrine. Sodium retention is common with diazoxide, and concomitant diuretic therapy is generally advisable. Hyperglycemia also occurs in most patients as a result of the effects of the drug in inhibiting insulin release. However, because of the short periods over which diazoxide is used, neither sodium retention nor hyperglycemia represents a clinically important side effect.

TABLE 6-1 Drugs in the Treatment of Hypertensive Crisis

Drug	Usual Adult Dose	Route	Onset of Action (min)	Duration of Action	Common Side Effects
Diazoxide (Hyperstat)	300 mg	Intravenous (bolus)	1	3–12 hr	Angina, fluid retention, hyperglycemia
Methyldopa (Aldomet)	250–500 mg	Intravenous	10–60	2–8 hr	Somnolence, parkinsonian-type syndrome
Reserpine (Serpasil)	1.0–2.5 mg	Intramuscular	45–90	3–8 hr	Somnolence, parkinsonian-type syndrome
Hydralazine (Apresoline)	10–40 mg	Intravenous	5–30	1–6 hr	Angina, palpitation, headache
Furosemide (Lasix)	40–120 mg	Intravenous	15–60	3–24 hr	Electrolyte imbalance
Trimethaphan (Arfonad)	1–10 mg/min	Intravenous (infusion)	1	1–5 min	Hypotension, ileus, urinary retention
Pentolinium (Ansolysen)	1–10 mg	Intramuscular	5–15	4–8 hr	Hypotension, ileus, urinary retention
Nitroprusside (Nipride)	0.05–0.2 mg/min	Intravenous (infusion)	1	1–5 min	Hypotension, nausea, muscular irritability
Phentolamine (Regitine) (For patients with pheochromocytoma)	2.5–10 mg	Intravenous (infusion may be required)	1	5–60 min	Hypotension, palpitation

Source: Chobanian, A. V., and Lanzoni, V. Current concepts of the drug therapy of hypertension. *Medical Counterpoint, March, 1971.*

TABLE 6-2 Physiologic Effects of Parenteral Antihypertensive Drugs

Drug	C.O.	H.R.	T.P.R.	R.B.F.	C.B.F.
Diazoxide	++	+++	---	+	+
Hydralazine	+	++	--	+/-	+/-
Methyldopa	+/-	-	-	-	+/-
Reserpine	+/-	-	-	-	+/-
Trimethaphan	--	+/-	-	---	-
Sodium nitroprusside	+	+	-	-	-

+++ = marked increase; ++ = moderate increase; + = mild increase; +/- = inconsistent effect; - = mild decrease; -- = moderate decrease; --- = marked decrease.

SODIUM NITROPRUSSIDE This compound is an exceedingly potent agent which acts as a direct peripheral vasodilator. Unlike diazoxide, it also produces some venodilation and peripheral pooling of blood. Venous return to the heart is reduced, as is cardiac output. The drug therefore may be of particular value in patients with ischemic heart disease in whom diazoxide is contraindicated. However, it has the disadvantage of a very brief duration of action, and constant monitoring of the patient is therefore required. Nitroprusside is converted to thiocyanate, and with prolonged infusions of greater than 48 to 72 hours, mental confusion and other neurological symptoms may develop. Thiocyanate levels in the blood should be measured with such long-term therapy.

TRIMETHAPHAN Trimethaphan is a potent ganglionic blocking drug with a very brief duration of action. It will generally produce a decrease in cardiac output and is therefore of particular value in patients with dissecting aortic aneurysms. It also induces peripheral venous pooling of blood and may be useful in cases of severe hypertension and pulmonary edema that are refractory to the other approaches.

PHENTOLAMINE This alpha receptor–blocking agent is the preferred drug in patients with hypertensive emergencies secondary to pheochromocytoma. The duration of action is brief and prolonged infusions may be required.

SLOW-ACTING DRUGS

METHYLDOPA AND RESERPINE These drugs are moderately effective and well-tolerated agents which inhibit sympathetic nerve activity. Their potencies are similar, although parenteral methyldopa is generally preferable to reserpine because of its somewhat more rapid onset of action. The drugs may cause marked somnolence and thus make evaluation of the comatose patient difficult. The compounds have a prolonged duration of action and are particularly useful when relatively rapid, but not instantaneous, decrease of blood pressure is deemed desirable.

HYDRALAZINE Hydralazine is a direct peripheral vasodilator which is of value in eclampsia or in acute clinical situations where the potency of diazoxide or nitroprusside is not required. It produces a reflex increase in cardiac output and is therefore contraindicated in patients with ischemic heart disease.

FUROSEMIDE Potent diuretics such as furosemide represent an important adjunct to therapy and should be administered to almost all patients in hypertensive crisis. Most patients with accelerated hypertension have increases in plasma and extracellular volume. Furosemide not only has an antihypertensive action of its own but also potentiates the effects of the other drugs.

GENERAL APPROACH TO THERAPY

The most important consideration in the treatment of hypertensive emergencies is the prompt reduction of blood pressure. Because these patients are severely ill, medications should be given parenterally. When a single agent proves to be ineffective, additional drugs should be used. Refractoriness to combined medications is very rare. Careful monitoring of blood pressure is essential. An arterial line may be desirable in some persons but is not required in most. Monitoring of urine volume and of the electrocardiographic tracing is essential. Whenever possible, the treatment should be carried out in an intensive care unit.

The level to which blood pressure should be lowered varies with the type of hypertensive crisis. In order to prevent vascular complications and renal insufficiency, the diastolic pressure generally should be maintained above 90 mHg during the acute phase of treatment, although at times, as with aortic dissections, a lower blood pressure may be preferred.

The complications of therapy will vary with the drug used. The important clinical complications observed in our experience at Boston City Hospital from 1968 to 1973 are summarized in Table 6-3. The commonest side effect was the rise in blood urea nitrogen level which was present to some degree in most patients but to a marked extent in approximately one-fourth of the group. Hypotension was relatively infrequent. Myocardial ischemia developed primarily in those patients receiving either diazoxide or hydralazine. Despite the marked reductions in blood pressure which were achieved, strokes or cerebrovascular insufficiency were surprisingly uncommon. The low incidence of cerebral manifestations may have reflected adequate cerebral autoregulation in most of the patients. No treatment failures were apparent in this group.

Although complications of acute antihypertensive therapy were relatively infrequent, we continue to be cautious in the use of parenteral antihypertensive drugs. Such therapy should be restricted to situations involving hypertensive crisis or to patients with moderate or severe hypertension who are unable to take oral medications. The relatively asymptomatic hypertensive patient should not be treated with parenteral drugs irrespective of the level to which the blood pressure is elevated.

TABLE 6-3 Complications of Parenteral Antihypertensive Therapy in 50 Consecutive Patients with Hypertensive Crisis at the Boston City Hospital

Complication	Incidence (%)
Hypotension requiring pressor drugs	8
Renal impairment (BUN ↑ >20 mg%)	28
Myocardial ischemia	8
Cerebrovascular insufficiency	6
Mesenteric vascular insufficiency	2
Treatment failure	0

TABLE 6-4 Guidelines to the Specific Treatment of Hypertensive Crisis

Type of Crisis	Indicated Drugs	Contraindicated or Less Desirable Drugs
Hypertensive encephalopathy	Diazoxide Sodium nitroprusside Trimethaphan Furosemide	Reserpine Methyldopa Hydralazine
Eclampsia	Hydralazine Furosemide Methyldopa	Diazoxide* Sodium nitroprusside*
Pulmonary edema	Furosemide Sodium nitroprusside Diazoxide Methyldopa	
Dissecting aneurysm	Trimethaphan Methyldopa Reserpine Propranolol Furosemide	Diazoxide Hydralazine
Intracranial hemorrhage	Furosemide Sodium nitroprusside Trimethaphan Hydralazine Methyldopa	Reserpine Methyldopa
Myocardial ischemia	Furosemide Sodium nitroprusside Methyldopa	Diazoxide Hydralazine
Renal failure	Furosemide Diazoxide Hydralazine Methyldopa Sodium nitroprusside	Trimethaphan

* Unapproved use of the drug.

A general guide to the treatment of specific forms of hypertensive crisis is given in Table 6-4. Depending on the specific clinical situation, drugs other than those in the recommended list can also be of value in the management of the hypertensive emergency.

REFERENCES

1. Byron, F. B. *The Hypertensive Vascular Crisis.* New York: Grune & Stratton, 1969.
2. Skinhoj, E., and Strandgaard, S.   Pathogenesis of hypertensive encephalopathy. *Lancet* 1:461–462, 1973.
3. Sellers, E. M., and Koch-Weser, J.   Protein binding and vascular activity of diazoxide. *N. Engl. J. Med.* 281:1141–1145, 1969.

JEROME S. BRODY
MICHAEL E. WHITCOMB

IN THIS CHAPTER we will deal separately with three major types of acute respiratory failure: (1) that occurring in patients with obstructive pulmonary disease; (2) that occurring in patients with the lung disease of acute pulmonary edema, the adult respiratory distress syndrome (ARDS); and (3) that occurring in patients with relatively normal lungs, i.e., nonpulmonary respiratory failure. The therapeutic approach to each group of patients is different, although it is not unusual for there to be pathophysiologic overlap, e.g., a patient with emphysema who has respiratory failure as a result of cardiogenic pulmonary edema (a form of ARDS) or as a result of respiratory depression following pain medication (a form of nonpulmonary respiratory failure). Because the therapeutic emphasis differs in each type of respiratory failure, it is extremely important to identify as quickly as possible the specific cause of respiratory failure in each patient.

COMMON PRINCIPLES AND FORMS OF THERAPY

DEFINITION

Respiratory failure is defined as an acute, potentially life-threatening fall in arterial oxygen tension (Pa_{O_2}) and/or increase in arterial carbon dioxide tension (Pa_{CO_2}). The latter is, by definition, caused by alveolar hypoventilation, i.e., ventilation inadequate to meet the metabolic demands of the body. In the absence of supplemental oxygen (O_2), hypoventilation results in both hypercapnia and hypoxemia. Patients who have been or are receiving supplemental O_2, however, may have normal or even elevated Pa_{O_2} with severe hypercapnia and acidosis.

    Pa_{O_2} can be decreased in conditions where the Pa_{CO_2} is normal or low. This picture is characteristic of patients with ARDS in whom severe ventilation perfusion imbalance or shunt-like flow occurs, in patients with

115

asthma, and in patients with normal lungs who have muscle weakness and cannot raise secretions or sigh and cough effectively.

RECOGNITION

Recognition of respiratory failure depends on measurement of arterial blood gas tensions and pH, since clinical signs of hypoxia and hypercapnia are notoriously imprecise and misleading. Sudden CO_2 elevation may be associated with early vasodilatation (warm, flushed, tachycardia) followed by neurogenic signs (mental depression, increased deep tendon reflexes, tremulousness, and asterixis) and ultimately cardiovascular and central nervous system depression (hypotension and coma), but absence of these signs does not rule out hypercapnia. Patients with chronic hypercapnia frequently have no symptoms at all, suggesting that many of the Pa_{CO_2}-related clinical findings are due to changes in pH. Signs and symptoms of hypoxemia are equally vague and nonspecific. Cyanosis is not consistently recognized until arterial saturation is less than 85%. Symptoms include restlessness, personality change, confusion, and ultimately coma.

ARTERIAL BLOOD GASES

When a patient is suspected of having acute respiratory failure, arterial blood should be drawn slowly (over 1 to 2 minutes) in a heparinized syringe (barrel coated and only dead space filled with heparin). The blood should be kept on ice until analyzed.

The blood gas sample can provide information about the duration of Pa_{CO_2} changes by careful evaluation of pH and bicarbonate (HCO_3). Chronic hypoventilation with associated renal HCO_3 retention is not life-threatening and should not be corrected immediately, since rapid return of the Pa_{CO_2} to normal will result in severe alkalosis and may lead to convulsions and death. Figure 7-1 shows pH and HCO_3 values expected for various levels of Pa_{CO_2} in pure acute or chronic respiratory failure. Such a diagram will also be helpful in recognition of associated metabolic acid-base derangements which may have precipitated respiratory failure, e.g., metabolic alkalosis decreasing respiratory drive. Polycythemia or pulmonary hypertension and right ventricular hypertrophy may indicate that hypoxia has been present for a considerable period of time. However, the most accurate method of judging duration of blood gas alterations is to have a prior set of blood gas determinations available for comparison. Thus, any patient who has been in respiratory failure should have a baseline study done prior to discharge from the hospital.

There are several important ancillary bits of information that one can gather from blood gas determinations. When the patient is breathing room air, the partial pressure of O_2 and CO_2 in alveolar air should equal approximately 140 mHg. The difference between 140 and Pa_{O_2} plus Pa_{CO_2} equals the alveolar-arterial (A-a) O_2 gradient and indicates efficiency of O_2 gas exchange. The A-a O_2 gradient is 5 to 15 mHg in normal young people and 15 to 25 mHg in the elderly. A patient in respiratory

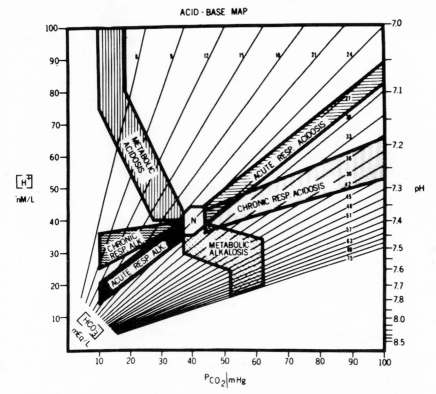

FIGURE 7-1   Acid-base map to show the normal compensatory range of pH, P_{CO_2}, and HCO_3 in simple acid-base disorders. Values on the ordinate represent blood H^+ concentration (left) in nanomoles per liter or pH (right). Abscissa is P_{CO_2} in mHg. Diagonal lines represent isopleths for blood HCO_3^- concentration in mEq per liter. Clear area in the center of the graph is the range of normal. Points which fall between boxes on map represent mixed disturbances. (From McCurdy, D. K. *Chest* 62:36S, 1972.)

failure with normal lungs might have a $Pa_{O_2} = 60$ mHg and a $Pa_{CO_2} = 70$ mHg. Because the A-a O_2 gradient is only 10 mHg, one can assume that this patient has relatively normal lungs and has pure hypoventilation problems. In contrast, a patient with pulmonary edema might be seen with a $Pa_{O_2} = 60$ and a $Pa_{CO_2} = 20$. This patient has a large A-a O_2 gradient (60 mHg) and severe gas exchange problems.

By having the patient perform several simple maneuvers at the bedside, one can frequently evaluate the mechanism of blood gas abnormalities. If a patient can voluntarily hyperventilate and lower Pa_{CO_2} values significantly, lack of central respiratory drive is a likely cause of hypoventilation. If by having the patient take several deep breaths or sighs (either voluntarily or with a respirator) the Pa_{O_2} is dramatically increased, ventilation maldistribution problems such as might be seen with secretions of early airway closure are a major problem.

Oxygen Therapy

Severe hypoxemia must be the first priority of treatment in respiratory failure, since hypoxemia may cause death or irreversible cerebral or myocardial damage. Hypercapnia, unless associated with pH values below 7.00, is not life-threatening. While the appropriate therapy for hypoxemia depends on the cause (i.e., normal lung hypoxemia might best be treated with mechanical ventilation alone, atelectasis by bronchoscopy and suction, and pulmonary edema with diuretics), most patients will require some form of supplemental O_2.

Table 7-1 lists types of O_2 therapy and the range of concentration to be expected. The Venturi masks provide the only constant O_2 concentration that needs not be monitored. With all other forms of O_2 therapy, inspired O_2 should be measured with some type of O_2 analyzer, making certain that the O_2 concentration is measured as close to the patient as possible. The appropriate form of O_2 therapy depends on the type of patient being treated. The Venturi masks are most useful in patients who need controlled forms of low O_2 concentrations, but simpler forms of therapy more acceptable to the patient are sufficient in most instances.

Oxygen should be used as if it were a potentially toxic drug. The patient should receive enough to achieve the desired goal, and no more. There is no reason that any patient should have superphysiologic Pa_{O_2} values, and indeed, for most patients a Pa_{O_2} of 60 to 70 mHg is sufficient. The toxic effects of O_2 are direct (e.g., capillary endothelial damage or decreased mucociliary clearance) and indirect (e.g., atelectasis or decreased respiratory drive; see Table 7-2). The end result of direct O_2 toxicity is an ARDS type of picture with severe progressive hypoxia refractory to further O_2 therapy.

Intubation

Intubation is of value in patients with excessive or difficult to mobilize bronchial secretions, intractable hypoxemia, or severe hypoventilation. The indications for intubation vary, depending on the condition being

TABLE 7-1 Forms of Oxygen Therapy

Equipment	Flow (L/min)	O_2 Concentration (%)
Nasal cannula	1–6	24–40
Face mask	6–8	30–45
	10–12	45–65
Partial rebreathing mask	6–8	40–80
Nonrebreathing mask	6–8	80–100
Venturi masks—24 or 28%	4	24 or 28
35 or 40%	8	35 or 40
T-tube adapter for use with endotracheal or tracheostomy tubes (with or without afterburner)	Can vary to achieve any concentration	

Table 7-2 Adverse Effects of Oxygen

Effect	Concentration (%)	Time (hr)	Manifestation
Cellular toxicity	100	36–48	Falling vital capacity
	90	48–72	and Pa_{O_2} ultimately
	80	72–96	leading to pulmo-
	70	96–120	nary edema
	<60	None	
Impaired mucociliary function	100 May occur at lower concentrations	6–12	Decreased particle clearance
Impaired alveolar macrophage function	100 May occur at lower concentrations	>48	Decreased particle and bacterial clearance
Atelectasis	>95	At any time	Sudden hypoxia, x-ray changes
Hypoventilation	May occur with any increase in O_2, only in patients with elevated Pa_{CO_2} and HCO_3	Immediate	Mental depression, coma, death

treated. A patient with normal lung respiratory failure due to myasthenia gravis should be intubated when the vital capacity has dropped below one liter or when hypoxemia occurs, even though the Pa_{CO_2} is normal; a patient with asthma should have intubation as soon as the Pa_{CO_2} begins to rise; but a patient with chronic obstructive lung disease might not require intubation with a Pa_{CO_2} of 70 or 80 mHg. The mode of intubation depends in part on its projected duration. If a patient clearly will require intubation for longer than 2 weeks, tracheostomy should be performed initially, but even in this instance, it is preferable to perform the tracheostomy over an endotracheal tube in order to ensure control of secretions and adequate oxygenation during the procedure. Orotracheal intubation is somewhat easier to perform than nasotracheal intubation, especially in an emergency, but it is less well tolerated and may produce more tracheal damage. All endotracheal tubes that are to be left in place for more than a few hours should be equipped with low pressure cuffs and the cuffs should be inflated only enough to provide an airtight seal. A chest x-ray picture should be taken after placement of the tube in order to ensure that it sits above the carina. Laryngeal damage is most frequently associated with traumatic and repeated intubation.

ARTIFICIAL VENTILATION

The two main indications for artificial ventilation are intractable hypoxemia and severe hypoventilation. Not all patients who have intubation need to be put on ventilators, but all patients on ventilators need to have intubation. There are two main types of ventilators—pressure-cycled and volume-cycled machines. The pressure-cycled ventilators reach a certain preset inspiratory pressure and then allow expiration to occur independent of the volume delivered. The volume-cycled machines provide a preset inspired volume independent of the inspiratory pressure required. As the lung becomes more or less compliant or more or less obstructed, the volume delivered to the patient varies with pressure-cycled respirators, and one must compensate by raising or lowering inspired pressure; however, volume delivered remains relatively constant in volume-cycled machines in these circumstances. As a rule, the worse the lung disease and the more labile the patient, the more important it is to use a volume-cycled machine. Thus, all patients with ARDS or severe obstructive lung disease should be placed on volume-cycled machines, whereas patients with nonpulmonary respiratory failure may be adequately ventilated with pressure-cycled machines.

After choosing the appropriate ventilator, one must consider the major ventilator settings and determine appropriate flow, respiratory rate, and volume or pressure levels. These decisions depend on what type of patient one is treating and what one is trying to accomplish with the ventilator. Assuming use of a volume ventilator, major decisions to be made are as follows:

ASSIST OR CONTROL By increasing sensitivity, one allows the patient to trigger the respirator more easily. If one wants the patient to determine his or her respiratory rate (a useful approach in most circumstances), the dial should be turned to a sensitivity which just allows patient triggering of each breath. If sensitivity is increased too much, the machine will trigger in response to movement or other nonrespiratory factors. If the sensitivity dial is turned off, the patient will be unable to trigger the machine. The rate dial can be set at a relatively low level in order to provide a safety backup system if the patient fails to initiate respiration at a specific rate. If the rate setting is too high, the machine rather than the patient will determine this parameter. In general, it is best to control totally patients who are extremely restless and uncooperative or who have such excessive respiratory drive that they do not allow the respirator to function in a mechanically efficient fashion. If the patient does not follow the respirator, one can hyperventilate the patient to diminish respiratory drive, sedate the patient with 4 to 10 mg morphine I.V., or paralyze the patient with pancuronium bromide (Pavulon), 0.04 mg/kg I.V. loading dose plus half the initial dose every hour.

MINUTE VENTILATION In a patient with normal lungs, minute ventilation can be set at a level of approximately 80 to 100 ml/kg. In patients with abnormal lungs and increased physiologic dead space, minute ventilation should be set at 100 to 140 ml/kg. If metabolic rate is increased, e.g., with fever, these values should be increased. If one also wishes to lower the Pa_{CO_2}, ventilation should be increased in proportion to the rate at which the Pa_{CO_2} is to be changed. With chronic CO_2 retention, Pa_{CO_2} should be decreased slowly (over 24 to 48 hours) in order to allow renal excretion of HCO_3, thus preventing severe metabolic alkalosis.

With acute CO_2 retention, the Pa_{CO_2} can be returned to normal immediately.

TIDAL VOLUME In normal persons, tidal volume should be set at 8 to
10 ml/kg; in patients with increased dead space or when slow rates of
ventilation are desired, 10 to 14 ml/kg is a reasonable level.

INSPIRATORY FLOW RATE The inspiratory flow setting should be in the
mid-range, i.e., 50 to 60 liters/min, except in situations in which a pattern
of slow deep breaths will provide more efficient gas exchange (e.g., in
a patient with emphysema). Flow rate may be increased in patients
who are breathing rapidly. It is important to remember that inspiration
should be 50% or less of each respiratory cycle in order to prevent diminished venous return and subsequent hypotension. Diminished blood
pressure following initiation of artificial ventilation may occur in patients with intravascular volume depletion, even when the inspiratory-
expiratory ratio is normal.

Once the patient has been set up on a respirator, one must follow the
clinical course and keep records in an orderly fashion. Initially, one must
remeasure arterial blood gases at relatively frequent intervals in order to
determine the effectiveness of the therapy. At each point, inspired O_2
concentration, tidal volume, minute ventilation, and respirator peak pressure should be measured and recorded. As the patient's condition stabilizes, blood gases can be drawn less frequently; but other respiratory
values should be recorded every 2 hours.

WEANING

There are several basic principles associated with weaning from the respirator (Table 7-3). However, each weaning problem must be dealt
with on an individual basis. In general, a patient must have a vital capacity in the range of 8 to 12 ml/kg and be able to trigger the respirator
prior to succesful weaning. Careful observance of symptoms, ventilatory
patterns, and blood gases is of major importance in the weaning process.
A rapid rise in Pa_{CO_2} on weaning suggests ineffective respiratory drive or

TABLE 7-3 Principles of Weaning from the Respirator

1. The longer on, the harder to wean
2. Precipitating problem must have been corrected
3. Blood gases (especially Pa_{CO_2}) should be at a level patient can maintain when off ventilator
4. Patient must be able to trigger machine and have vital capacity of at least 8–12 ml/kg
5. Respiratory drive intact (watch sedatives and other drugs, correct meta-bolic alkalosis)
6. Initial weaning during day for short periods, rest at night
7. Psychological factors and general support

lung-chest mechanics. A rapid drop in Pa_{O_2} without a rise in Pa_{CO_2} suggests airway closure and atelectasis. The latter may respond to weaning positive end-expiratory pressure breathing (PEEP).

SPECIFIC TYPES OF ACUTE RESPIRATORY FAILURE

OBSTRUCTIVE LUNG DISEASE

In patients with obstructive lung disease one is usually dealing with a chronic problem, exacerbated by one of a number of potential hazards. As a rule, identification of the precipitating event is important in deciding on specific therapy, but in many patients with chronic obstructive pulmonary disease (COPD), no single event can be identified and a broad general approach to airway management must be initiated.

The major events precipitating acute respiratory failure in patients with obstructive pulmonary disease, and thus the approaches to diagnosis and therapy, are multiple (Table 7-4). A carefully taken history from either the patient or relatives is usually the most important clue to what the initiating problem might have been. Frequently, a series of interrelated events has occurred so that one must treat several problems simultaneously.

Bronchial infection and pneumonitis need not be associated with peripheral leukocytosis and fever in patients with COPD. Often, a change in sputum quantity or consistency and the finding of white cells and increased macrophages on sputum examination are the only indications of infection. The initial Gram stain is of great importance in deter-

TABLE 7-4 Factors Precipitating Acute Respiratory Failure in Patients with Obstructive Lung Disease

Problem	Method of Diagnosis*	Therapy
Infection	Wet mount of sputum and Gram stain	Antibiotics (after Gram stain and culture)
Secretions	Observation	Hydration, suction, physical therapy
Bronchospasm	Physical examination	Bronchodilators
Congestive heart failure (myocardial infarction?)	Physical examination, ECG	O_2, digitalis, diuretics
Respiratory drive	Review medication, electrolytes, pH	Cl^-, H^+, acetazolamide, ventilate
Miscellaneous (pulmonary emboli, pneumothorax, rib fracture, upper airway obstruction)	Physical examination and laboratory tests	Varies with cause

* In each instance, a good history from patients or relatives will provide the best clue as to the precipitating event.

mining the potential causative organism. If infection is suspected, ampicillin or other antibiotics which will affect both pneumococci and *Hemophilus influenzae* should be started. Secretions are a major problem in such patients, and aggressive attempts at drainage frequently reverse the pattern of failure rapidly. Altered central nervous system (CNS) respiratory drive may be a major precipitating event either because the patient has been given a sedative or because diuretics have produced metabolic alkalosis with secondary hypoventilation. Thus, one must always approach these patients with the thought that something has changed to precipitate respiratory failure and that defining the event will be important in reversing the process.

The initial approach to patients with COPD revolves around oxygenation and the need to intubate and ventilate. In general, those patients with normal or near normal Pa_{CO_2} values can be given any form of O_2 therapy, while those patients who have elevated Pa_{CO_2} levels, particularly on a chronic basis, have a greater tendency to hypoventilate when their hypoxic ventilatory drive is removed. Thus, a Venturi mask with an appropriate O_2 concentration is of value in such persons.

Those patients who are in coma or have Pa_{CO_2} values greater than 80 mHg on an acute basis should have immediate intubation and be given ventilatory support. However, most patients should be approached initially in a conservative fashion, with O_2 and appropriate aggressive therapy. One can then follow the clinical trend of the patient before intubation is instituted. Small or even moderate elevations of Pa_{CO_2} are not life-threatening and are tolerable if the patient's oxygenation and clinical status is improving. Pa_{CO_2} values of 70 or 80 mHg do not require intubation if the clinical trend is one of overall improvement. However, a Pa_{CO_2} of 60 mHg might require intubation if the patient is clinically deteriorating and was admitted with a normal or low initial value. Often intubation alone with better management of secretions will suffice, and not all such patients need to be placed on a ventilator.

Patients with bronchial asthma usually are seen with hypoxemia and hypocapnia, i.e., evidence of considerable hyperventilation. As the process worsens or the patient begins to tire, the Pa_{CO_2} level begins to rise, an indication for early intubation. In general, if a patient has asthma and a high Pa_{CO_2} level, he either has associated COPD or is in severe status asthmaticus, and should have immediate intubation and be placed on a ventilator.

As with COPD, a good history and review of possible common precipitating factors (Table 7-4) will help to determine what specific precipitating events one might treat. One must pay particular attention to the sputum smear as an index of infection and state of hydration. Sympathomimetic agents are the first line of treatment, although many patients will have used these agents excessively prior to admission. Initial attempts at therapy should begin with epinephrine, 0.2 to 0.5 ml of 1 : 1,000 solution, given subcutaneously. This can be repeated at 15- to 20-minute intervals. Isoproterenol, 0.5 ml of a 1 : 200 solution given by aerosol, is an effective bronchodilator and can be given as often as every 1 to 2 hours in patients without cardiovascular disease. At this time, beta-2 adrenergic agents that have bronchodilating but few cardiovascular effects and are longer acting than isoproterenol are just becoming available in the United States.

Methylxanthines are effective bronchodilators which affect the adenyl cyclase-cyclic 3':5' AMP system at a different site than sympathomimetic drugs, and thus act with them in a synergistic fashion. Aminophylline should be given as a 350- to 500-mg intravenous bolus over 5 to 15 minutes and then as a continuous drip of 0.7 mg/kg/hr. Corticosteroids have proved to be of value in asthma as anti-inflammatory agents and as stabilizers of adenyl cyclase. Steroids should be used intravenously in high doses, maintained until the attack clears, and then tapered. Appropriate doses of hydrocortisone are 400 to 600 mg/24 hr.

ADULT RESPIRATORY DISTRESS SYNDROME

A growing number of cases of acute respiratory failure in the adult occur in persons with little or no underlying lung disease. The term *adult respiratory distress syndrome* (ARDS) has been used to describe those persons with this complex clinical and pathophysiologic syndrome who have the most severe derangement of pulmonary gas exchange. In this discussion, ARDS will be used in a general manner to indicate the presence of respiratory failure associated with diffuse lung injury irrespective of the severity of the gas exchange defect. A number of clinical entities have been associated with the development of this syndrome (Table 7-5). Although the mechanism of lung injury is apparent in some of these diseases, in the majority of cases the factors contributing to the pathogenesis of this syndrome have not been identified.

The major manifestations of ARDS are progressive dyspnea, clinical and roentgenographic evidence of diffuse bilateral alveolar infiltrates, and impairment of oxygenation. It is important to categorize correctly patients with this syndrome, since the principles governing their evaluation and management are distinct from those used in patients with exacerbations of chronic airway disease, status asthmaticus, or nonpulmonary respiratory failure.

PATHOPHYSIOLOGY The basic insult to the lung in ARDS results in distortion of the lung parenchyma and disruption of the alveolar-capillary

TABLE 7-5 Causes of Adult Respiratory Distress Syndrome

Aspiration pneumonitis
Viral or mycoplasma pneumonitis
Fat embolization
Hemorrhagic pancreatitis
Postperfusion lung injury
"Shock lung"
Drugs (heroin, methadone, etc.)
O_2 toxicity
Cardiogenic pulmonary edema
Smoke inhalation

membrane. As a result, there are two major pathophysiologic abnormalities in persons with this syndrome: uneven distribution of ventilation with subsequent airway closure and atelectasis, and an increase in extravascular lung water. Both conditions cause a reduction of the functional residual capacity (FRC) of the lung, a decrease in pulmonary compliance, and a mismatching of ventilation and perfusion. These abnormalities lead to an increase in the work of breathing and impairment in systemic oxygenation.

The defect in oxygen exchange is caused both by diffuse ventilation-perfusion (V/Q) mismatching, and an increase in the pulmonary shunt volume. The V/Q mismatching is due not only to distortion of the lung parenchyma but also to the extravasation of fluid into the lungs through the damaged alveolar-capillary membrane. The shunt lesion is determined by the severity of parenchymal involvement and by the decrease in the functional residual capacity of the lung. In severe disease the shunt lesion is the dominant factor affecting systemic oxygenation. When the right-left shunt through the lungs approximates 30% of the cardiac output, raising the inspired O_2 concentration above 60% has only a slight effect on the Pa_{O_2} .This observation is of great significance in the management of these patients.

EVALUATION The evaluation of patients with ARDS is directed toward defining the severity of the oxygenation defect and identifying potentially reversible factors. From a practical clinical standpoint, the severity of the defect in oxygenation can be ascertained by measuring the arterial Po_2 after the patient has been breathing from a mask delivering high inspired oxygen concentrations for 15 to 20 minutes. If the Pa_{O_2} becomes excessively elevated, then it is apparent that the defect in gas exchange is of only moderate severity, and that at least during the initial stage of the disease, conventional methods of oxygen therapy can be employed. If an acceptable Pa_{O_2} (>70 mHg) cannot be achieved, the gas exchange defect is severe and intubation and mechanical ventilation will most likely be required.

An equally important aspect of the evaluation of patients with ARDS is an assessment of their pulmonary hemodynamics. Because leakage of fluid across the damaged alveolar-capillary membrane is a basic component of the pathophysiology of this syndrome, maintenance of fluid balance in these patients is critical. It is clear that left ventricular decompensation is frequently present in such patients and that it is often impossible to determine this on clinical grounds alone. Therefore, in patients with progressive respiratory failure, pulmonary artery and pulmonary wedge pressure should be measured with a Swan-Ganz catheter. Fluid therapy can then be intelligently guided by serial measurements of the pulmonary wedge and mean pulmonary artery pressures, and mixed venous oxygen tension.

In evaluating the patient with ARDS, emphasis must be placed on assuring adequate oxygenation. Only after an acceptable Pa_{O_2} has been attained should attention be directed toward investigation of the etiology of the lung disease or definition of the hemodynamic status.

MANAGEMENT As has been emphasized, severe hypoxemia must be corrected as rapidly as possible. There is no rationale for instituting therapy with nasal prongs or a Venturi mask, since these oxygen delivery systems provide only small increases in the inspired oxygen concentrations (Table 7-1). If an acceptable Pa_{O_2} cannot be achieved by the proper use of a mask with a reservoir bag, intubation and mechanical ventilation should be undertaken. If a mask system proves satisfactory, frequent arterial blood gas measurements should be performed to determine if a satisfactory Pa_{O_2} is being maintained. Because of the dynamics of the pathophysiology in this syndrome, rapid deterioration in gas exchange may occur during the course of this disease.

The proper use of mechanical ventilators has been discussed earlier. However, several principles warrant reemphasis. Because ARDS is characterized by stiff, noncompliant lungs, a volume-cycled respirator should be used for providing ventilatory assistance. Although the specifics of the use of a ventilator must be individualized in each case, large tidal volumes and the use of an inspiratory plateau are frequently beneficial in providing optimal oxygenation. In patients with severe hypoxemia who have large right-left shunts, positive end-expiratory pressure ventilation may also be required. PEEP exerts its major effect on gas exchange by increasing the FRC. As the FRC is raised, the magnitude of the right-left shunt decreases and the Pa_{O_2} level increases. As a general rule, the inability to maintain a Pa_{O_2} level greater than 60 mHg using an inspired oxygen concentration of 80% is an indication to institute PEEP.

Ideally, monitoring of pulmonary hemodynamics and mixed venous Po_2 should be available whenever PEEP is employed. Swan-Ganz catheterization provides critical information about the underlying pathophysiology prior to institution of PEEP, and allows assessment of the effects of PEEP on cardiac output. A decrease in cardiac output commonly occurs when PEEP is employed. If the cardiac output falls significantly, the increase in arterial Po_2 may not lead to an increase in tissue oxygen delivery, a sequence of events which can be detected by monitoring central venous Po_2. One should also be aware of the possibility that PEEP may result in unilateral or bilateral pneumothorax.

Intelligent management of fluid therapy also requires monitoring central hemodynamics. Serial measurements of the pulmonary wedge pressure and mixed venous Po_2 provide important information about the functional status of the left ventricle and its response to fluid therapy. Some patients with ARDS have relative hypovolemia and will become hypotensive when mechanical ventilation is instituted. The cardiac output in these patients will respond to volume loading. Conversely, because patients receiving ventilatory support tend to retain fluid, volume overload may easily occur during the course of therapy and lead to a deterioration of pulmonary gas exchange. It should be remembered that patients receiving no caloric intake should lose 300 to 600 gm of body weight each day. Failure to do so represents positive fluid balance. Because tissue oxygenation is a function of O_2 delivery and tissue requirements, one should be certain that the hemoglobin level is normal, that alkalosis or other causes for left-shifted oxyhemoglobin dissociation curves are not present, and that fever and other causes for increased tissue O_2 demands are controlled.

NONPULMONARY RESPIRATORY FAILURE

Nonpulmonary respiratory failure is caused by diseases which suppress the central nervous system control of ventilation or interfere with effective function of the chest cage. Suppression of the central control of ventilation is usually due to trauma or drug ingestion, while ineffective function of the chest cage is most often caused by trauma or neuromuscular disease.

In each of these conditions, respiratory failure is characterized by progressive hypoventilation resulting in hypoxemia and hypercapnea. However, in the presence of ineffective ventilation, a variety of pulmonary parenchymal complications may occur and cause an additional defect in oxygenation. Atelectasis, aspiration, and infection are the commonest complications in this clinical setting.

The management of patients with nonpulmonary respiratory failure is aimed at maintaining adequate ventilation for gas exchange and preventing complicating parenchymal disease. Intensive chest physiotherapy and mechanical ventilatory support are the most important aspects of the therapy of these patients. Because the parenchymal complications are related to ineffective clearance of secretions, good pulmonary toilet is extremely important. Indeed, it may be necessary to perform a tracheostomy for optimal management of secretions, even though mechanical ventilatory support is not required.

If the patient's ventilation is inadequate to maintain satisfactory arterial blood gases, ventilatory assistance will be required. In those patients with progressive loss of chest cage function caused by neuromuscular diseases, serial measurements of the vital capacity and peak inspiratory and expiratory pressures are useful in anticipating the requirement for ventilatory assistance.

There are no unique features of mechanical ventilation in these patients. Good general nursing care and attention to the basic fundamentals of mechanical ventilation are the key factors in their management.

The duration of the requirement for ventilatory assistance is determined by the primary disease. In certain settings, such as with drug ingestion, the need for ventilatory assistance might be quite short, whereas with trauma or neuromuscular disease, a prolonged course can be anticipated.

SELECTED READINGS

Campbell, E. G.   The management of acute respiratory failure in chronic bronchitis and emphysema. *Am. Rev. Respir. Dis.* 96:626, 1967.

Pontoppidan, H.   Acute respiratory failure in the adult. *N. Engl. J. Med.* 287:690, 1972.

Williams, M. H.   Ventilatory failure, etiology and clinical forms. *Am. J. Med.* 48:477, 1970.

MANAGEMENT OF ACUTE FLUID AND ELECTROLYTE PROBLEMS

Edward A. Alexander

THE THERAPEUTIC PLAN for the management of patients with fluid and electrolyte disorders must be based on a thorough understanding of the pertinent pathophysiology and the total clinical situation. "Cookbook" therapy is frequently hazardous. Although an approximation of the total body fluid or electrolyte imbalance is necessary to begin therapy, it must be understood that the initial calculation of imbalance is only an estimate that must be continually reevaluated during treatment and corrected as the effect of treatment becomes clear and the clinical situation changes. Fluid and electrolyte disorders are rarely life-threatening and seldom require instantaneous therapy. However, the conditions considered below may occasionally be severe enough to warrant immediate treatment. It is also important not to plan total immediate correction of the imbalance but to plan only enough to remove the patient from that relative "emergency" state to one in which normal body mechanisms may make the final correction.

DISORDERS OF POTASSIUM METABOLISM

The normal body content of potassium is about 40 to 50 mEq/kg of body weight, most of which is located within cells. The concentration within cells is 150 to 160 mEq/liter, while in the extracellular fluid the concentration is 4 to 5 mEq/liter. This high concentration gradient is maintained by active transport of K^+ into cells and passive diffusion outward. Alterations in acid-base balance will markedly affect the distribution of K^+: the more acid the extracellular fluid, the more K^+ shifts from the intra- to the extracellular space and vice versa. Potassium is important as a cofactor in many enzyme systems and for the maintenance of the transmembrane potential, which is primarily determined by the intracellular to extracellular K^+ concentration. Plasma concentration of K^+ and total body K^+ are generally related at both normal and reduced levels, because potassium deficits lead to hypokalemia. However, this is often not a linear relationship and frequently may be a completely erroneous guideline. Hyperkalemia rarely, if ever, implies excess total body K^+ but represents a shift in the intra- to extracellular distribution.

HYPERKALEMIA

The important causes of hyperkalemia may be classified as (1) *inadequate renal excretion* because of acute renal failure, terminal chronic renal failure, adrenocortical insufficiency, and drugs such as spironolactone; (2) *excess potassium load* because of hypercatabolism, tissue destruction, internal hemorrhage, severe acidosis, and excess ingestion or infusion of potassium; and (3) *pseudohyperkalemia* (serum only) because of release of potassium from platelets and white cells of clotted blood.

The major clinical features of hyperkalemia are largely due to the depolarization of cardiac and skeletal muscle causing interference with normal excitability. The electrocardiographic changes include peaking of T waves, widening of the QRS complex and increasing P-R interval, loss of P wave, and finally ventricular arrhythmias culminating in arrest. ECG changes are frequently related to the plasma level of potassium, but this is not always true. Hence, therapy must not be restricted to only those patients with ECG alterations.

In determining therapy, it is helpful to classify hyperkalemia according to severity, depending on both plasma level and ECG (Table 8-1). For minimal hyperkalemia, cation exchange resins such as sodium polystyrene sulfonate may be administered orally, 15 to 20 gm 3 to 4 times a day, together with 20 ml of 70% sorbitol and 100 ml of tap water. Resins may be given repeatedly. For moderate hyperkalemia, immediate intravenous therapy is indicated. One liter of 10% glucose is administered, usually with the addition of 88 to 132 mEq of sodium bicarbonate (2 to 3 ampules). About ⅓ of this is given during the first hour and the remainder over the next 2 to 3 hours. Reduction in plasma potassium usually begins within 30 minutes, and the infusion may be repeated as long as the patient has adequate renal function.

TABLE 8-1 Treatment of Hyperkalemia

Classification	Plasma Potassium Level (mEq/L)		ECG	Treatment
Minimal	5.5–6.5	and	Normal	Cation exchange resin
Moderate	6.5–7.5	or	Peaked T waves	Glucose and/or bicarbonate, I.V.
Severe	>7.5	or	Absent P wave, widened QRS complex, ventricular arrhythmia	Begin with calcium infusion followed by bicarbonate and glucose

In severe hyperkalemia, calcium infusion is effective within 5 to 10 minutes. Ten to 30 ml of calcium gluconate is infused at a rate of 2 ml/ min with continuous ECG monitoring. Hypercalcemia decreases threshold potential and hence opposes the effect of hyperkalemia, which lowers the resting potential toward threshold. Since the effect of calcium is short-lived, administration of glucose and bicarbonate should immediately follow the calcium infusion. Hemodialysis and peritoneal dialysis require several hours to effectively remove potassium; hence this mode of therapy is restricted to prophylaxis.

HYPOKALEMIA

The major causes of hypokalemia are (1) *gastrointestinal loss* because of diarrhea, vomiting, laxative abuse, ureterosigmoidostomy, etc.; (2) *urinary loss* because of diuretics, adrenal steroids, renal tubular impairment, etc.; and (3) *inadequate intake*.

Hypokalemia usually occurs gradually, and symptoms and signs are unusual until the depletion is severe (<3.0 mEq/liter), and even then may be absent. Most commonly, fatigue, malaise, and irritability occur, but if the deficit is acute or very severe, muscle weakness, hyporeflexia, and eventually flaccid paralysis and cardiac arrest may occur. ECG abnormalities include U waves and broadening of the Q-T interval. The total body potassium deficit may be estimated from the plasma concentration and blood pH. A reduction in plasma potassium of 1 mEq/liter occurs with a total body deficit of approximately 125 to 150 mEq. However, if plasma potassium is below 2.0 mEq/liter, the total body deficit is impossible to predict, since there may be little further decrease in plasma concentration. In addition, the plasma concentration of potassium may be strikingly affected by the acid-base status of the patient. For every 0.1 pH unit plasma potassium may vary from 0.5 to 1.0 mEq/liter, increasing with acidemia and decreasing with alkalemia.

Treatment is best managed by the oral route if possible and is usually adequate for patients without cardiac or neuromuscular abnormalities. If intravenous therapy is required, the rate should not exceed 10 mEq/hr at a concentration of not more than 30 mEq/liter, with the total amount not to exceed 200 mEq/day. If treatment is urgent, potassium may be given at a rate of 40 mEq/hr at a concentration of 60 mEq/liter along with continuous ECG monitoring.

ACID-BASE DISORDERS

Disorders of acid-base balance are common problems occurring as complications of many disease states. Occasionally the acid-base abnormality may be so severe as to be life-threatening. The major concern is with the gain or loss of hydrogen ions. There is no meaningful way to define total body hydrogen ion content, since hydrogen ion exists in dissociated form in small amounts in extracellular and intracellular fluid but in far larger quantities as undissociated acids, e.g., $H_2PO_4^-$, H_2CO_3, etc., or bases such as HPO_4^{--} or HCO_3^-. The capacity of the body fluids to liberate or bind hydrogen ions is referred to as buffering, and the buffering capacity of the body prevents large changes in hydrogen ion concentration. The body fluids are far more effective in buffering against the addition of acid (acidosis) than against the loss of acid (alkalosis).

Acidosis results whenever acid production exceeds acid excretion and is identified by an increase in blood hydrogen ion concentration above the normal level of 40 nEq/liter (fall in pH below 7.40). If acidosis results from impaired pulmonary excretion there will be an elevation in blood Pco_2, that is, an addition of carbonic acid. If acidosis results from an increase in hydrogen ion production or failure of renal excretion, then acids other than carbonic will accumulate in the extracellular fluid and bicarbonate concentration will fall. This also occurs with the direct loss of bicarbonate (actually CO_2 content, but for clinical purposes the two are not different).

Alkalosis results whenever acid elimination exceeds acid production and is identified by a decrease in blood hydrogen ion concentration below 35 nEq/liter (elevation in pH above 7.45). If alkalosis is caused by overbreathing, Pco_2 will be low. If alkalosis results from excess loss of acid, bicarbonate concentration will be elevated. Excess intake of exogenous alkali also raises bicarbonate.

A careful clinical history and bedside observation will usually suggest both the presence and the cause of acid-base disturbances. Blood measurements are then needed to confirm and assess the severity of the problem.

METABOLIC ACIDOSIS

Metabolic acidosis is the commonest acid-base disorder requiring emergency therapy. It is etiologically best divided into those situations which increase the unmeasured anions, and those in which the unmeasured anions are normal. The unmeasured anions may be defined as the plasma sodium concentration minus the sum of the chloride and bicarbonate concentrations. This total normally does not exceed 12.

The principal causes of metabolic acidosis are shown in Table 8-2. Exogenous or endogenous acids account for the increase in unmeasured anions, whereas hyperchloremia is associated with a normal anion gap.

The symptoms and signs of metabolic acidosis are dependent upon the rapidity of onset and the severity of the disorder. They include anorexia, malaise, fatigue, dyspnea, stupor, coma, and shock. Characteristically the blood pH and plasma bicarbonate are reduced and at the extreme may be below 7.0 and 5 mEq/liter respectively. Maximal compensatory hyperventilation may lower Pco_2 to 10 mm Hg. Immediate therapy is indicated if the blood pH is below 7.2 or the plasma bicarbonate below 7 mEq/liter. To calculate bicarbonate deficit, multiply 0.4 × body weight (kg) × (desired minus actual) bicarbonate concentration. This amount should be infused as sodium bicarbonate. Sodium bicarbonate is provided in ampules of 44 mEq in 50 ml, or 880 mEq/liter. It should never be infused undiluted, because fatal cardiac arrhythmias may occur. Correction should be aimed at raising bicarbonate to about 15 mEq/liter, with half the correction achieved in 6 to 12 hours. If acidosis is severe or the patient is

TABLE 8-2 Causes of Metabolic Acidosis

Increased Unmeasured Anions
1. Renal Failure
2. Ketoacidosis
        diabetes mellitus
        starvation
        alcoholic
3. Lactic Acidosis
4. Exogenous acids
        methyl alcohol
        ethylene glycol
        paraldehyde
        salicylate
        cationic amino acids

Normal Unmeasured Anions
1. Diarrhea
2. Renal tubular acidosis
3. Ureterosigmoidostomy
4. Acidifying agents
        ammonium chloride
        carbonic anhydrase inhibitors

acutely ill, half the correction should be achieved in 2 hours. It is particularly important to evaluate the effect of therapy every 2 to 3 hours, since calculated deficits may be grossly underestimated or continued production of endogenous acid, e.g., lactic acid, may require massive bicarbonate infusions even to keep up with production.

Occasionally patients with severe acidosis may also have renal or cardiac failure and thus be likely to become fluid overloaded when the necessary sodium bicarbonate is given. Such patients should be treated with dialysis.

The commonest cause of acute severe metabolic acidosis is probably uncontrolled diabetes mellitus. The acidosis results from the increased production of acetoacetic and beta-hydroxybutyric acids. Production of acid varies widely among patients, and repeated measurements of blood acid-base and potassium levels are essential for proper treatment of the electrolyte imbalance. Excess production of lactic acid occurs in several clinical situations in which the supply of oxygen is insufficient, e.g., exercise, shock, or anoxia, or when there is interference with oxygen utilization, e.g., by phenformin. Many cases of idiopathic lactic acidosis have also been reported. Because studies of blood lactate concentration are often not readily available, a presumptive diagnosis can often be made by exclusion of the other known causes of large anion gap acidosis. In addition, massive rapid requirements of bicarbonate (>500 mEq in 8 to 12 hours) after initiation of treatment seldom are produced by any other cause.

Rapid diagnosis of acidosis caused by ingestion of methyl alcohol, ethylene glycol, and aspirin is particularly important, because these agents are dialyzable. In addition, the blindness that sometimes follows methyl alcohol intoxication may be prevented by maintenance of a moderate blood level of ethyl alcohol, achieved by infusing 50 ml of 95% ethyl alcohol in 500 ml of 0.9% NaCl over 30 to 60 minutes. Diagnosis of these ingestions is confirmed by blood concentration but must be suspected in any undiagnosed acidosis. Oxalate crystals in the urine are suggestive of ethylene glycol ingestion, whereas a positive ferric chloride test is helpful in the diagnosis of salicylate overdose. Acidosis is rare in adults with salicylate overdose. Treatment with bicarbonate should be initiated in these situations while the patient is being prepared for peritoneal dialysis or hemodialysis.

METABOLIC ALKALOSIS

It is extremely unusual for metabolic alkalosis to require emergency treatment. However, hypokalemia, often severe, usually occurs concurrently and may require urgent treatment (see above). Metabolic alkalosis is produced by the loss of nonvolatile acid, an excess intake (oral or intravenous) of alkali, or from extracellular volume contraction caused by loss of sodium and chloride.

The signs and symptoms of metabolic alkalosis are rare and are difficult to separate from those of hypokalemia. They include apathy, malaise, confusion, and slight respiratory depression. Tetany may occasionally occur, especially if the onset of alkalosis is rapid.

Metabolic alkalosis is most commonly found because of loss of stomach acid either spontaneously or by gastric suction. Contraction of extracellular fluid from excess diuretics is also a frequent cause. Less common causes include mineralocorticoid excess, rapid reduction in hypercapnia in patients with respiratory acidosis, and excessive intake of alkali.

Therapy is rarely urgent, and the imbalance usually responds readily to removal of the causative factor. The major therapeutic thrust is usually correction of the hypokalemia and the NaCl deficit. However, occasionally, for example in postoperative patients requiring continuous gastric drainage, the pH may remain consistently over 7.6 and intravenous acid therapy may be necessary. The amount of hydrogen ions necessary to return the patient to a safer pH may be estimated by attempting to reduce plasma bicarbonate to below 40 mEq/liter. To calculate hydrogen ion deficit multiply 0.4 × body weight (kg) × (actual minus desired) concentration. If the patient does not have liver disease, this may be infused as 0.9% ammonium chloride which contains 169 mEq/liter of hydrogen ion. Recently we have successfully utilized 0.1 normal hydrochloric acid, which contains 100 mEq/liter of hydrogen ion. HCl must be infused into a large central vein, because extravasation will cause tissue necrosis.

HYPONATREMIA

One of the commonest abnormalities observed in the hospitalized patient, hyponatremia rarely requires emergency treatment. Because sodium and its salts contribute the bulk of osmotically active particles, serum osmolality can be approximated as $2 \times Na^+$ concentration $+ 10$. A more accurate measure includes consideration of glucose and urea when they are elevated.

$$\text{Serum OSM} = 2\,[Na^+]\,mEq/\text{liter} + \frac{\text{glucose mg}/100\,\text{ml}}{18}$$

$$+ \frac{\text{BUN mg}/100\,\text{ml}}{2.8}$$

Because all cells except those in the kidney, which respond to antidiuretic hormone (ADH), are always freely permeable to water, extracellular fluid (ECF) osmolality will equal intracellular fluid (ICF) osmolality. Any imbalance between ECF and ICF osmolality is immediately corrected by the movement of water along osmotic gradients. It should be clear then that the concentration of sodium in serum and the absolute total body sodium content are distinctly different entities. Sodium concentration describes the relative amounts of sodium and water in ECF and is unrelated to sodium intake and output. Sodium content is directly related to ECF volume and unrelated to serum concentration. Thus, hyponatremia represents a relative increase in the ratio of water to solutes. It must be emphasized that the concentration of sodium in the serum, per se, is not a measure of the state of hydration, because total body water may be increased, normal, or decreased in the presence of hyponatremia. It is likewise not a measure of total body sodium, because total body sodium may be increased, normal, or decreased in the presence of hyponatremia. What the finding of hyponatremia does represent is an imbalance of total body water to total body sodium, i.e., an excess of water for the body solutes present. The ability to excrete a water load is dependent on (1) the absence of ADH; (2) the delivery of adequate quantities of sodium-containing fluid to the distal diluting sites; (3) a functional solute reabsorptive mechanism at the diluting site; and (4) maintenance of distal nephron water impermeability in the absence of ADH. Any abnormality in these functions will impair the ability to excrete a water load and hence may lead to hyponatremia.

ECF CONTRACTION (SODIUM DEPLETION)

When a normal person loses excessive sodium because of perspiration, vomiting, or diarrhea, ECF contracts as a result of sodium and water loss. The intravascular volume participates in the ECF reduction, and this decrease in effective intravascular volume sets off a number of appropriate physiologic responses to combat this loss and retain fluid. A consequence of these protective reactions is hyponatremia. Volume depletion lowers the glomerular filtration rate (GFR), stimulates proximal reabsorption, and increases the release of ADH. Although this situation of total body salt depletion occurs most frequently in association with gastrointestinal losses, it is also seen in hypoadrenalism, the excessive use of diuretics, and renal salt wasting. The clinical picture is that of decreased ECF. Skin turgor is poor, eyeballs are sunken and soft, blood pressure is somewhat low, and pulse and hematocrit levels are elevated. Orthostatic hypotension is also common. Blood urea nitrogen (BUN) and creatinine levels are slightly elevated. Any water ingestion at this time will aggravate the hyponatremia. Clearly the appropriate therapy is the provision of sufficient saline to replace the deficit.

ECF Expansion (Sodium Excess)

The disorders most commonly associated with ECF expansion are congestive heart failure and hepatic cirrhosis. There is no question that the problem is not one of too little sodium, because there is clearly too much sodium in the body. These patients are edematous and the edema is ECF containing sodium. However, the pathophysiologic mechanisms are similar to those of the patient with ECF depletion. These patients have an "ineffective intravascular volume." Although the total plasma volume may be increased the relative intravascular volume may be diminished. Whatever the stimulus, the body responds as if there were true volume depletion. Although GFR may or may not be decreased, proximal reabsorption is probably enhanced and there is again a diminished distal fluid load. Even in the face of serum hypotonicity ADH is almost certainly circulating, and although there may be maximal stimulation for removal of tubular solutes (hyperaldosteronism), excess reabsorption of water prevents the excretion of a dilute urine. Retention of additional ingested water then aggravates the hyponatremia. The clinical hallmarks of this condition are edema and little sodium in the urine. The treatment for the hyponatremia is water restriction. Treatment with diuretics to reduce total body sodium will often worsen the hyponatremia (see below) unless negative water balance is carefully maintained.

Drugs

The number of drugs known to affect water excretion is rapidly increasing. Although it is appreciated that narcotics, barbiturates, anesthetic agents, and nicotine impair water excretion, their specific mechanism of action is unclear. Oral hypoglycemic drugs such as chlorpropamide appear to potentiate the action of ADH. Cyclophosphamide, demeclocycline, and vincristine have also been reported recently to cause hyponatremia.

The most widely used drugs impairing excretion of a water load are the diuretics, including furosemide, ethacrynic acid, and the thiazides, all of which impair NaCl transport in the ascending limb and/or the distal tubule, thereby blocking the manufacture of solute free fluid. In addition, volume depletion secondary to diuretics sets into motion all the mechanism mentioned above under ECF Contraction.

Pseudohyponatremia

Normal serum is about 93% water by weight, while the rest is composed of protein and lipids. The hospital laboratory routinely reports sodium concentration in mEq/liter of serum. Therefore, actual sodium concentration in serum water = $[Na^+]$ (serum)/0.93. When the laboratory reports $[Na^+]$ = 140 mEq/liter, it is actually 140/0.93 = 150 mEq/liter. We regularly factor for this error and accept it. However, when plasma lipid or protein concentration increases significantly, e.g., if serum water content is reduced to 80% and Na concentration equals 150 mEq/liter, it would be reported as 120 mEq/liter (120/0.8 = 150). Lipids seldom affect serum Na concentration unless neutral fat is elevated, and the serum is lactescent. A similar correction is necessary for elevation in serum proteins.

Hyperglycemia also produces hyponatremia, because glucose is largely restricted to the ECF and an increase in glucose concentration draws water out of cells. This is, in fact, true hyponatremia but not hypoosmolality, for the glucose replaces the Na as an osmotically active constituent of plasma. To estimate what the actual serum sodium will be after the glucose has been metabolized, assume an increase of 1.6 mEq/liter in serum sodium for every 100 mg/100 ml decrease in glucose.

Syndrome of Inappropriate ADH (SIADH)

The primary disorder is an excess of ADH causing water retention. It should be clear that this diagnosis cannot be entertained unless all known mechanisms which impair water excretion are ruled out. As was pointed out above, these include endocrine, cardiac, hepatic, or renal dysfunction, volume depletion, drugs, and physical or emotional stress. As a practical matter, if these possibilities are excluded, then in any patient with hypotonic serum the urine should be diluted to an osmolality of <100 mOsm/kg H_2O and not to just some level less than the plasma osmolality. The inability to dilute the urine maximally under these conditions, then, virtually always implies inappropriate ADH secretion. As a clinical rule of thumb, patients with BUN >15 mg/100 ml rarely have this syndrome.

In this condition, ingested water is retained, expanding total body water. Expansion of ECF inhibits tubular reabsorption of sodium and a natriuresis ensues. This combination of obligatory water reabsorption and sodium excretion results in hyponatremia. Despite the hyponatremia there will always be significant amounts of sodium in the urine. From a clinical point of view, the salient features of this syndrome are (1) hyponatremia; (2) urinary excretion of significant amounts of sodium despite hyponatremia; (3) absence of clinical edema; (4) absence of volume depletion; (5) normal adrenal, renal, hepatic, and cardiac fr.ction; and (6) improvement by fluid restriction.

The causes of the syndrome are numerous and include a variety of central nervous system diseases (head injuries, brain abscess, tumor, inflammatory diseases, etc.), pulmonary lesions (small cell carcinoma, tuberculosis, pneumonias), malignancies (some of which make an ADH-like material), myxedema, and acute porphyria. As previously stated, water restriction will return the serum sodium toward normal. However, elimination of the primary cause of the ADH secretion is necessary for cure of the syndrome.

TREATMENT

ECF CONTRACTION Volume deficits should be replaced with isotonic saline solution unless serum sodium is below 115 mEq/liter, in which case 3 to 5% NaCl may be used initially.

ECF EXPANSION Water should be restricted to insensible loss (~500 ml) plus 300 to 500 ml/day. Do *not* treat with hypertonic saline solution unless the patient has symptoms, i.e., difficulty concentrating, anorexia, headache, apathy, nausea, and vomiting. (Coma and perhaps generalized convulsions may occur but they are rare.) These symptoms are very unusual unless the sodium concentration falls below 115 mEq/liter or the fall in concentration has been very rapid. The problem is too much water, not too little sodium.

If hypertonic saline treatment is deemed an emergency, an attempt should be made to increase the serum sodium to about 120 mEq/liter with the infusion of 5% NaCl. Multiply 0.6 × body weight (kg) × (desired-actual) sodium concentration. There are 85 mEq of NaCl/100 ml of 5% saline solution.

SELECTED READINGS

Bartter, F. C., and Schwartz, W. B.   The syndrome of inappropriate secretion of antidiuretic hormone. *Am. J. Med.* 42:790–806, 1967.

Fuisz, R. E.   Hyponatremia. *Medicine* 42:149–170, 1963.

Garella, S., Dana, C. L., and Chazan, J. A.   Severity of metabolic acidosis as a determinant of bicarbonate requirements. *N. Engl. J. Med.* 289: 121–126, 1973.

Kassirer, J. P.   Serious acid-base disorders. *N. Engl. J. Med.* 291:773–776, 1974.

Leaf, A.   The clinical and physiologic significance of the serum sodium concentration. *N. Engl. J. Med.* 267:24–30, 72–83, 1962.

Levinsky, N. G.   Hyperkalemia, the Clinical Spectrum. In *Clinician*. Chicago: Searle, 1973. Pp. 58–64.

Maxwell, M. H., and Kleeman, C. R.   *Clinical Disorders of Fluid and Electrolyte Metabolism.* 2d ed. New York: McGraw-Hill, 1972.

Rector, F. C., Jr. (Ed.).   Symposium on acid-base homeostasis. *Kidney Int.* 1:273, 1970.

Rector, F. C., Jr., and Knochel, J. P.   Hypokalemia. In *Clinician*. Chicago: Searle, 1973. Pp. 42–57.

Waters, W. C., Hall, J. D., and Schwartz, W. B.   Spontaneous lactic acidosis: The nature of the acid-base disturbance and considerations in diagnosis and management. *Am. J. Med.* 35:781–793, 1963.

Weiner, M. W., and Epstein, F. H.   Signs and symptoms of electrolyte disorders. *Yale J. Biol. Med.* 43:76–109, 1970.

LEAH M. LOWENSTEIN

ACUTE RENAL FAILURE is the rapid deterioration of renal function, characterized by a fall in glomerular filtration rate, oliguria, and the harmful accumulation of substances normally excreted in the urine. Emergency conditions that arise during the course of acute renal failure include hypervolemia, hypovolemia, hyperkalemia, acidosis, hypertension, cardiac arrythmias, convulsions, and infection. The most important and immediate task of the physician is to determine whether the acute renal failure is due to extrarenal or to renal causes. The second most important task is to plan treatment to prevent the acute complications of acute renal failure. The third most important task is to identify and treat the complications that arise.

CLINICAL PATTERNS

The major causes of acute renal failure are listed in Table 9-1. They are divided into three categories: prerenal, renal, and postrenal conditions. It is important to identify in which category the patient's renal failure occurs, because in the prerenal and postrenal conditions immediate treatment is needed to avoid renal parenchymal damage.

PRERENAL AZOTEMIA

Prerenal azotemia occurs following severe hypovolemia, congestive heart failure, or hypotension. Renal function is impaired by renal ischemia, which is severe enough to cause a reduction in glomerular filtration rate and an increase in the tubular reabsorption of urea (Table 9-2) but not severe enough to lead to parenchymal damage.

* Supported in part by PHS Grants AM 17713 and No 1-AM-4-2212.

TABLE 9-1 Causes of Acute Renal Failure

───

Prerenal causes (prerenal azotemia)
  Dehydration
  Hypotension
  Congestive heart failure
Renal causes (parenchymal disease)
  Acute tubular necrosis
    Nephrotoxins
      Antibiotics
      Organic chemicals, pesticides, myoglobin
      Heavy metals
    Ischemia
      Hypotension
      Severe renal vasoconstriction
      Thrombi, emboli
  Glomerular diseases
    Acute glomerulonephritis
    Goodpasture's syndrome
    Lupus nephritis
    Eclampsia
  Acute interstitial diseases
    Hypersensitivity reactions
    Antibiotics
    Severe pyelonephritis
Postrenal causes
  Acute obstruction of the ureters or urethra
    Stones
    Prostatic disease
    Tumors
    Fibrosis

───

ACUTE TUBULAR NECROSIS

Acute tubular necrosis is a self-limited condition that can be divided into three phases. (1) In the initial phase, which lasts about 36 hours, the clinical manifestations are usually the result of the initial cause of acute renal failure, e.g., hypotension or drug toxicity. During this phase, the urine output is variable, and may be low (50 ml/day) or normal. (2) The oliguric phase begins between the second and the fifth day. Unlike the first phase, the symptoms and signs of the oliguric phase are due to renal damage and are usually independent of the cause of the renal failure. The urine output varies between 50 and 400 ml a day. Clinically, the pattern varies from patient to patient, depending upon the degree of retention of fluid, electrolytes, and nitrogenous substances. Anorexia, nausea, and vomiting may be present. Fluid overload may result in congestive heart failure, with high venous pressure, increased blood flow, and cardiac arrythmias. Neurological signs include muscle cramps and twitching, lethargy, and convulsions. (3) The diuretic phase occurs after an average of 1 to 3 weeks, with a progressive increase in urine volume heralding the recovery of renal function. During this time the daily urine volume often doubles each day until one liter is excreted. Massive diure-

TABLE 9-2 Differential Diagnosis in Acute Renal Failure

Condition	Urine Volume (ml/24 hr)	Urine Na+ Concen- tration (mEq/L)	GFR* (ml/min)	Serum BUN-Cr* Ratio	Urine- Plasma Cr Ratio
Prerenal azotemia	<400†	<20	>10	>10/1	>20/1
Nonoliguric ATN*	>400	>20	2–10	10/1	<20/1
Oliguric ATN	<400†	>20	<1	10/1	>20/1
Acute postrenal obstruction	Variable	<20	Variable	>10/1	>20/1

* Abbreviations: ATN: acute tubular necrosis; GFR: glomerular filtration rate; BUN: blood urea nitrogen (concentration); Cr: creatinine.
† Conditions associated with complete anuria: cortical necrosis, bilateral complete obstructive uropathy, bilateral renal artery occlusion.

sis may occur, caused by fluid overloading during the oliguric phase, with major losses of sodium, potassium, and water. However, with adequate fluid balance during the oliguric phase, the diuretic phase usually results in only moderate losses of fluid and electrolytes.

NONOLIGURIC ACUTE TUBULAR NECROSIS

Acute tubular necrosis may occur in a more benign form, without oliguria. The parenchymal renal damage is less severe than in the oliguric form, but the causes of both are the same, with surgical procedures and nephrotoxins as frequent culprits. The daily urine volume is greater than 400 ml/day, but is still limited in amount so that fluid overload can readily occur. The course is usually less prolonged than that of the oliguric form, but the mortality rate is still high, at 25%.

ACUTE GLOMERULAR OR INTERSTITIAL DISEASE

Acute glomerular and interstitial diseases vary widely in their symptoms. Patients with acute renal failure caused by glomerulonephritis may be seen with oliguria, edema, and hypertension. Interstitial nephritis may also be characterized by acute renal failure. The emergency complications in acute renal failure caused by these conditions are similar to those of acute tubular necrosis, except that hypertension occurs more frequently and may be a special problem.

ACUTE URINARY TRACT OBSTRUCTION

Acute renal failure follows complete bilateral obstruction or unilateral obstruction superimposed on chronic renal disease, e.g., uric acid stones and chronic uric acid nephropathy. The symptoms vary from severe (e.g., renal colic) to none at all, and the course varies from the rapid development of renal failure with complete anuria to a slower development (over weeks) if the obstructive lesion slowly occludes the lower urinary tract. After the obstruction is relieved, a massive diuresis can occur, over several days, with loss of up to 10 liters of urine daily. Massive losses of sodium and potassium also occur. Immediate quantitative replacement of the losses is necessary to prevent severe circulatory collapse.

DIFFERENTIAL DIAGNOSIS

For adequate emergency treatment, the three major categories of acute renal failure must be differentiated from one another.

CLINICAL FINDINGS

The clinical picture is important in determining the cause of the acute renal failure, especially in the first 24 hours, when complications have not blurred the original findings. Dehydration, hypotension, or congestive heart failure indicates that prerenal azotemia may be present. One of the many causes of acute parenchymal damage may be evident.

URINE SEDIMENT

In prerenal azotemia, hyaline and finely granular casts are present in moderate numbers. In acute tubular necrosis, medium brown granular casts, and tubular epithelial cells and casts, are present in large numbers. In acute glomerular diseases and vasculitis, red blood cells and occasional red blood cell casts are present. In postrenal obstruction the sediment is sparse, with few cells and casts.

URINE COMPOSITION

Measurement of the urine volume and of sodium and creatinine concentrations is paramount in identifying the different types of renal failure (see Table 9-2). Urine sodium concentration is low (<20 mEq/liter) in prerenal and postrenal failure, and high (>20 mEq/liter) in acute tubular necrosis. In prerenal azotemia the urine is concentrated, with a urine-plasma creatine ratio of >20 : 1. In acute tubular necrosis, this ratio is usually low. The urine-plasma ratio of osmolality is similarly affected. Values over 2 : 1 indicate prerenal azotemia; values under 1.1 : 1, acute tubular necrosis.

BLOOD UREA AND CREATININE VALUES

Studies of blood urea and creatinine are also helpful in the differential diagnosis (see Table 9-2).

RADIOGRAPHY

Radiography is important if (1) acute renal failure is to be distinguished from chronic renal failure, and (2) a suspicion of acute postrenal obstruction exists. The kidneys may be seen on a plain flat film of the abdomen. The kidneys are normal-sized in acute renal failure and may be small in chronic renal failure. Intravenous pyelography is useful in the diagnosis of obstruction. Even with acute renal failure and serum creatinine levels of 10 mg/100 ml, the kidneys will usually be visualized and the dilated calyces of acute obstruction detected. Laminography and films taken several hours after the dye injection will increase the degree of visualization. Retrograde pyelography, to determine the patency of one ureter, should only be performed if the diagnosis of obstruction is probable and intravenous pyelography is not helpful.

DIFFERENTIATION OF PRERENAL AZOTEMIA FROM ACUTE TUBULAR NECROSIS

There are several diagnostic cum treatment steps that help to differentiate prerenal azotemia from acute tubular necrosis. After the patient is rehydrated, a single trial can be given of (1) 25 gm of mannitol intravenously over a 15- to 30-minute period, (2) furosemide, 80 to 200 mg, given rapidly intravenously, (3) both 12.5 gm mannitol and 80 mg of furosemide together for their additive effect, or (4) one liter of saline solution infused rapidly over 30 minutes. An increase in urine volume within 2 hours to over 40 ml/hr after any of these trials indicates that the acute renal failure is probably due to prerenal azotemia rather than to intrinsic renal disease. However, these tests may not differentiate the two groups of patients because (1) some patients with prerenal azotemia caused by dehydration respond very little until their fluid volume is replaced, whereas (2) some patients with acute tubular necrosis do respond with an increase in urine output. It has not been demonstrated in man that mannitol or diuretics prevent acute tubular necrosis once it begins.

TREATMENT

Treatment of acute renal failure consists of prevention of the fluid, electrolyte, and metabolic abnormalities and the treatment of the abnormalities that do arise. In patients with prerenal azotemia caused by hypovolemia, replacement of fluid volume until clinical signs of dehydration disappear and blood pressure is adequately maintained will result in the return of blood urea nitrogen levels to normal, often within a day or two.

Treatment without dialysis can be successfully used to prevent all of the emergency complications of acute renal failure. The following general measures should be taken.

All fluid losses should be accurately tabulated and replaced. Insensible loss is calculated as approximately 500 ml daily plus 50 ml/day for each degree of temperature rise above 99°F. The patient should be weighed, preferably twice daily, as an aid to gauging fluid replacement. A diet of at least 100 gm of glucose and 10 to 20 gm of protein is desirable for patients who can eat. Parenteral alimentation with commercially available solutions of amino acids, glucose, and electrolytes is desirable for patients unable to eat [1].

COMPLICATIONS

FLUID OVERLOAD Fluid overload, leading to congestive heart failure and hypertension, occurs in patients who are improperly managed or who are overloaded with salt and water when they come to the hospital. Salt and water should be restricted, and, if necessary, digitalization with digoxin should be done. However, digitalization should be avoided if at all possible, since wide variations in serum potassium concentrations lead to digitalis toxicity. The maintenance dose is decreased according to the impairment in renal function (Table 9-3).

HYPERKALEMIA Occurring during renal failure, because the excretion of potassium is limited, hyperkalemia follows the eating of excess potassium, the release of potassium from cells in hemolysis or trauma, and from drugs; death occurs from its cardiac effects. Twice daily electrocardiograms should be obtained. Hypokalemia can occur during the diuretic phase, with increased potassium losses in the urine. The treatment of these conditions is discussed in Chapter 8.

ACIDOSIS Acidosis in acute renal failure is usually not severe. It is advisable not to treat it unless the bicarbonate concentration is less than 12 mEq/liter. The bicarbonate concentration may then slowly be brought up to 12 with intravenous sodium bicarbonate. The amount to be given is discussed in Chapter 8.

INFECTION Because infection is one of the major causes of death in patients with acute tubular necrosis, it is important to identify the sites of infection and to treat with the proper antibiotic agent. The doses of antibiotic drugs for treatment should be adjusted to the degree of im-

TABLE 9-3 Effect of Acute Renal Failure on the Maintenance Dose Intervals of Commonly Used Drugs [3]

Drug		None	Degree of Renal Failure		
			Mild C_{Cr}: 50–80 ml/min	Moderate C_{Cr}: 10–50 ml/min	Severe C_{Cr} <10 ml/min
Cardiovascular					
Diazoxide	HP	I.V. bolus	No change		
Digoxin		q 12 h	2*	2–3	3–4
Guanethidine		q 24 h	1	1.5	1.5–2
Lidocaine		I.V. drip	No change		
Methyldopa	HP	q 6 h	1	1.5–2	2–3
Procainamide		q 3 h	1	1.5–2	2–3
Propanolol		q 6 h	No change		
Quinidine	HP	q 6 h	1	1.5–2	2–3

TABLE 9-3 (*continued*)

Drug		None	Mild C_{Cr}: 50–80 ml/min	Moderate C_{Cr}: 10–50 ml/min	Severe $C_{Cr} < 10$ ml/min
			Degree of Renal Failure		
Diuretic					
Acetazolamide		q 6 h	1	2	avoid
Aminophylline		q 6 h		No change	
Ethacrynic acid		q 6 h	1	avoid	avoid
Furosemide		q 6 h		No change	
Antimicrobial					
Ampicillin	H	q 6 h	1	1	1–2
Carbenicillin	HP	q 4 h	1	1.5–3	3–4
Cephaloridine	HP	q 6 h	1	2	4–6
Cephalothin	HP	q 6 h	1	1	1.5–2
Cloxacillin		q 6 h		No change	
Erythromycin		q 6 h		No change	
Gentamicin	H	q 8 h	1.5	1.5–3	6
Isoniazid	HP	q 8 h	1	1.5	1.5–2
Kanamycin	HP	q 8 h	3	3–9	9–12
Methicillin		q 4 h	1	1	2–3
Nafcillin		q 6 h		No change	
Neomycin		q 6 h	1	2	3–4
Oxacillin		q 6 h	1	1	1.5–2
Penicillin G		q 8 h	1	1	1.5
Streptomycin	HP	q 12 h	2	2–6	6–8
Tetracycline		q 6 h	1.5–2	6–8	12
Vancomycin		q 6 h	4–12	12–40	40
Analgesic and sedative		normal	<2.5	2.5–8	>8
Acetaminophen		q 4 h	1	1	avoid
Acetylsalicylic acid	HP	q 4 h	1	1.5	2–3
Chlordiazepoxide		q 8 h	1	1.5	1.5–3
Diazepam		q 8 h		No change	
Morphine		q 4 h		No change	
Phenobarbital	HP	q 8 h	1	1	2
Phenothiazine		q 6 h	1	1.5–2	2–3
Miscellaneous					
Allopurinol		q 8 h	1	1.5	1.5–3
Azathioprine	H	q 12 h	1	1.5	2
Crystalline (regular) insulin		q 6 h	1	1.5–2	2–4
Diphenylhydantoin	H	q 8 h		No change	
Heparin		q 4 h		No change	
Phenformin		q 8 h	1	avoid	avoid
Tolbutamide		q 8 h	1	1.5	1.5–2

* Factor by which the usual time interval between doses should be multiplied.
C_{Cr}: Creatinine clearance.
H: Known to be removed by hemodialysis.
P: Known to be removed by peritoneal dialysis.

pairment of renal function, as shown in Table 9-3. A major site of infection is the urinary tract. Indwelling catheters should not be used unless necessary (e.g., with prostatic obstruction), and urine cultures should be obtained daily. Prophylactic antibiotics should be avoided. Tetracycline and sulfonamides should not be used because of their potential for increasing renal damage. Gentamicin and kanamycin should be used only if other antibiotic drugs are not appropriate, because they increase renal damage if the dosage is not strictly controlled (see Table 9-3).

CONVULSIONS Convulsions may occur during the course of acute renal failure as a complication of (1) the uremic syndrome, (2) the disequilibrium syndrome after hemodialysis, and (3) cerebral hemorrhage caused by severe uremia. Diphenylhydantoin (100 mg) and diazepam (5 to 10 mg) I.V. generally stop the convulsions.

DIALYSIS

In patients who are treated conservatively, the indications for peritoneal dialysis or hemodialysis are (1) severe uremia, with stupor, vomiting, and muscle twitching, (2) fluid overload, (3) severe hypertension associated with fluid overload, (4) pericardial friction rub, and (5) severe acidosis. However, frequent treatment with hemodialysis and peritoneal dialysis is now widely used to (1) prevent the complications cited above, (2) enable the patient to receive adequate protein to prevent malnutrition, and (3) avoid the unpleasant symptoms of uremia. Hemodialysis and peritoneal dialysis can be performed twice weekly or more frequently if the complications mentioned above occur. Dialysis probably does not alter the course or mortality of acute renal failure.

Peritoneal dialysis is a relatively simple technique, needing only dialysis catheters and solutions. It can be performed in most hospitals with little training of personnel. Hemodialysis is preferable to peritoneal dialysis only if a nephrotoxin to be removed is better removed by hemodialysis (see Chapter 1, Drug Overdoses and Poisonings), or if technical difficulties prevent the performance of peritoneal dialysis (postoperative abdominal drainage sites, abdominal adhesions, localized intra-abdominal abscess). Peritonitis is not a contraindication. The procedure for peritoneal dialysis at Boston City Hospital is outlined in Table 9-4. Thirty to 36 exchanges (2 liters per exchange) are generally used during each dialysis. Potassium is added to give a dialysate concentration of 4 mEq/liter. Since digitalized patients may develop serious cardiac arrhythmias when their blood potassium levels are lowered, the potassium concentration in the dialysate of patients on digitalis should be maintained at 5 mEq/liter.

Clearances with peritoneal dialysis include creatinine, 15 ml/min; urea, 26 ml/min; and potassium, 21 ml/min [2].

Although many of the emergency complications can be well controlled by prompt treatment and dialysis, the mortality rate in acute renal failure is still high (50%). Patients usually die of infection or from their underlying condition, with the damaged kidney inaccurately named as the agent of death.

TABLE 9-4 Orders for Peritoneal Dialysis at Boston City Hospital

1. Plan _____ exchanges.
2. Each exchange equals 2 liters of 1½% glucose solution. Always use the 1½% glucose concentration unless specifically ordered to use the 7% glucose solution.
3. To 2 liters only of each exchange add:
   (a) _____mEq KCl. (_____ ml. of KCl solution).
   (b) _____mg. heparin (_____ units). Add to the first _____ exchanges.
   (c)
   (d)
4. Label bottles of each exchange with the number of the exchange.
5. Label the bottle of each exchange to which medication was added with the ingredients.
6. Warm dialysate solution in hot water in the hot water basin to body temperature (so that it feels neither hot nor cold to touch).
7. Infuse the dialysate solution as rapidly as possible. (Should take approximately 10 min. If more than 15 min are required, notify house officer.)
8. Near the end of the infusion, clamp tubing before air enters it in order to prevent air entering the abdominal cavity.
9. Leave the dialysate solution in the abdomen for _____ min.
10. Using the collecting bag, empty abdomen as rapidly as possible. The air trap above collecting bag must be perpendicular at all times to prevent retrograde contamination and peritonitis. Draining should take about 15 to 30 min.
11. If drainage is difficult:
   Crank up head of bed to _____ degrees.
   Turn patient onto _____ side.
   Try manual compression of abdomen.
12. Keep a record of the dialysis on a peritoneal dialysis data sheet. Note that the balance is positive when the fluid remains in the patient and negative when more fluid is removed on drainage than was instilled. (Notify house officer if balance is greater than 500 ml on any single exchange or greater than 750 ml total.)
13. Try to maintain zero balance. Try to remove 2,000 ml with each exchange unless otherwise directed.
14. BP, P, R, every hour. Temp. every 2 hours. Notify house officer promptly if BP less than _____, pulse greater than _____, temperature greater than _____, abdominal pain or leakage.
15. Weigh patient daily.
16. Save used bottles of dialysate solution in patient's room until end of dialysis.
17. Culture first bottle and every 6th bottle afterward.
   If any questions, call house officer or the renal fellow.
   Renal Fellow: _____
   Phone Numbers: _____

The 3 most important steps are: (1) adding correct amount of KCl to each exchange; (2) maintenance of sterile technique; (3) removing proper amount of fluid with each exchange.

REFERENCES

1. Dudrick, S. J., Steiger, E., and Long, J. M. Renal failure in surgical
   patients: Treatment with intravenous essential amino acids and hypertonic glucose. *Surgery* 68:180, 1970.
2. Boen, S. T. *Peritoneal Dialysis in Clinical Medicine.* Springfield, Ill.:
   Thomas, 1964.
3. Bennett, W. M., Singer, I., and Coggins, C. J. A guide to drug therapy
   in renal failure. *J.A.M.A.* 230:1544, 1974.

DIAGNOSIS AND MANAGEMENT OF ENDOCRINE EMERGENCIES

ROBERT M. LEVIN

THE MAJOR ENDOCRINE emergencies that one may encounter in clinical medicine include thyrotoxic crisis (also called thyroid storm), myxedema coma, acute adrenal insufficiency, hypercalcemic crisis, diabetic ketoacidosis, and hypoglycemia. The latter two emergencies are discussed separately in the following chapter of this text. Each of the above endocrine emergencies should be avoidable if the underlying endocrine abnormality is considered, diagnosed, and treated properly during its early manifestations (if the patient seeks medical advice at an early stage of the disease). However, such is not always the case, and each of these endocrine disorders can become so severe as to become life-threatening.

THYROID STORM

Thyroid storm, or thyrotoxic crisis, may result from the inadequate treatment of a patient with a diffuse toxic goiter (Graves' disease) in the following situations: (1) during the intraoperative or postoperative period in a patient improperly medically prepared for thyroidectomy, (2) following a therapeutic dose of radioactive iodine, which may produce a severe irradiation thyroiditis and the resultant release of large amounts of preformed hormone from the damaged gland, and (3) following the too abrupt discontinuation of antithyroid drugs, particularly if iodine was part of the medical regimen. In addition, it may occasionally be seen in a patient who has never received any treatment for his thyrotoxicosis and who is now exposed to a stressful situation such as an infection, diabetic ketoacidosis, toxemia of pregnancy, a traumatic incident (including a surgical emergency), or severe psychological trauma. The pathophysiology of this condition is poorly understood. There is no evidence that the serum level of thyroid hormones is any higher during the storm than it was a few days before the crisis. This has led to the speculation that this condition is due to a "decompensation" of the peripheral organs and tissues from the effects of the excess thyroid hormones. Although one cannot afford the luxury of performing all the desired diagnostic tests and awaiting their results prior to instituting therapy of a patient in storm, one should certainly draw blood for serum thyroxine and triiodothyronine levels prior to starting therapy.

Diagnosis

The clinical picture of a severely thyrotoxic patient should allow the proper diagnosis to be made at the bedside if one looks carefully for evidence of exophthalmopathy, the characteristic pretibial dermopathy, the presence of a goiter, hyperactive deep tendon reflexes, tachycardia, and tremulousness. Thyrotoxic storm presents an exaggerated picture of thyrotoxicosis. The excessive hypermetabolism is characterized by fever, which may be as high as 106°F, and skin which is warm, flushed, fine in texture, and very moist from profuse sweating. The cardiovascular, gastrointestinal, and central nervous systems are particularly involved and may present a variable and occasionally very confusing clinical picture. Cardiovascular findings may include a marked tachycardia which is excessive for the body temperature, supraventricular arrhythmia, and congestive heart failure. Gastrointestinal findings include diarrhea, abdominal pain, nausea, vomiting, and an enlarged liver with abnormal liver function tests that may include an elevated serum bilirubin. Central nervous system findings include marked restlessness, tremor, emotional lability, psychotic behavior, and progression to apathy, stupor, and coma.

Treatment

Treatment should be started as soon as possible and may be directed at the following areas: (1) controlling the increased synthesis and secretion of thyroid hormones, (2) combatting the metabolic effects of thyroid hormones already circulating in the blood and present in the tissues, (3) diagnosing and beginning treatment of any underlying infection or other precipitating illness, and (4) providing general supportive care (Table 10-1).

Large doses of antithyroid drugs should be administered immediately in order to block organification of iodide within the gland. Propylthiouracil in doses of 200 mg (or methimazole, 20 mg) every 4 to 6 hours is effective within one hour after oral or nasogastric tube administration. Although propylthiouracil is not expected to give prompt clinical benefit, it is important to begin this medication before administration of iodide. The iodide, a major therapeutic agent which will be discussed below, should not be started before the propylthiouracil because it will accumulate within the gland and may be used to make new thyroid hormone. Propylthiouracil has the added advantage of blocking the peripheral deiodination of thyroxine, thereby lowering the serum triiodothyronine level.

Iodide should be started one hour after the propylthiouracil has been given. It acts rapidly and effectively in blocking the release of preformed

TABLE 10-1 Summary of Treatment of Thyroid Storm

---

1. Control thyroid hormone synthesis
   a. Propylthiouracil, 200 mg every 4 to 6 hr p.o., *or*
   b. Methimazole, 20 mg every 4 to 6 hr p.o.
2. Control thyroid secretion rate
   a. Lugol's solution, 30 drops daily p.o., *or*
   b. Sodium iodide, 1 gm I.V. every 8 hr by slow drip
3. Combat ongoing metabolic effects of thyroid hormones
   a. Propranolol hydrochloride, 1 to 2 mg I.V. slowly every 4 to 6 hr, *or*
      20 to 40 mg p.o. every 4 to 6 hr, *or*
   b. Reserpine, 1.0 to 2.5 mg I.M. every 4 to 6 hr, *or*
   c. Guanethidine sulfate, 50 to 150 mg p.o. each day
4. General Supportive measures
   a. Fluids, glucose, electrolytes, and vitamins
   b. Ice packs, fans, and refrigerated mattresses
   c. Hydrocortisone phosphate (or hydrocortisone sodium succinate), 200
      to 300 mg I.V. daily

---

hormone from the gland. Lugol's (strong iodine) solution, 30 drops daily by mouth, or sodium iodide, 1 gm I.V. every 8 hours by slow drip, is adequate.

To block the metabolic effects of thyroid hormones that have already been released from the gland, beta-adrenergic blocking agents or drugs that deplete the catecholamines are very effective. Although the exact relationship between thyroxine and the catecholamines remains unsettled in this condition, it is clinically suspected that many of the symptoms of thyrotoxicosis are either caused by or worsened by the sympathetic amines. Reserpine, 2.5 mg every 4 to 6 hours I.M., may lead to marked clinical improvement within 4 to 8 hours. Propranolol, 1 to 2 mg given intravenously slowly over 5 to 10 minutes and repeated every 4 to 6 hours, is also very effective in controlling the cardiac and the psychomotor manifestations of thyrotoxicosis. The effects may last up to 4 hours after intravenous administration and up to 8 hours after the oral administration of 20 to 40 mg every 4 to 6 hours. The dose of propranolol needed to slow the pulse, reduce the tremor and excess sweating, slow intestinal motility, and in general lower the oxygen consumption by the body is quite variable. Up to 240 to 320 mg daily may be needed in younger patients. The serum levels of the thyroid hormones are not affected by either reserpine or propranolol. Although propranolol is very well tolerated by thyrotoxic patients, caution should be used in patients with heart failure or bronchial asthma. In such persons, it may be advisable to use reserpine or guanethidine. Guanethidine is effective within 24 hours in oral doses of 50 to 150 mg, but the maximal effect of the drug may not be reached for a few days. Reserpine is also very well tolerated in thyrotoxicosis, although its onset of action is somewhat slower than that of propranolol. Side effects that may be encountered with reserpine include central nervous system depression and diarrhea.

The general supportive measures that are important in a patient with thyroid storm include dextrose and water intravenously to correct the fluid losses from the excessive sweating and to supply the caloric needs of the body. Electrolytes should be replaced as needed. B complex vitamins are often added. A high body temperature should be treated with fans, ice packs, or refrigerated mattresses. Aspirin, which can theoretically increase even further the metabolic rate in these patients, should probably be avoided. Digitalis and diuretics may be needed if the patient develops heart failure. Adrenal corticosteroids are indicated because of the increased metabolism and turnover and secretion rates that occur in this condition. The patient is obviously under great stress, and it is theoretically possible that his adrenocortical reserve may be exceeded. It is advisable to administer 200 to 300 mg of hydrocortisone sodium succinate intravenously daily as long as the patient remains critically ill.

Despite these heroic measures, the mortality rate in thyroid storm is still 20 to 50 percent.

MYXEDEMA COMA

Myxedema coma will probably be seen with increasing frequency because of the current popular use of radioactive iodine in the treatment of thyrotoxicosis. Although myxedema coma was rarely seen in patients under 50 in the 1950s and 1960s, the recent trend toward treating younger and younger thyrotoxic patients with radioiodine should be a warning to all clinicians to consider myxedema as a cause of coma. Most of the cases have been noted to appear during the winter months and, indeed, exposure to cold is a precipitating factor. However, in over half the reported cases of myxedema coma, the patient lapsed into coma after admission to the hospital. This circumstance often occurs after the unfortunate administration of a sedative, analgesic, or anesthetic that the myxedematous patient is unable to metabolize adequately. In general, myxedema coma occurs most often in patients with long-standing, often neglected hypothyroidism (failure to seek medical advice because of the insidious course of the disorder) which occurs in chronic thyroiditis or following surgical or radioiodine ablation of a thyrotoxic gland.

Diagnosis

In most cases, the diagnosis is not difficult to make at the bedside if one remembers to consider it. Helpful findings include an anterior neck scar and evidence of prior thyrotoxic disease (e.g., exophthalmopathy and pretibial myxedema). The usual clinical picture is that of an elderly female who gave her admission history in a deeply pitched hoarse voice and who has dry skin, thin coarse hair, marked pallor, excess body weight, eyelid edema, a slow pulse, abdominal distension, and a delayed relaxation phase in her deep tendon reflexes. Hypothermia is not infrequent, and temperatures as low as 75°F (24°C) have been reported. A temperature less than 90°F (34°C) is a serious prognostic finding. Hyponatremia, hypoglycemia, and respiratory acidosis are associated complications. The electrocardiogram may reveal low voltage, flattened or inverted T waves, and a very slow rate. Effusions of the pericardium, pleura, and joints should be looked for.

TREATMENT

Treatment should be directed at (1) replacing most of the patient's extrathyroidal hormone pool, (2) treating the precipitating factor(s), and (3) treating the complications of the disorder (Table 10-2). Carbon dioxide narcosis is a serious and often fatal complication of myxedema coma. This respiratory complication is the result of one or more of the following factors: a large tongue may lead to upper airway obstruction; chest wall muscle infiltration and mucopolysaccharide deposition may lead to a deficient bellows action of the chest; pleural effusions and ascites may impair ventilation; and direct suppression of the respiratory center in the medulla by drugs may lead to slow and shallow respirations. An endotracheal tube or even a tracheostomy may be required. Frequent arterial blood gas and pH determinations should be made.

Prompt replacement of the extrathyroidal hormonal pool is the key to a successful outcome. Although the recommended treatment for an ambulatory patient with severe myxedema is to begin with very small doses of levothyroxine (for example, the equivalent of ¼ grain [15 mg] of thyroid daily) and to increase by similar amounts every week or two, one must be more aggressive in treating myxedema coma. An initial intravenous dose of 300 to 500 μg levothyroxine should be administered, followed by 25 to 30 μg I.V. daily until the patient is awake and can take medications orally. One then very gradually increases doses as noted above for the ambulatory patient. This intravenous loading dose is not surprising when one considers that a euthyroid patient may have, for example, a serum L-thyroxine level of 10 μg/100 ml of blood, or 100 μg per liter, or 500 μg per 5 liters of blood. The patient with hypothyroidism

TABLE 10-2 Summary of Treatment of Myxedema Coma

1. Thyroid hormone replacement
   a. The extrathyroidal hormonal pool in hypothyroidism approximates ·360 μg/1.73 mm^2
   b. Therefore, give 300 to 500 μg L-thyroxine I.V. as initial dose
   c. The fractional turnover rate of 7% in hypothyroidism necessitates giving 25 to 30 μg of L-thyroxine daily
2. Treat reduced pulmonary ventilation
3. Treat hypotension with L-thyroxine before determining need for vasopressors
4. Treat hyponatremia with fluid restriction
5. Treat hypoglycemia with I.V. glucose
6. Avoid rapid external warming
7. Treat precipitating event (e.g., infection, GI bleeding, myocardial infarction)
8. Hydrocortisone phosphate, 200 to 300 mg I.V. daily

does have a considerably smaller extrathyroidal hormonal pool (about 360 μg) than the euthyroid person, and, therefore, should receive a loading dose that is closer to 300 than 500 μg. The fractional turnover rate of thyroxine averages 7% per day (compared to 11% in the euthyroid person) and, therefore, the initial daily replacement dose is only about 25 to 30 μg. Additional therapeutic measures should include management of the hypotension. Treatment should be started with L-thyroxine before vasopressors are used because the blood pressure may rise with thyroid alone. The hyponatremia will respond to L-thyroxine and fluid restriction. It is rarely necessary to administer intravenous saline solution unless, of course, the patient's serum sodium is less than 115 mEq per liter and the blood pressure does not respond to the aforementioned therapy. Rapid external warming should be avoided and, in fact, can lead to increased oxygen consumption and peripheral vascular collapse. The precipitating event should be treated, whether that be a gastrointestinal bleed, myocardial infarct, stroke, or infection. The use of steroids in this condition is controversial. However, the pituitary reserve of corticotropin (ACTH) may be less than normal and the administration of intravenous steroids is suggested. The equivalent of 200 to 300 mg of hydrocortisone phosphate should be administered daily during the patient's critical period. Despite the fact that well over 90% of all hypothyroidism is due to primary thyroid disease, there remains the small chance that the patient has pituitary insufficiency as the underlying disease. Therefore, since the administration of steroids for just a few days is quite safe, their use during these first few days of therapy may be life-saving.

ACUTE ADRENAL INSUFFICIENCY

It is estimated that over 5 million people in the United States are receiving steroids in doses sufficient to suppress the pituitary-adrenal axis, that is, doses in excess of the equivalent of 50 mg of cortisone acetate daily for at least 10 days. Steroids are now used quite commonly in patients with poison ivy, asthma, rheumatoid arthritis, and a wide variety of other conditions. These patients are susceptible to the development of acute adrenal insufficiency within the 6- to 12-month period following cessation of their steroid therapy, should they become acutely stressed. For example, adrenal insufficiency should be suspected in patients who become acutely hypotensive in the following clinical situations: during the induction of anesthesia; during a protracted bout of gastroenteritis associated with nausea, vomiting, and diarrhea; and during the course of a serious infection. Of course, adrenal insufficiency can also develop in patients with primary involvement of the adrenal glands, such as by tuberculosis, blastomycosis, and hemorrhage into the adrenals secondary to anticoagulant therapy. Patients with known adrenal insufficiency in whom, during an acute illness, the dose of steroids is not increased appropriately may also develop adrenal insufficiency.

The classic picture of adrenal insufficiency is that of weakness, anorexia, weight loss, and hypotension. These patients may, in addition, complain of nausea and vomiting, abdominal pain, craving for dietary salt, and areas of increased skin pigmentation. Coma is rarely the presenting manifestation of the patient with adrenal insufficiency. The findings in adrenal insufficiency are due to the deficiency of cortisol and aldosterone, the two major materials made by the adrenal gland. Aldosterone deficiency leads to an impaired ability to retain salt, which leads to extracellular fluid volume depletion. This explains the postural syncope, hypotension, azotemia, and hyperkalemia that may be seen in these patients. The deficiency of cortisol leads to a decrease in gluconeogenesis and symptomatic hypoglycemia, the inability to excrete a water load, and hyperpigmentation. The increased pigmentation, best seen over the creases of the palms, and the nipples, oral mucosa, knees, and elbows, is a result of the absence of cortisol's negative feedback on the pituitary and, therefore, increased production of ACTH and melanocyte-stimulating hormone (MSH). Scars of recent duration should also be carefully examined for increased pigmentation.

TREATMENT

The successful treatment of the patient with acute adrenal insufficiency is dependent upon early diagnosis, prompt institution of parenteral steroid medication and intravenous fluids, and recognition and therapy of the precipitating factor(s) (Table 10-3). Although one cannot afford to await the results of confirmatory tests proving the presence of adrenal insufficiency, serum should be drawn for the determination of cortisol, electrolytes, sugar, and urea nitrogen prior to starting therapy. An initial intravenous dose of 100 mg of hydrocortisone phosphate (or succinate esters) should immediately be given, followed by a total dose of no less than 300 mg over the first 24 hours. This will provide a circulating level of hydrocortisone similar to that of an acutely stressed patient with intact adrenal function. The initial bolus should be followed by an intravenous infusion of hydrocortisone phosphate administered at a rate of 15 mg/hr over the first 24 hours. This large amount of hydrocortisone contains sufficient mineralocorticoid effect so that additional deoxycorticosterone acetate rarely need be given. Simultaneously, 5% dextrose and saline solution should be started I.V. Over 20% of the extracellular fluid volume is often depleted in patients with hypotension and adrenal insufficiency, and rapid correction is necessary. Assuming that the patient does not have serious cardiovascular disease or chronic renal failure, the first liter of 5% dextrose and saline solution should be administered over 30 to 60 minutes. The next 2 to 3 liters should be given over the next few hours.

TABLE 10-3 Summary of Treatment of Acute Adrenal Insufficiency

1. Hydrocortisone phosphate (or succinate esters), 100 mg I.V. stat followed by infusion of hydrocortisone at 15 mg/hr over the first 24 hours
2. 5% dextrose and saline solution, first liter to be infused over 30 to 60 min and next 2 to 3 liters over next few hours
3. Treatment of the precipitating factor(s)

Intravenous fluids are extremely important in the acute phase of therapy, not only to replace volume but also to deliver the proper electrolytes that are required and to correct any hypoglycemia. The occasional patient whose adrenal insufficiency is associated with hypercalcemia will respond to intravenous saline solution with a marked hypercalciuria.

When the emergency situation is over, the steroids may be gradually tapered by giving intramuscular or oral hydrocortisone or cortisone acetate every 6 to 8 hours. The eventual maintenance daily regimen will usually consist of a combination of glucocorticoid and mineralocorticoid. For example, an effective regimen is 20 mg of hydrocortisone (or 25 mg of cortisone acetate) in the morning with 0.5 mg of fluorohydrocortisone and an additional 10 mg of hydrocortisone (or 12.5 mg of cortisone) in the early evening.

HYPERCALCEMIC CRISIS

It is not surprising that the serum calcium may be elevated by a large number of conditions (see Table 10-4). The serum calcium is normally well controlled within the relatively narrow range of 8.8 to 10.5 mg/100 ml. If one considers that the total blood volume is approximately 5 liters, then there are roughly only 500 mg of calcium within this compartment. This is a rather trivial quantity compared to the 1,000 gm of calcium that are contained in the body, over 99% within the skeleton. Approximately 4,000 mg of this bone calcium is readily available to the extracellular fluid compartment for exchange. The mechanism whereby this bone source of calcium can be called upon is described below. When the serum calcium falls, the parathyroid glands release more parathyroid hormone (PTH), which stimulates the kidney to synthesize an increased

TABLE 10-4 Causes of Hypercalcemia

1. Excess parathyroid hormone
   a. Primary hyperparathyroidism
   b. Tertiary hyperparathyroidism
   c. Pseudohyperparathyroidism
2. Excess vitamin D or abnormal sensitivity
   a. Vitamin D intoxication
   b. Sarcoidosis
   c. Idiopathic hypercalcemia of childhood
3. Increased bone turnover
   a. Metastatic cancer to bone
   b. Multiple myeloma
   c. Lymphoma, leukemia, reticulum cell sarcoma
   d. Thyrotoxicosis
   e. Immobilization
4. Miscellaneous
   a. Milk-alkali syndrome
   b. Adrenal insufficiency
   c. Thiazide diuretics
   d. Prolonged use of tourniquet prior to drawing blood

amount of 1,25-dihydroxycholecalciferol. This active vitamin D metabolite is then released and carried to the gut, where calcium reabsorption is increased, and to the bone, where increased bone resorption occurs. When the serum calcium then begins to rise into the high normal range, this negative feedback signal effects the suppression of PTH release.

The 24-hour urinary calcium is normally between 80 and 200 mg and is not much changed by alterations in the dietary intake of calcium. Marked increases in dietary calcium are reflected by a linear increase in fecal calcium. In general, on a normal diet, which contains about 1,000 mg of calcium daily, only 15 to 20% is absorbed. This percent may, however, increase considerably with a low calcium diet.

SYMPTOMS AND SIGNS

Hypercalcemia is being identified with increasing frequency because of the introduction of multiphasic screening tests currently being performed in many hospitals and clinics. These previously unrecognized elevations of the serum calcium may be seen with any of the following symptoms and signs: (1) general malaise, fatigue, lassitude, and weakness; (2) renal colic, polyuria, polydipsia, and nocturia; (3) constipation, epigastric pain, anorexia, nausea, and vomiting; and (4) lethargy, muscle weakness, drowsiness, confusion, psychosis, stupor, and coma. Although recurrent kidney stones may alert the physician to obtain a serum calcium determination, many of the above symptoms do not readily suggest hypercalcemia as their cause when they are randomly presented to the physician. When the serum calcium exceeds 16 mg/100 ml, a true emergency exists and the prompt diagnosis of hypercalcemia must be made and treatment started or the prognosis is gloomy. Parathyroid or hypercalcemic crisis is characterized by intractable nausea and vomiting, abdominal pain, lethargy, oliguria, myocardial necrosis, circulatory collapse, and even cerebral thromboses. Once the calcium reaches levels approximating 20 mg/100 ml, the prognosis is bleak.

CAUSES

In the clinical practice of medicine, the causes of hypercalcemia that are most commonly encountered are metastatic cancer to bone (especially breast cancer) and multiple myeloma (55%), primary hyperparathyroidism (20%), and pseudohyperparathyroidism (15%) (Table 10-4). The differentiation of these entities can be made if one performs a skeletal radiographic survey or bone scan (which is even more sensitive) and a measurement of the serum immunoreactive parathyroid hormone level. An elevated PTH level rules out metastatic disease to bone but may not differentiate primary hyperparathyroidism from pseudohyperparathyroidism. Pseudohyperparathyroidism refers to the presence of nonparathyroid gland tumors that produce a PTH-like material. Hypernephromas and bronchogenic carcinomas account for 60% of these neoplasms, with many of the remaining 40% being caused by tumors involving the urogenital tract, liver, pancreas, lymph nodes, esophagus, colon, and parotid gland. However, the following features

TABLE 10-5 Manifestations of Primary Hyperparathyroidism

1. Hypercalcemia
   a. Neuropsychiatric, e.g., lassitude, decreased recent memory, irritability, depression, and personality changes
   b. Peptic ulcer symptoms
2. Abnormal deposition of calcium in the tissues
   a. Renal calculi and nephrocalcinosis
   b. Band keratopathy
   c. Calcifications in capsules around joints and in tendons
   d. Chondrocalcinosis
   e. Pancreatitis
3. Skeletal findings
   a. Osteitis fibrosa cystica
   b. Osteoporosis
   c. Osteomalacia
   d. Osteosclerosis
   e. Subperiosteal erosions
   f. Bone cysts

strongly favor a diagnosis of pseudohyperparathyroidism: unexplained weight loss, anemia, cachexia, urinary calcium over 500 mg per day, a markedly elevated sedimentation rate, an increased alkaline phosphatase level (in the presence of a normal bone scan), and the presence of a metabolic alkalosis. These patients often fail to have a history of renal calculi or bone disease because they do not live long enough to develop these complications of long-standing hypercalcemia. The clinical features that favor a diagnosis of primary hyperparathyroidism are listed in Table 10–5.

TREATMENT

SALINE SOLUTION The treatment of hypercalcemia depends upon the level of the serum calcium and the patient's clinical condition (Table 10-6). If

TABLE 10-6 Summary of Treatment of Hypercalcemic Crisis

1. Hydration and natriuresis
   a. Normal saline solution, 3 liters, if cardiorenal function permits, alternating with 5% D/W, 1 liter. Infusion rate is determined by urinary flow rate
   b. Potassium replacement as determined by urinary K^+ measurements and ECG monitoring
   c. Furosemide, 40 to 100 mg I.V. every 4 to 6 hr
2. Phosphate (Inphos), 0.5 to 1.0 gm p.o. every 6 hr, or 50 to 100 mmol I.V. over 8 to 12 hr
3. Prednisone, 20 mg every 6 hr p.o.
4. Mithramycin, 25 μg/kg body weight I.V. over 10 min and may be repeated in 24 to 48 hr
5. Hemodialysis

the patient is not acutely ill and serum calcium is less than 13 mg/100 ml, hydration with normal saline solution may be all that is necessary to lower the serum calcium level and maintain the patient until the proper diagnostic tests are performed. However, moderate or severe hypercalcemia in a patient with symptoms must be treated more aggressively and without delay. These more severely hypercalcemic patients usually have quite severe volume depletion by the time they enter the hospital. The elevated serum calcium leads to polyuria by its effect on the basement membrane of the renal tubular cell, causing an impairment of concentration of the urine. The patient is often unable to maintain an adequate fluid intake to keep up with this excessive loss of salt and water by the kidney because of associated symptoms of anorexia, nausea, and vomiting. This results in contraction of the extracellular space and further increase in the concentration of the serum calcium and phosphate. Calcium-phosphate crystals (microthrombi) may then precipitate in small vessels throughout the body, producing pancreatitis, pulmonary thromboses, and even focal neurological abnormalities. Therefore, intravenous saline solution should be started promptly. The first few liters should be given rather rapidly, with monitoring of the patient's central venous pressure and urinary output. This fluid results in a marked natriuresis, which promotes a proportional increase in urinary calcium. Furosemide may also be given in doses up to 100 mg I.V. to produce further increases in urinary sodium and calcium. In one published study of 8 hypercalcemic patients, 100-mg doses of furosemide resulted in a mean drop in the serum calcium of 3.1 mg/100 ml and the excretion of 0.7 to 2.7 gm of calcium (see report by Suki et al.). Urine volumes should be measured hourly in order to determine the infusion flow rate. Urinary sodium and potassium determinations should be made every 4 hours. The first hourly urine volume may contain up to 90 to 120 mEq of sodium and 10 to 20 mEq of potassium. Appropriate intravenous electrolyte replacement therapy must be given; for example, 4 liters of physiologic saline solution with 20 mEq of potassium chloride followed by one liter of 5% dextrose and water.

PHOSPHATE THERAPY   The aforementioned regimen may have to be supplemented with phosphate therapy, again dependent upon the rate of fall of the serum calcium level. Oral phosphate therapy (2 to 4 gm daily in divided doses) or intravenous phosphate (Inphos, disodium monopotassium phosphate) can be utilized. Each 100 mmol of Inphos contains 162 mEq of potassium and 3.1 gm of phosphorus. It is recommended that one begin with 50 mmol of Inphos diluted in one liter of 5% dextrose and water delivered over 8 to 12 hours. The serum calcium must be measured at frequent intervals. Maximal benefit should be expected within 6 to 24 hours from the onset of the infusion. The serum calcium level may begin to rise again after 24 hours, but it may stay down for up to 4 to 6 days. There is no way of predicting the response in a given patient. Subsequent infusions of Inphos may have to be increased up to 100 mmol per liter of dextrose and water. One should start with a lower dose of intravenous phosphate in order to avoid complications such as heart failure (caused by the too rapid drop of myocardial calcium, which causes a decrease in myocardial contractility), phlebitis, and soft tissue and vascular calcifications. Hyperphosphatemia is a relative contraindication to phosphate therapy. Of course, oral phosphate therapy has a lesser chance of causing any of the above complications. However, if the patient is acutely ill, has a very high serum calcium level, and has cardiac and/or kidney failure, intravenous phosphate therapy is indicated. Phosphates apparently promote the deposition of calcium into the skeleton and soft tissues.

OTHER THERAPEUTIC AGENTS Steroids are important therapeutic agents in those patients whose hypercalcemia is associated with vitamin D intoxication, sarcoidosis, or some malignancies. Up to 80 mg of prednisone per day in divided doses is required. However, the rate of response to steroids is so variable that, in an emergency situation, saline solution and phosphates are the preferred therapy. The maximal hypocalcemic effect from steroids may take anywhere from a few days to several weeks.

Mithramycin, a cytostatic antibiotic useful in the treatment of testicular tumors, may be given as a single intravenous dose of 25 μg/kg of body weight and repeated in 24 to 48 hours. However, as with the steroids, the response to mithramycin is variable and unpredictable. One cannot predict either the onset of action or the duration of its hypocalcemic effect. In addition, mithramycin is potentially a dangerous drug and is capable of causing bleeding problems. Its use should probably be limited to those patients with malignancies or to those who have been unresponsive to the other regimens noted above.

Calcitonin has been tried in the emergency treatment of hypercalcemia. Because of its inhibition of bone resorption, high hopes were entertained that calcitonin would be a valuable therapeutic tool. However, like steroids and mithramycin, unpredictability and variability have made it a little-used drug for treating hypercalcemia.

Disodium ethylenediaminetetraacetate (EDTA) is a potent hypocalcemic agent, but its nephrotoxicity from high doses (a total dose of over 3 gm is dangerous) or from prolonged administration has discouraged its use.

SELECTED READINGS

Breuer, R. I., and LeBauer, J.   Caution in the use of phosphates in the treatment of severe hypercalcemia. *J. Clin. Endocrinol. Metab.* 27:695–698, 1967.

Canary, J. J., Schaaf, M., Benedict, J. D., Jr., and Kyle, L. H.   Effects of oral and intramuscular administration of reserpine in thyrotoxicoses. *N. Engl. J. Med.* 257:435–442, 1957.

Goldsmith, R. S., and Ingbar, S. H.   Inorganic phosphate treatment of hypercalcemia of diverse etiologies. *N. Engl. J. Med.* 274:1–7, 1966.

Grossman, W., Robin, N. I., Johnson, L. W., Brooks, H., Selenkow, H. A., and Dexter, L.   Effects of beta blockade on the peripheral manifestations of thyrotoxicosis. *Ann. Intern. Med.* 74:875–879, 1971.

Ivy, H. K., Wahner, H. W., and Gorman, C. A.   T$_3$ toxicosis. *Arch. Intern. Med.* 128:529–534, 1971.

Lafferty, F. W.   Pseudohyperparathyroidism. *Medicine* 45:247–260, 1966.

Mackin, J. F., Canary, J. J., and Pittman, C. S.   Thyroid storm and its management. *N. Engl. J. Med.* 291:1396–1398, 1974.

McArthur, J. W., Rawson, R. W., Means, J. H., and Cope, O.   Thyrotoxic crisis: Analysis of 36 cases seen at Massachusetts General Hospital during past 25 years. *J.A.M.A.* 134:868–874, 1947.

Melby, J. C.   Systemic corticosteroid therapy: Pharmacology and endocrinologic considerations. *Ann. Intern. Med.* 81:505–512, 1974.

Muggia, F. M., and Heinemann, H. O.   Hypercalcemia associated with neoplastic disease. *Ann. Intern. Med.* 73:281–290, 1970.

Perlia, C. P., Gubisch, N. J., Walter, J., Edelberg, D., Dederick, M. M., and Taylor, S. G., III.   Mithramycin treatment of hypercalcemia. *Cancer* 25:389–394, 1970.

Saberi, M., and Utiger, R. D.   Serum thyroid hormone and thyropin concentrations during thyroxine and triiodothyronine therapy. *J. Clin. Endocrinol. Metab.* 39:923–927, 1974.

Sterling, K., Brenner, M. A., Newman, E. S., Odell, W. D., and Bellebarba, D.   The significance of triiodothyronine in maintenance of euthyroid status after treatment of hypothyroidism. *J. Clin. Endocrinol. Metab.* 33:729–731, 1971.

Stock, J. M., Surks, M. J., and Oppenheimer, J. H.   Replacement dosage of L-thyroxine in hyperthyroidism, *N. Engl. J. Med.* 290:529–533, 1974

Suki, W. N., Yium, J. J., Von Minden, M., Saller-Hebert, C., Eknoyan, G., and Martinez-Maldonado, M.   Acute treatment of hypercalcemia with furosemide. *N. Engl. J. Med.* 283:836–840, 1970.

Volpe, R., Edmonds, M., Lampi, L., Clarke, P. V., and Row, V. V. The pathogenesis of Graves' disease. *Mayo Clin. Proc.* 47:824–834, 1972.

Werner, S. C., and Ingbar, S. H. (Eds.).   *The Thyroid.* 3d ed. New York: Harper & Row, 1971.

Williams, R. H. (Ed.).   *Textbook of Endocrinology.* 5th ed. Philadelphia: Saunders, 1974. Pp. 270–274.

11   DIABETIC KETOACIDOSIS AND NONKETOTIC HYPEROSMOLAR HYPERGLYCEMIC COMA

S. Edwin Fineberg
Robert M. Levin

DIABETIC KETOACIDOSIS (DKA) is generally a disorder of explosive onset, marked by polyuria, polydipsia, air hunger, and prominent musculoskeletal and abdominal pains. Nausea, vomiting, and diarrhea are additional frequent symptoms. The patient appears fatigued. His skin is dry and with poor turgor, his eyeballs soft and sunken, and his pulse weak and rapid. Depending on the duration of his symptoms before he seeks medical attention, he may already be hypotensive and obtunded. The common clinical features noted in diabetic ketoacidosis are listed in Table 11-1. This acute emergency most often occurs in young adult diabetics who have been receiving insulin and develop an infection (particularly urinary tract, pulmonary, and skin infections) or who have neglected to take their insulin. It is quite unusual for new adult diabetics to be seen first with DKA, and probably less than 15% are seen in this manner. The mean age of this latter group of patients is 38 years. Conditions such as malignancy, myocardial infarction, or pancreatitis may also precipitate this endocrine emergency.

In recent years, DKA has been reported to be associated with an overall mortality rate of 3 to 10%. The prognosis is worsened by old age, increased duration of the acidosis and/or coma, a very high blood sugar level, hypotension, and the severity of the associated conditions. Myocardial infarction and septicemia are the two major contributors to death in DKA. Fetal survival during ketoacidosis in pregnancy is extremely poor (70% fetal loss), and the maternal mortality rate is 10%. Pancreatitis complicating DKA may be difficult to detect because of the modest elevation of amylase and the abdominal pain which occur commonly in DKA. Severe acidosis and hyperglycemia are particularly ominous signs in hemorrhagic pancreatitis. DKA occurring in a uremic individual is extremely difficult to manage, and death caused by fluid overload is common. Rarely, cerebral edema and electrolyte disorders (hyper- and hypokalemia) will lead to death in DKA. However, these conditions are usually preventable and will be discussed below.

163

TABLE 11-1 Clinical Features of Diabetic Ketoacidosis

Anorexia, nausea, and vomiting

Dehydration
    Soft, sunken eyeballs; dry mucous membranes; inelastic skin; tachy-
    cardia; hypotension

Pain
    Crampy musculoskeletal pain; diffuse abdominal pain (not peritoneal in
    type); pleural pain

Deep, rapid respiration (when pH <7.2; may be depressed when pH
    <6.9)

Weakness and malaise

Decreased muscle tone (especially if decreased serum K^+ is present)

CNS depression
    Headaches; drowsiness; decreased DTR; stupor; dilated pupils; coma

PATHOPHYSIOLOGY

The basic biochemical defect underlying DKA is a relative or absolute
deficiency of insulin (Fig. 11-1). Severe insulin deficiency is associated
with increased lipolysis, making free fatty acids (FFA) and glycerol
available for hepatic ketogenesis, which is greatly increased by glucagon
excess during DKA. Because muscle is less able to oxidize ketoacids with
severe insulin lack, these strong organic acids (especially acetoacetic and
beta-hydroxybutyric acid) dissociate and soon lead to a metabolic acidosis. Amino acids, which are released from muscle at an increased rate
during insulin deficiency, provide added substrate for hepatic gluconeogenesis. Glucagon excess enhances gluconeogenesis and augments glycogen breakdown. This increased glucose production by the liver occurs
in the face of a decreased ability of muscle and adipose tissue to utilize
glucose for oxidation and fuel storage (as glycogen and fat). The glucose
concentration soon exceeds its renal threshold and leads to an osmotic
diuresis with concomitant water and electrolyte losses. Profound volume loss may lead to hypotension and shock. Glucose concentrations
will not exceed 600 mg/100 ml unless there is a contraction of fluid volume with a degree of prerenal azotemia. Because thirst is not impaired
in DKA, extreme hyperglycemia is seldom seen. However, hyperosmolarity of a mild to modest severity is a regular feature of DKA and has recently been invoked as a causative factor in the acute neurological dysfunction that occurs.
    Sodium depletion is often masked because water loss is usually in ex-
cess of solute. Because of the large urinary losses of potassium induced by
the osmotic diuresis, potassium depletion is often severe but may be
poorly reflected by the serum levels. This is because, in the presence of
acidosis, hydrogen and sodium ions shift into the intracellular space
in exchange for potassium. Consequently, patients with high serum potassium levels upon admission may still have moderately diminished
potassium stores, whereas persons with normal and low serum potassium

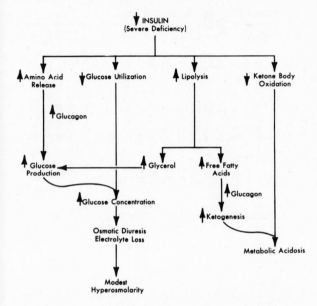

FIGURE 11-1   Pathogenesis of diabetic ketoacidosis.

levels have profound potassium depletion. Often neglected in DKA are deficits in magnesium and phosphate. Magnesium loss may lead to neuromuscular irritability and alterations in consciousness, including seizures. Phosphate depletion may lead to a depletion of red blood cell 2,3-diphosphoglycerate, thus altering hemoglobin-oxygen binding affinity.

DIFFERENTIAL DIAGNOSIS

In addition to DKA, acute central nervous system dysfunction in diabetes mellitus may be associated with a number of disorders, including (1) hypoglycemia, (2) nonketotic hyperosmolar hyperglycemic coma (NKHHC), (3) alcoholic ketoacidosis, and (4) lactic acidosis. Neurological dysfunction can vary from confusion to deep coma. Occasionally bizarre behavior and overt psychosis are observed with hypoglycemia and NKHHC. The clinical and laboratory features of these disorders are summarized in Tables 11-2 to 11-4. Alcohol-related ketoacidosis (AKA) in the nondiabetic, a phenomenon now recognized with increasing frequency, metabolic acidosis caused by poisoning, and disorders such as uremia and strokes which not infrequently occur in diabetics must also be included in the differential diagnosis of neurological dysfunction.

Hypoglycemia, the commonest of the aforementioned disorders, should be suspected clinically in an individual who has signs of sweating, tachycardia, dilated pupils, and altered mental status. Some diabetic patients may lack such signs of sympathetic discharge and may only have the neurological dysfunction. This diagnosis can be made by a rapid

TABLE 11-2 Differential Diagnosis of Coma Occurring in the Diabetic Patient

Condition	Onset	History	Drug History	Physical Signs and Laboratory Results
Hypoglycemia	Sudden	Sweating, faintness, personality changes, behavior disturbances	Insulin or oral hypoglycemic agents Alcohol ingestion	Dilated pupils, sweating, tachycardia Confusion to coma Hypoglycemia
Diabetic ketoacidosis	1–24 hr	Polyuria, polydipsia, nausea, vomiting, diarrhea, abdominal pain	Insulin-requiring diabetics, newly discovered diabetics (15%)	Deep sighing rapid respirations Moderate dehydration Confusion to deep coma Blood sugar 675 ± 17 Serum acetone: >4+ at 1 : 1 dilution Arterial pH 7.07 (6.92–7.22) Osmolarity 323
Nonketotic hyperosmolar hyperglycemic coma	24 hr–2 wk	Inadequate fluid intake, increasing somnolence, polyuria	Noninsulin-using diabetics, newly discovered diabetics (40%) Steroids, diazoxides, and antimetabolites Peritoneal dialysis	Profound dehydration Obtunded to deep coma Often localizing neurological signs (focal seizures) Blood sugar 1,096 (400–2,760) Serum acetone: <2+ at 1 : 1 dilution Arterial pH 7.26 (6.81–7.53) Osmolarity 405 (348–456)
Lactic acidosis	1–24 hr	Increasing obtundation, preexistent liver, cardiac, or renal disease	Phenformin	Warm skin, vasodilation Deep sighing respirations Deep coma Large anion gap without significant ketonemia
Alcoholic ketoacidosis	24 hr	Omission of solid food for 24–72 hr preceded by intake of large amounts of alcohol	Alcohol excess	Large liver Minimal or no dehydration Blood sugar 162 (25–235) Serum acetone: up to 3+ undiluted Arterial pH 7.25 (7.09–7.28) Osmolarity 299

TABLE 11-3 Clinical Features Distinguishing Diabetic Ketoacidosis from Hypoglycemia

Clinical Features	DKA	Hypoglycemia
Anorexia, nausea, and vomiting	+	−
Dehydration	+	−
Rapidity of onset of coma	Slow	Rapid
Depth of respirations	Deep	Normal or shallow
Sweating	−	+
Nervousness	−	+
Glucose content of fresh urine specimen	+	−
Reagent test for glucose (Dextrostix)	↑ Glucose	↓ Glucose
Response to I.V. glucose (give only after glucose sample is obtained)	−	Usually prompt unless hypoglycemia is long-standing

determination of blood glucose with a fresh Dextrostix (Ames). Significant dysfunction does not occur unless blood glucose is below 50 mg/100 ml. Lack of response to intravenous glucose is not sufficient to disprove this diagnosis, because neurological abnormalities may persist for up to one week after an episode with eventual recovery. However, if hypoglycemia is clinically suspected, a tube of blood should be drawn for blood sugar determination and the patient immediately treated intravenously with 50 to 100 ml of 50% glucose followed by an infusion of 10%

TABLE 11-4 Comparison of Patients with Diabetic Ketoacidosis and with Nonketotic Hyperosmolar Hypoglycemia

Clinical Features	DKA	NKHHC
Prodroma	Less than 24 hr	3–5 days
Median age	38	61
No history of diabetes	15%	40%
Anorexia, nausea, vomiting	+	−
Crampy musculoskeletal pain	+	−
Neurological abnormalities (esp. seizures)	Uncommon	Common
Kussmaul respiration	+	−
Hypotension	15%	30%
Av. initial blood sugar (mg/100 ml)	675	1,096
Ketonemia	Marked	Moderate to none
Free fatty acid level	Elevated	Normal
Av. plasma osmolality (mOsm/L)	323	405
Severe acidosis	Common	Uncommon
Insulin needs	Large	Less than ⅔ that of DKA
Mortality rate	3–10%	40–70%

dextrose and water. A helpful adjunct to therapy is the intramuscular injection of 1 mg of glucagon. However, glucagon alone should not be administered because it will be effective only if hepatic glycogen is still present. Hypoglycemia associated with oral hypoglycemic agents may recur for several days after the drug is discontinued. This is especially true with chlorpropamide, which has a biologic half-life of 36 hours. Patients whose hypoglycemia is due to use of the oral hypoglycemic drugs should be hospitalized and given constant infusions of 10% dextrose and water until their blood sugar levels are clearly normal.

Because increased respiratory exchange and acute neurological dysfunction are seen in other disorders, a diagnosis of DKA must be based on its biochemical features: (1) significant ketonemia (serum acetone strongly reactive at a 1 : 2 dilution or greater of plasma); (2) acidosis (arterial pH <7.25, HCO_3^- <15 mEq/liter); and (3) elevated blood glucose. An atypical picture can be seen with alcohol ingestion. Under such circumstances, the blood glucose concentrations can be near normal along with a decreased serum ketone reaction. Alcohol metabolism leads to an inhibition of glucose production and a reduction of acetoacetate to betahydroxybutyrate. With hypotension or prolonged acidosis of unusual severity, acetoacetate may also be reduced to betahydroxybutyrate. Because Acetest tablets detect only acetone and acetoacetate, this shift will reduce serum ketone concentrations measurable by this test. In this case, ketone body excess may be detectable only by direct enzymatic measurement, which is not readily available.

Nonketotic hyperosmolar hyperglycemic coma can be differentiated from DKA by the following features: longer prodrome, older age of the patient, profound dehydration, absence of Kussmaul respirations, presence of localizing neurological findings, much higher blood sugar and osmolarity, only mild acidosis, and relatively minimal ketonemia (see Tables 11-2 and 11-4). It is not uncommon for the maturity-onset diabetic to be first seen by the physician with the clinical picture of NKHHC. Moreover, to complicate matters even more, the patient may have a mixed picture of both DKA and NKHHC.

Lactic acidosis in diabetes can occur in a pure form or as mixed acidosis with ketoacidosis (see Table 11-2). The latter is a diagnosis of exclusion which should be suspected when a patient has a profound acidosis with a large, unexplained anion gap. Glucose concentrations are usually normal. Pure lactic acidosis alone, in the absence of circulatory insufficiency, is associated with a mortality rate in excess of 90%. Death usually results from cardiac failure or hepatic insufficiency.

Alcoholic ketoacidosis can easily be confused with DKA (see Table 11-2). A clue to its presence is the clinical setting of severe acidosis occurring in a nondiabetic, chronic alcoholic patient. These patients frequently have a 24- to 72-hour history of food deprivation preceded by the intake of large amounts of alcohol. They may or may not have the clinical stigmata of chronic liver disease. Their blood chemistries are quite unlike those of DKA. They usually have a normal to slightly elevated blood sugar, a normal osmolarity, and undetectable or mild ketonemia because of the reduction of acetoacetate to betahydroxybutyrate (which is not measured by the Acetest tablet).

DIABETIC KETOACIDOSIS

INITIAL EVALUATION

Prior to beginning therapy, a rapid clinical examination must be made, during which time other causes of coma and ketoacidosis are considered and a bedside assessment of the degree of dehydration is made. Poor tissue turgor, soft, sunken eyeballs, and postural blood pressure changes are helpful bedside findings. Blood should be obtained promptly for a complete blood count, glucose, urea nitrogen, creatinine, electrolytes, amylase, and arterial blood gases, including pH. The serum acetone determination can be performed in the emergency room by applying a drop or two of serum onto a crushed nitroprusside (Acetest) tablet. The reaction may be decreased in undiluted serum and, therefore, testing at a 1 : 1 dilution is mandatory to demonstrate ketonemia. The serum dilution at which the nitroprusside tablet turns from strongly positive to moderate should be carefully noted because this will serve as an important guide to insulin dosage, as noted below. However, the nitroprusside tablet–serum reaction measures primarily acetoacetate and, to a lesser extent, acetone. Beta-hydroxybutyrate, the principal ketone body present in ketoacidosis, is not measured at all. When DKA is complicated by alcohol ingestion or shock, acetoacetate is reduced to β-hydroxybutyrate, and the serum ketones may be nondetectable. In uncomplicated DKA, the ratio of betahydroxybutyrate to acetone to acetoacetate acid is 3 : 2 : 1.

In addition to the serum potassium level, an electrocardiogram should be taken before therapy is begun. The lead with the best visualized T waves should be noted and that lead repeated every 20 to 30 minutes during the early phase of the treatment period in order to follow the patient's potassium status. An ECG flow sheet should be posted at the bedside with a few complexes cut out and taped to the sheet. This should be repeated at frequent intervals, as noted above, and each tracing labeled with the time it was taken. Thus, therapeutic changes in the administration of potassium can be made as frequently as necessary without having to wait for the serum level results to return from the laboratory. Examples of the electrocardiographic changes that occur in hypo- and hyperkalemia are noted in Figure 11-2. A chest x-ray should be obtained as soon as the aforementioned measures are completed and a complete urinalysis performed as soon as the patient is able to void. A diabetic ketoacidosis flow sheet should be started (Fig. 11-3) onto which hourly blood test results, fluids administered, medications given, urinary output, and the patient's vital signs should be recorded.

TREATMENT

Prolonged acidosis may lead to insulin resistance and possible irreversible enzyme damage. The treatment of diabetic ketoacidosis must therefore be started promptly (Table 11-5). The most important aspects of therapy are the administration of sufficient insulin and fluids, the prevention of hyperkalemia or hypokalemia, and the avoidance of the consequences of overtreatment with alkali or insulin. Avoidance of overcorrection of aci-

HYPERKALEMIA

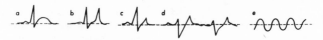

a. Normal

b. Tall peaked T wave; tent-like narrow base

c. T wave of normal amplitude; peaked, narrow base

d. P-R and QRS lengthen; P and R amplitude decrease

e. QRS loses angularity and may assume sign wave shape

HYPOKALEMIA

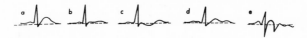

a. Normal

b. Flattened T wave; depressed ST segment

c. ST segment depressed; prolongation of QT interval

d. Biphasic P; prominent U wave; prolonged QT

e. Inverted T; U wave prominent

FIGURE 11-2   Electrocardiographic changes in hyperkalemia and hypokalemia

dosis by bicarbonate will prevent complications caused by alkalosis such as respiratory depression, "paradoxical" cerebrospinal fluid (CSF) acidosis, and alteration of hemoglobin affinity for oxygen. The blood glucose should be expected to decrease by 90 mg/100 ml/hr once insulin therapy is begun; early more drastic falls in glucose are usually due to hemodilution. Ketonemia of a modest degree (strongly positive when diluted 1 : 2) may persist up to 36 hours after the patient's entry into the hospital because of the slow clearing of the serum acetoacetate.

Once the initial blood studies are drawn, an intravenous infusion of half-normal saline solution should be started, oxygen administered nasally, and gastric lavage performed if gastric dilatation is present or if there is persistent vomiting. Bladder catheterization should be avoided unless the bladder becomes distended or unless monitoring of urinary output is essential for the management of shock.

INSULIN The initial insulin dosage is determined by the clinical and biochemical estimate of the severity of the ketoacidosis. This dose will vary from 50 units in the patient who is alert and only mildly acidotic, and whose blood glucose concentration is modestly elevated, to 300 units of regular insulin in a patient who is in shock and severely acidotic, and whose glucose concentration is greater than 800 mg/100 ml. Insulin should be given intravenously whenever circulatory insufficiency with decreased absorption of insulin is a possibility. Guidelines are suggested in Table 11-6.

TIME		CLINICAL STATE						BLOOD							URINE		OUTPUT		THERAPY INTAKE				REMARKS
Date, Hour	Mental State*	Rectal Temp.	Pulse	Resp. Rate	Resp. Depth**	B.P.	BUN	Blood Sugar	CO_2	Cl	Na	K	Serum Acetone	Sugar	Acetone	Urine	Other	P.O.	IV.Type	KCl	Insulin (IV or SQ)		REMARKS
																		Vol.	Vol.	mEq	Units		
TOTAL																Vol.	Vol.	Vol.	Vol.	mEq	Units		

*1. Alert
2. Drowsy
3. Stuporous
4. Comatose

**1. Normal
2. Moderately Deep
3. Very Deep

FIGURE 11-3 Diabetic ketoacidosis flow sheet used at Boston City Hospital.

TABLE 11-5 Treatment of Diabetic Ketoacidosis

1. Insulin therapy
    a. 100 to 300 units regular insulin initially (depending on serum ace-
       tone), half I.V. and half S.C. (all I.V. if hypotension exists or if the
       patient has marked volume depletion)
    b. Second dose of regular insulin should be given 60 to 90 minutes later,
       dose to be determined by serum acetone and blood sugar levels
       (1) If no change in blood sugar, ketones, or clinical condition, initial
           dose should be repeated
       (2) If the blood sugar level increases or fails to fall within a few hours,
           one should begin doubling the dose
       (3) Subsequent doses depend on serum glucose and ketone levels and
           pH
    c. Average dose of insulin patient should receive by the time the blood
       sugar level falls below 200 mg is 500 U
    d. Every effort should be made to start patient on an intermediate-acting
       insulin (NPH, Lente) within 24 to 48 hours of admission
2. Gastric lavage (for gastric dilatation or persistent vomiting)
3. Restoration of circulating volume
    a. A liter of normal saline solution should be given rapidly over the first
       30 to 60 minutes depending on degree of volume depletion and the
       cardiorenal status. Average deficit in total body water is 5 to 15%.
       Most of the volume deficit is best replaced with half normal saline
       solution
    b. Pressors and/or plasma expanders may be necessary to restore circula-
       tory integrity
4. Correction of acidosis
    a. If serum HCO_3^- is >10 mEq/liter, bicarbonate therapy is probably not
       required unless patient is hypotensive or in coma
    b. HCO_3^- should not be given initially if serum K^+ is low or there is
       ECG evidence of hypokalemia
    c. If HCO_3^- is 5 to 10 mEq, calculate deficit on basis of 50% body weight
    d. If HCO_3^- is <5, severe acidosis is present; calculate deficit at 2 ×
       body weight
    e. Do not correct beyond 15 mEq/liter
5. Replacement of potassium
    a. No need to replace initially unless initial serum K^+ is <3.5 mEq/liter
       or ECG reveals hypokalemic changes. Be certain that the urinary
       output is satisfactory before giving K^+
    b. No more than 40 mEq of K^+ should be put in each liter unless severe
       hypokalemia is present
    c. The usual total body K^+ deficit is 300 to 400 mEq
    d. Once the patient is no longer receiving hourly insulin and HCO_3^- I.V.,
       the remaining deficit can be replaced orally
    e. An ECG strip should be obtained every 30 minutes (or sooner if indi-
       cated) to note early hypokalemic changes in the T waves. The date
       and hour should be marked and the strip taped to an ECG flow sheet
       at foot of the bed. Persistent hypokalemia may need to be treated
       with up to 80 mEq of K^+ in each liter of fluids with frequent ECG
       monitoring
6. Miscellaneous
    a. Proper cultures should be obtained and antibiotics started if an infec-

TABLE 11-5 (*continued*)

tion is identified. Treatment may be based on the Gram stain findings
b. Oxygen should be given nasally
c. Magnesium deficit should be replaced—estimated to be 0.8 mEq/kg of body weight
d. A central venous pressure line should be considered if cardiac failure is suspected
e. Urethral catheterization should be avoided if at all possible. Definite indication is presence of a distended bladder and patient unable to void

In mildly ill patients, one-half of the initial dose of insulin should be repeated every 4 hours (with serum glucose, acetone, and electrolytes observed at the same time). In moderately ill patients, insulin and laboratory follow-up should be repeated every 2 hours, and in the severely ill, every hour. If serum glucose levels and ketones increase, insulin resistance should be suspected. The initial dose of insulin should then be doubled, with a doubling dose of insulin hourly. Blood glucose concentrations should fall at a rate of about 30 mg/100 ml/hr. When glucose concentrations fall to below 300 mg/100 ml, insulin should be discontinued and intravenous 5% dextrose and water begun. Additional insulin may not be needed for many hours. At this point in the treatment, the patient should be given one-quarter of his usual daily dose every 6 hours subcutaneously. Up to this point, only regular insulin should be administered; however, a long-acting insulin can be given in the morning of the second day of therapy.

The following experimental regimens of therapy in DKA have recently been reported: (1) a constant infusion of 8 to 12 U of insulin per hour in saline solution to which 1% serum albumin is added; (2) multiple intramuscular injections of insulin, beginning with 10 to 15 U and repeating 5 to 10 U hourly; and (3) multiple subcutaneous injections of 5 U every 30 minutes. These protocols have not been widely tested as yet but seem to hold promise for treatment of DKA in those patients in whom there is no unusual insulin resistance. Low dose therapy seems remarkably free from late treatment complications of hypokalemia and hypoglycemia. There are a number of advantages of low dose, constant

TABLE 11-6 Insulin Administration in Ketoacidosis

Clinical Severity	Initial Insulin Dose (units)	Serum Acetone	Blood Glucose (mg/100 ml)	Mental Status
Mild	50–100 (half S.C. and half I.V.)	Strongly + to 1 : 2	300–600	Alert to confused
Moderate	100–200 (I.V.)	Strongly + to 1 : 8	600–800	Obtunded
Severe	200–300 (I.V.)	Strongly + to 1 : 8	800	Comatose

intravenous infusion of insulin: (1) a straightforward protocol can be followed obviating the need for multiple hourly decisions to be made about the blood sugar level, severity of the acidosis, route of administration of the insulin, and dosage; (2) there is ample evidence that the rate of decline of the blood sugar in uncontrolled diabetes is steady and rapid with serum insulin concentrations of 20 to 200 μU/ml (results achieved with infusion rates of 2 to 12 units per liter); and (3) hypokalemia and hypoglycemia are less likely to develop during this treatment protocol.

FLUID AND ELECTROLYTES (Table 11-7) The safest initial fluid therapy in DKA is normal saline solution. Potassium (K^+) and bicarbonate (HCO_3^-) should not be added unless the serum K^+ is less than 3.5 mEq/liter or if there is electrocardiographic evidence of hypokalemia (see Fig. 11-2). Four percent of the patients with DKA have a serum K^+ of less than 3.5 mEq/liter, whereas 22% have levels greater than 6.0 mEq/liter. The intravenous administration of HCO_3^- may cause a rapid shift of K^+ into cells, in exchange for hydrogen, and lead to a rapid decline in the serum K^+. When hypokalemia is present initially, the total body K^+ deficit is severe and requires replacing 80 to 100 mEq of potassium chloride hourly with nearly constant electrocardiographic monitoring and frequent determinations of the serum K^+. Patients who are treated with the largest doses of insulin and HCO_3^-, and sustain the greatest fall in serum glucose, are the likeliest candidates for hypokalemia. On the other hand, because many patients with DKA may be seen with profound acidosis and hyperkalemia, the administration of K^+ is to be avoided until (1) an electrocardiogram has been done in order to evaluate the T waves, (2) a serum K^+ determination is done, and (3) an adequate urinary output has been demonstrated, i.e., over 25 ml/hr. The rapid infusion of K^+ into a hyperkalemic patient can lead to lethal K^+ intoxication.

Hypotension requires rapid volume repletion. A central venous pressure catheter should be inserted and normal saline solution infused at one liter every 45 to 90 minutes until the hypotension is corrected. Frequent measurements of the central venous pressure and urinary output

TABLE 11-7 Fluid and Electrolyte Deficit and Replacement

Fluid or Electrolyte	DKA		NKHHC*	
	Replacement†	Deficit‡	Replacement	Deficit
Water	6 L (0–18)	80 ml/kg	12 ± 3.5 L (SD)	9 ± 3
Potassium	165 mEq (0–620)	5 mEq/kg	215 ± 83	137
Sodium	530 mEq (0–1,460)	6 mEq/kg	512 ± 161	407
Phosphate	—	0.7 mM/kg	—	—
Magnesium	—	0.6 mEq/kg	—	—

* From Arrieff [2].
† From Beigelman [4].
‡ From Butler [6].

will determine the rate of fluid administration. If the rapid infusion of saline fails to raise the blood pressure and the central venous pressure is rising, then pressor therapy should be considered. The presence of Kussmaul respirations suggests that the arterial pH is less than 7.2 and intravenous HCO_3^- should be administered. Attempts should be made to correct severe acidosis prior to starting vasopressors.

CORRECTION OF ACIDOSIS Acidosis need not be corrected if the serum HCO_3^- is above 10 mEq/liter or the Pco_2 is greater than 18 mm. In modest acidosis, the HCO_3^- space is 100% of the total body water (50% of weight in kilograms). The amount of HCO_3^- required for correction in a 70-kg man with a serum HCO_3^- of 8 to 15 mEq/liter can be determined as follows: the deficit of 7 mEq/liter is multiplied by 50% of the body weight, or 35 kg (liters). However, only half of this 245 mEq of HCO_3^- should be given over the initial 6 hours of therapy. An HCO_3^- of 5 mEq/ liter or less, or a Pco_2 of 10 to 12 mm/liter, indicates the presence of severe acidosis. This requires prompt, large dose therapy with bicarbonate using an HCO_3^- distribution space equal to 200% of total body water. Each ampule of $NaHCO_3$ contains 44 mEq of Na, which may contribute to fluid overload if given too rapidly. Because patients with DKA will "self-correct" the acidosis when properly treated, it is essential to avoid overcorrection of acidosis. Late alkalosis often results from infusion of unnecessarily large amounts of HCO_3^-. Such alkalosis can lead to respiratory depression and, because of the low red blood cell levels of 2,3-diphosphoglycerate, an increased binding affinity of oxygen by hemoglobin.

WATER DEFICIT AND REPAIR Dehydration in DKA can amount to 5 to 15% of total body water. A useful estimate of the degree of water loss in a 70-kg man who is severely dehydrated is as follows: total body water is 50% of 70 kg, or 35 kg (liters) × 15%. This 5.2 liter deficit can also be calculated by simply multiplying the body weight in kilograms by the average water deficit in DKA, or 70 kg × 80 ml/kg = 5,600 ml. Rehydration can be rapid in DKA, with replacement of the water deficit over 12 hours.

PHOSPHATE AND MAGNESIUM THERAPY Phosphate and magnesium deficits are substantial in DKA (see Table 11-7). Phosphate and potassium can be replaced simultaneously by the infusion of potassium phosphate (a mixture of dibasic and monobasic phosphates), 5 mM/liter, in lieu of potassium chloride. Such replacement will speed the regeneration of red blood cell 2,3-diphosphoglycerate. Magnesium cannot be replaced until urinary flow is adequate. Furthermore, sulfate solution cannot be added to intravenous fluids containing sodium (insolubility of Na_2SO_4 leads to precipitation). Magnesium sulfate (50% solution) can be added to each liter of dextrose and water. Up to 64 mEq of $MgSO_4$ can be replaced in 24 hours. Magnesium sulfate can also be given as intramuscular injections every 4 hours. The serum magnesium level should be checked each day during replacement therapy.

Resistance to therapy may be related to such underlying problems as septicemia, myocardial infarction, and pancreatitis. Any pulmonary infiltrate should make the physician suspect tuberculosis, which is often atypical in location. A bloody nasal discharge with periorbital edema may represent the first manifestations of mucormycosis which occurs in diabetics and persons with various debilitating illnesses.

NONKETOTIC HYPEROSMOLAR HYPERGLYCEMIC COMA

Nonketotic hyperosmolar hyperglycemic coma, like DKA, begins at some point with decreased insulin action or decreased insulin availability (Fig. 11-4). Important in the understanding of the pathophysiology of NKHHC is that it takes approximately 3 to 5 times as much insulin to block glucose production and enhance glucose transport across cell membranes as it does to block peripheral lipolysis. In the person who is able to secrete some insulin as glucose concentrations increase, insulin secretion is enhanced. This in turn leads to blockade of lipolysis. If this individual then is able to ingest enough water, his glucose concentrations will stabilize at about 400 to 600 mg/100 ml in the presence of a normal renal threshold for glucose. However, persons who eventually go on to develop NKHHC at some point begin to restrict their fluid intake, or renal impairment must be present. This combination of a hyperglycemic osmotic diuresis and fluid restriction leads inexorably to a volume-depleted patient. Hyperosmolarity, per se, has a further effect on blocking peripheral lipolysis and blockade of insulin secretion.

Whereas blood glucose concentrations during DKA range on the aver-

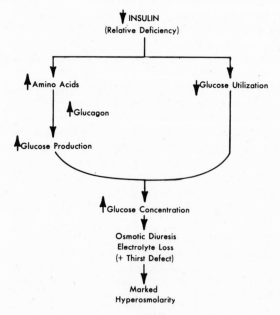

FIGURE 11-4　Pathogenesis of NKHHC.

age between 300 and 600 mg/100 ml the blood glucose in NKHHC generally exceeds 600 mg/100 ml and sometimes is as great as 2,000 mg/100 ml. Profound acidosis is uncommon, and serum ketones are absent or small in concentration. Persons who develop NKHHC are generally elderly. Most notable are the various neurological signs seen in these patients, including focal seizures. Nonketotic hyperosmolar coma has been reported in association with various forms of medical therapy, including drugs (steroids, dilantin, and diazoxide), treatment of patients with extensive burns, hyperalimentation therapy, and peritoneal dialysis. A comparison of the findings in DKA and NKHHC is made in Tables 11-2 and 11-4. Only a minority of these persons turn out to be insulin-dependent diabetic patients. The outcome in NKHHC is far different from that of DKA, with mortality rates being reported between 40 and 70%. Most deaths are due to septicemia or a life-threatening disorder such as carcinoma or myocardial infarction. Gram-negative pneumonia has been reported in up to 15% of the patients. However, death attributable to the hyperosmolar state, per se, has been reported in approximately 20% of patients. The mortality rate increases with the duration of the hyperosmolarity.

TREATMENT

INITIAL THERAPY INCLUDING INSULIN Since volume depletion is virtually universal in NKHHC, fluid therapy should be started with saline solution (Table 11-8). Effective osmolarity should then be calculated (see above), so that persons who are not hyperosmolar can be identified. Such persons are extremely sensitive to the hypoglycemic actions of insulin and have minimal to no neurological deficit. They require no more than 25 to 50 U of insulin, administered every 2 to 4 hours. Rapid reduction of plasma glucose to normal in such a patient may lead to shock and renal insufficiency. These patients are at special risk for water intoxication. In hyperosmolar persons, initial insulin therapy can be simply estimated by Arrieff's formula of 10% of the plasma glucose as units of insulin (i.e., plasma glucose = 2,000 mg/100 ml; insulin = $2,000 \times 0.10 = 200$ U I.V.). Insulin can be safely administered, according to the given formula, every 2 hours intravenously. A rising blood glucose level indicates insulin resistance and is handled as described under DKA. When blood glucose concentrations fall to 30 mg/100 ml, dextrose and water should be started so that plasma glucose concentrations are maintained between 200 and 300 mg/100 ml. If hypotension is present, saline solution should be infused until the blood pressure rises and urine flow is restored or until the central venous pressure begins to rise; without an increase in urine flow, pressors should be used. Severe acidosis is occasionally present in NKHHC, and studies of arterial blood gases and pH should be done on admission. High-dose HCO_3^- as described above may be required.

FLUID AND ELECTROLYTES The water deficit in NKHHC can be calculated from the body weight and knowledge that the average water deficit is 25% of total body water. For example, a 70-kg man (whose total body water is 50%, or 35 liters) with an estimated water deficit of 25%

TABLE 11-8 Treatment of Nonketotic Hyperosmolar Hyperglycemic Coma

---

1. Insulin therapy
   a. No more than 50 U of insulin should be given per hour unless blood glucose level remains unchanged or begins to rise; then double the dose hourly. (Do not allow glucose to fall below 200 mg/100 ml during the first 12 hours of therapy)
2. Restoration of circulating volume
   a. Fluid therapy with normal saline solution should be given until blood pressure is restored or a calculation of osmolarity indicates that hyperosmolarity is present
   b. Calculation of osmolarity: $2 \times (\text{serum Na} + \text{K}) + \dfrac{\text{Blood glucose}}{18}$ (mg/100 ml)
   c. Correction of hyperosmolarity and water replacement. Replace about ½ of water deficit as hypotonic saline solution (½ normal saline solution) in 12 hours, the remainder in 24 to 36 hours. One should attempt to keep the patient slightly hyperosmolar during the first 12 hours of therapy, aiming for a calculated osmolarity of 305 to 315 mOsm/liter. (N.B.: A sudden fall in glomerular filtration rate during therapy may be due to a fall in osmolarity below normal)
3. Correction of acidosis. Severe acidosis may be present in this disorder and is treated as in DKA
4. Underlying disorder. Rule out any associated life-threatening disorders, especially Gram-negative septicemia

---

represents a need for 8.7 liters of water to be replaced. The average amount of water infused until osmolarity nears normal has been shown to be about 12 liters. Not more than one-half of the estimated water deficit plus urinary losses should be replaced during the first 12 hours of therapy. Half-normal saline solution is the fluid of choice. Potassium chloride is added to the regimen under the same circumstances as noted under DKA.

A critical problem in NKHHC is the osmolar state itself. Persistence of extreme hyperosmolarity will lead to death. However, a too rapid reduction in hyperosmolarity may lead to cerebral edema. The osmolarity should be calculated every 2 hours. When the plasma glucose falls below 300 mg/100 ml or the osmolarity falls below 310 to 320 mOsm/liter, dextrose and water should be infused. Only half of the water deficit (plus urinary losses) should be replaced during the first 12 hours and the remainder during the next 24 hours.

ALCOHOLIC KETOACIDOSIS

Severe metabolic acidosis associated with prolonged drinking of alcohol (especially binge drinking) and decreased food ingestion has recently been described with increasing frequency in the literature. Persons with this disorder have blood glucose concentrations which are usually 300 mg/100 ml or less, along with acidosis caused by increases in ketone bodies (mostly betahydroxybutyrate) and, to a lesser extent, lactic acid. Despite a number of similarities that may exist between DKA and alcoholic ketoacidosis (AKA), the therapy of the latter is quite different (see Table 11-2). Patients with AKA require only modest fluid replacement with fluids containing glucose and only modest amounts of HCO_3^-. Insulin therapy does not seem to improve recovery times. The recommended intravenous therapy in this disorder is one liter of 5% D/W containing 44 mEq of $NaHCO_3$ every 90 minutes unless severe acidosis is present. Potassium chloride should be added to the infusion when the urine flow is adequate. Electrocardiographic monitoring and serum potassium levels should be closely followed. Twenty-five units or less of regular insulin can be given every 4 to 6 hours if the blood glucose level is over 300 mg/100 ml. Most of these patients will require no insulin whatsoever after recovery from their acute illness. In general, AKA in the nondiabetic is a relatively benign disorder with a good outcome if the patient does not have an underlying hemorrhagic pancreatitis or septicemia.

LACTIC ACIDOSIS

Lactic acidosis should be vigorously treated with $\frac{1}{6}$ molar $NaHCO_3$. The amount of HCO_3^- needed should be calculated as described under DKA. There is no satisfactory therapy for this severe metabolic acidosis at present. One regimen for which success has been claimed is the simultaneous administration of 5% D/W, $NaHCO_3$, and insulin. Unless a correctable underlying disorder can be found the prognosis is most grave.

SELECTED READINGS

1. Alberti, K. G. M., Hockaday, T. D. R., and Turner, R. C. Small doses of intramuscular insulin in the treatment of diabetic coma. *Lancet* 2: 515–522, 1973.
2. Arrieff, A. I., and Carroll, H. J. Non-ketotic hyperosmolar coma with hyperglycemia: Clinical features, pathophysiology, renal function acid base balance, plasma-cerebrospinal fluid equilibria and the effects of therapy in 37 cases. *Medicine* 51:73–94, 1972.
3. Atchley, D. W., Loeb, R. F., Richards, D. W., Jr., Benedict, E. M., and Driscoll, M. E. On diabetic acidosis: A detailed study of electrolyte balance following insulin withdrawal and reestablishment on insulin therapy. *J. Clin. Invest.* 12:297–326, 1933.
4. Beigelman, P. M. Severe diabetic ketoacidosis (diabetic coma), 482 episodes in 257 patients: Experience of 2 years. *Diabetes* 20:490–500, 1971.
5. Beigelman, P. M. Potassium in severe diabetic ketoacidosis. *Am. J. Med.* 54:419–420, 1973.
6. Butler, A. M., Talbot, N. B., Burnett, C. H., Stanbury, J. B., and MacLachlan, E. A. Metabolic studies in diabetic coma. *Trans. Assoc. Am. Physicians* 60:102–109, 1947.
7. Cohen, A. S., Vance, V. K., Runyan, J. W., and Hurwitz, D. Diabetic

180   DIABETIC KETOACIDOSIS AND HYPERGLYCEMIC COMA

acidosis. An evaluation of the cause, course, and treatment of 73 consecutive cases. *Ann. Intern. Med.* 52:55–86, 1960.

8. Cooperman, M. T., Davidoff, F., Spark, R., and Pallotta, J.   Clinical studies of alcoholic ketoacidosis. *Diabetes* 23:433–439, 1974.
9. Fitzgerald, M. G., O'Sullivan, D. J., and Malins, J. M.   Fatal diabetic ketosis. *Br. Med. J.* 1:247–250, 1961.
10. Fulop, M., Tannenbaum, H., and Dreyer, N.   Ketotic hyperosmolar coma. *Lancet* 2:635–639, 1973.
11. Garella, S., Dana, C. L., and Chazan, J. A.   Severity of metabolic acidosis as a determinant of bicarbonate requirements. *N. Engl. J. Med.* 289: 121–126, 1973.
12. Kidson, W., Carey, J., Kraegen, E., and Lazarus, L.   Treatment of severe diabetes mellitus by insulin infusion. *Br. Med. J.* 2:691–694, 1974.
13. Marliss, E. B., Ohman, J. L., Jr., Aoki, T. T., and Kozak, G. P.   Altered redox state obscuring ketoacidosis in diabetic patients with lactic acidosis. *N. Engl. J. Med.* 283:978–980, 1970.
14. McCurdy, D. K.   Hyperosmolar hyperglycemic nonketotic diabetic coma. *Med. Clin. North Am.* 54:683–698, 1970.
15. Müller, W., Faloma, G. R., and Unger, R. H.   Hyperglucagonemia in diabetic ketoacidosis. Its prevalence and significance. *Am. J. Med.* 54:52–57, 1973.
16. Nabarro, J. D. N., Spencer, A. G., and Stowers, J. M.   Metabolic studies in severe diabetic ketosis. *Q. J. Med.* 21:225–248, 1952.
17. Page, M. McB., Alberti, K. G. M., Greenwood, R., Gumaa, K. A., Hockaday, T. D. R., Lowy, C., Nabarro, J. D. N., Pyke, D. A., Sönksen, P. H., Watkins, P. J., and West, T. E. T.   Treatment of diabetic coma with continuous low dose infusion of insulin. *Br. Med. J.* 2:687–901, 1974.
18. Semple, P. F., White, C., and Manderson, W. G.   Continuous intravenous infusion of small doses of insulin in the treatment of diabetic ketoacidosis. *Br. Med. J.* 2:694–698, 1974.
19. Smith, K., and Martin, H. E.   Response of diabetic coma to various insulin dosages. *Diabetes* 3:287–295, 1954.
20. Tranquada, R. E., Grant, W. J., and Peterson, C. R.   Lactic acidosis. *Arch. Intern. Med.* 117:192–202, 1966.
21. Young, E., and Bradley, R. F.   Cerebral edema with irreversible coma in severe diabetic ketoacidosis. *N. Engl. J. Med.* 276:665–669, 1967.

NELSON M. GANTZ

INFECTIOUS DISEASE medical emergencies are often life-threatening. Prompt recognition, identification of the causative agent, and selection of appropriate therapy are vital to the patient's survival. This section addresses the problem of identification of the agent by Gram stain and culture, followed by the clinical features and management of gram-negative bacteremia, acute bacterial endocarditis, acute bacterial meningitis, and bacterial pneumonias.

THE GRAM STAIN

Gram staining is the cornerstone of diagnostic bacteriology and divides organisms on the basis of their shape and staining characteristics into four groups: gram-positive rods, gram-positive cocci, gram-negative rods, and gram-negative cocci. Knowing to which group an infecting organism belongs provides important information concerning diagnosis, prognosis, and selection of antimicrobial agents.

To make Gram-stained smears:

1. Make a thin smear of the material, i.e., pus, sputum, spinal fluid, on a clean glass slide
2. Allow smear to dry at room temperature. Do not heat
3. Fix smear by passing slide once or twice through flame of a bunsen burner
4. Cover smear with crystal violet (blue color)
(There is no need to time these steps as stains act rapidly)
5. Rinse with water
6. Cover smear with Gram's iodine (brown color)
7. Rinse with water
8. Decolorize with alcohol until the *thinnest* areas of the smear have lost all blue color. Do not try to completely decolorize thicker areas

181

9. Rinse with water
10. Cover smear with safranin or basic fuchsin (red color)
11. Rinse with water
12. Dry smear by blotting with clean paper towel and examine with oil
    immersion lens

In an adequately Gram-stained smear, the nuclei of the polymorphonuclear leukocytes stain pink, whereas if they are underdecolorized, they
appear blue. With overdecolorization, organisms like cocci in clusters
which are obviously gram-positive stain pink. Another source of error is
interpreting precipitated Gram stain material as gram-positive cocci.
Poorly stained smears should be discarded.

HANDLING OF CULTURES

The aim is to deliver the clinical specimens to the laboratory uncon-
taminated and containing the same organisms, if any, that were removed
from the patient. These aims are achieved if the clinical specimens are
carried immediately to the bacteriology laboratory for inoculation on
appropriate media. Unfortunately, sometimes this is impossible or impractical. In circumstances where clinical specimens are first stored, special care must be taken for optimal results.

Specimens obtained using aseptic technique from an area of the body
which is normally sterile will contain either no organisms or pathogenic
organisms in pure culture. These specimens should be placed in an incubator at about 36°C while they await transportation to the bacteriology
laboratory. This allows the pathogenic organisms, if present, to multiply
so that they will be more readily identified when reaching the bacteriology laboratory. Examples of specimens which are handled in this manner
include blood cultures, cerebrospinal fluid, joint fluid, peritoneal fluid,
pleural fluid, and pericardial fluid.

Specimens from normally sterile areas of the body that cannot be
readily obtained without contamination, like urine, sputum, and specimens from the pharynx, skin, vagina, urethra, and cervix, must be handled to preserve pathogens if present without allowing other organisms
to overgrow these pathogens. These specimens should be put into a re-
frigerator at 4°C. At this temperature, most bacteria will neither multiply
nor die, so that the relative relationship of pathogens to normal organisms can be preserved for about 8 to 10 hours.

Many strains of *Neisseria gonorrhoeae* require an atmosphere with
increased carbon dioxide in order to begin growth. These specimens must
be immediately inoculated onto chocolate or Thayer-Martin agar and
incubated in a candle jar or carbon dioxide incubator. Specimens to be
examined for anaerobic organisms like *Bacteroides, Peptococcus,* and *Pep-
tostreptococcus* cannot survive in the presence of oxygen. When transporting to the laboratory specimens from sites where anaerobes are suspected, such as lung, abdominal, and pelvic abscesses, and empyemas,
there should be minimal contact with atmospheric oxygen. Also when

obtaining the sample, contamination by anaerobic bacteria normally present in the oropharynx and in the gastrointestinal and genitourinary tracts should be excluded. One simple method is to draw the pus or other material directly from the lesion into a syringe, excluding air bubbles. The specimen can then be carried to the laboratory in the sealed syringe or inoculated into an anaerobic tube.

GRAM-NEGATIVE BACTEREMIA

CLINICAL FEATURES

Bacteremia is the presence of bacteria in the bloodstream. The clinical spectrum varies from an abrupt onset of shaking chills and fever to hypothermia. When chills, fever, tachycardia, confusion, and hypotension are present, the condition is often called septicemia, septic shock, or sepsis. Temperature can be normal. Urinary or gastrointestinal symptoms and signs may call attention to the primary infection site. Clinical findings may be subtle, especially in the elderly, with only confusion and hyperventilation present. Shock occurs in about 40% of patients [1]. Gram-positive bacteremia with *Streptococcus* (*Diplococcus*) *pneumoniae* or *Staphylococcus* can produce shock despite their lack of endotoxin. Bleeding secondary to disseminated intravascular coagulation (DIC) may occur. A picture of shock should initiate a study to rule out septicemia as well as other causes of hypotension such as pulmonary embolism, hemorrhage, or myocardial infarction.

CAUSE

Gram-negative infections may be community- or hospital-acquired. Community infections are usually secondary to urinary, gastrointestinal, or biliary infections and less often to pneumonia. Organisms isolated include *Escherichia coli*, *Klebsiella*, Enterobacter, and *Proteus*. Other gram-negative organisms such as *Pseudomonas* and *Bacteroides* occur less frequently. *Bacteroides* species are usually traced to a bowel or genital focus. Hospital-acquired sepsis is usually related to instruments such as intravenous lines or urinary catheters, or follows surgical procedures such as bowel resection. Another source of bacteremia is pulmonary infections secondary to respirator use. Hospital-acquired organisms include those previously listed as well as *Pseudomonas* and *Serratia*. *Pseudomonas* infections are common in patients with leukemia or burns. The source of infection can be identified in about 90% of patients [1–3].

DIAGNOSIS

A history, physical examination, and appropriate Gram stains are important for prompt diagnosis in suspected bacteremia. The causative agent should be identified by Gram staining and culturing urine, sputum, stool, wound drainage, and other body fluids. Both aerobic and anaerobic blood cultures should be obtained. Clotting factors are frequently deficient because of DIC, but overt bleeding is uncommon [4]. In the absence of granulocytopenia and obstruction, fever if caused by a urinary tract infection is accompanied by pyuria. The limulus assay for endotoxin and the nitroblue tetrazolium (NBT) test have not proved useful [5, 6].

TREATMENT

Antibiotic agents are selected on the basis of Gram stains and known flora at the suspected primary focus of infection. Once cultures and susceptibilities are known, the least toxic and most effective antibiotic should be chosen. There is no place for "covering the waterfront" with a standard multiple antibiotic regimen in patients with sepsis. This practice leads to confusion, adverse reactions, and increased bacterial resistance. When gram-negative rods are suspected, select either kanamycin or gentamicin—the latter is effective against *Pseudomonas*. Ampicillin, tetracycline, and cephalothin do not have an adequate gram-negative spectrum and should be used only after the agent is identified. In patients with no identified primary infection site, i.e., a person with leukemia and fever, choose an agent effective against gram-positive organisms (nafcillin) and one suitable for gram-negative organisms (gentamicin) (Table 12-1). This combination, however, still "misses" enterococci and anaerobes. If these organisms are suspected, ampicillin and clindamycin or chloramphenicol can be used. A problem with the use of multiple antibiotic agents is that if a drug-related skin eruption develops, one does not know which drug to implicate.

In addition to antibiotics, a surgical procedure may be necessary to drain a septic site or relieve obstruction. Foreign bodies such as intravenous lines should be changed. Shock should be treated with fluids, central venous pressure monitored, and urine output measured hourly. The vasoactive drugs isoproterenol or dopamine may be needed if hypotension persists despite volume expansion. Complications which should be anticipated include hypoxia, electrolyte imbalance, acidosis, and disseminated intravascular coagulation (DIC). Administer heparin for bleeding due to DIC and treat other complications appropriately. Data regarding efficacy of corticosteroids are controversial, and therefore these drugs presently are not recommended.

The major determinant of prognosis is the underlying disease, the highest mortality from infection occurring with other diseases known to be rapidly fatal [1]. Also important in determining outcome is the selection of an appropriate antibiotic agent based on susceptibility testing [7]. Assuming that an organism is susceptible and the antibiotic drug reaches the infection site, there is no evidence for one antibiotic drug being superior to another. Because the mortality rate is about 40%, prevention is the key. Unnecessary use of antibiotic drugs should be avoided. Infection risk increases with the duration of bladder catheterization and with breaking the closed drainage system. Intravenous lines require daily examination and should be changed at least every 72 hours.

ACUTE BACTERIAL ENDOCARDITIS

CLINICAL FEATURES

Acute infective endocarditis usually begins abruptly with shaking chills and high fever. Normal heart valves are involved in about 50% of patients. A history of suppurative infection, frequently cutaneous, or intravenous drug use is common [8]. If the disease is right-sided, murmurs are absent (67%) and pulmonary manifestations predominate [9, 10]. Murmurs are frequent (67%) with left-sided disease and over time change in character [11]. Extracardiac manifestations secondary to embolization and abscess formation may also dominate. Thus, the outstanding extracardiac features may include brain abscess, meningitis, hemiplegia, and splenic or renal infarction with abscess formation. Heart failure caused by valve destruction can occur. Petechiae, splenomegaly, and Janeway lesions are helpful in making the diagnosis. Osler's nodes, splinter hemorrhages, and Roth's spots are rarely present but appear with increasing duration of the illness.

CAUSE

Staphylococcus aureus is the commonest organism isolated in acute endocarditis. Other causative bacteria include enterococci, gram-negative rods like *E. coli* or *Pseudomonas*, *Neisseria gonorrhoeae*, and *Streptococcus (Diplococcus) pneumoniae*. Fungi such as *Candida* also infect valves [12, 13].

DIAGNOSIS

Blood cultures are critical in identifying the causative agent and will be positive in 85 to 90% of patients [14, 15]. Because the bacteremia in endocarditis is continuous, the time of drawing the blood cultures is not crucial. However, aseptic technique in obtaining the cultures is essential. Contaminated blood cultures only confuse the picture. If acute endocarditis is suspected, 6 blood cultures should be obtained over a 2- to 3-hour period and then antimicrobial therapy should be started. In contrast, subacute endocarditis is not a medical emergency and blood cultures should be drawn over a 12- to 72-hour period before beginning therapy in order to increase the probability of isolating the organism. Gram stains of the buffy coat smears, of cerebrospinal fluid, or of cutaneous lesions may be helpful. Arterial blood cultures have no advantages over venous cultures. Leukocytosis is usually present. Positive blood cultures occur as frequently with right-sided cardiac involvement as with left-sided valvular infections.

TREATMENT

Therapy depends upon the agent and antibiotic susceptibilities of the organism isolated. A bactericidal agent is essential. If coagulase-positive staphylococci are suspected or isolated, a semisynthetic penicillin such

TABLE 12-1 Antimicrobial Therapy for Bacteremia with Normal and Impaired Renal Function

Organism	Antibiotic*	Dose and Route (Normal Renal Function)	Dosage Change with Increased Serum Creatinine Levels
Escherichia coli	Gentamicin	1.0–1.7 mg/kg q 8 h I.M. or I.V.	1.7 mg/kg q 8 × serum creatinine in hours†
	Kanamycin	7.5 mg/kg q 12 h I.M. or I.V.	7.5 mg/kg q 9 × serum creatinine in hours†
Klebsiella Enterobacter	Gentamicin	1.0–1.7 mg/kg q 8 h I.M. or I.V.	1.7 mg/kg q 8 × serum creatinine in hours
	Kanamycin	7.5 mg/kg q 12 h I.M. or I.V.	7.5 mg/kg q 9 × serum creatinine in hours
Serratia	Gentamicin	1.0–1.7 mg/kg q 8 h I.M. or I.V.	1.7 mg/kg q 8 × serum creatinine in hours
	Polymyxin B	0.8 mg/kg q 8 h I.V.	0.8 mg/kg q 72 h
Proteus mirabilis	Ampicillin	2 gm q 4 h I.V.	Not required, or more reduction
	Kanamycin	7.5 mg/kg q 12 h I.M. or I.V.	7.5 mg/kg q 9 × serum creatinine in hours
	Gentamicin	1.0–1.7 mg/kg q 8 h I.M. or I.V.	1.7 mg/kg q 8 × serum creatinine in hours
Proteus (indole positive)	Gentamicin	1.0–1.7 mg/kg q 8 h I.M. or I.V.	1.7 mg/kg q 8 × serum creatinine in hours
	Kanamycin	7.5 mg/kg q 12 h I.M. or I.V.	7.5 mg/kg q 9 × serum creatinine in hours
Pseudomonas aeruginosa	Gentamicin‡	1.0–1.7 mg/kg q 8 h I.M. or I.V.	1.7 mg/kg q 8 × serum creatinine in hours
	Polymyxin B	0.8 mg/kg q 8 h I.V.	0.8 mg/kg q 72 h
	Carbenicillin	5 gm q 4 h I.V.	1–2 gm q 6 h
Bacteroides fragilis	Clindamycin	600 mg q 6–8 h I.V.	Not required
	Chloramphenicol	1 gm q 6 h I.V.	Not required
Viridans streptococci	Penicillin ± streptomycin	2 million U q 4 h I.V. / 500 mg q 12 h I.M.	1 million U q 4 h I.V. / Avoid streptomycin
Enterococci	Penicillin + gentamicin	3 million U q 3 h I.V. / 1.0 mg/kg q 8 h I.M. or I.V.	1.0–1.5 million U q 3 h I.V. / 1.0 mg/kg q 8 × serum creatinine in hours†
Staphylococcus aureus (penicillinase positive)	Penicillinase resistant penicillin (nafcillin, oxacillin)	2 gm q 4 h I.V.	Not required
	Cephalothin	2 gm q 4 h I.V.	1.5 gm q 4 h
	Vancomycin	500 mg q 6 h I.V.	1 gm q 7 days

Staphylococcus (coagulase negative)	Penicillinase resistant penicillin	2 gm q 4 h I.V.	Not required
	Cephalothin	2 gm q 4 h I.V.	1.5 gm q 4 h
	Vancomycin	500 mg q 6 h I.V.	1 gm q 7 days†

* Useful antibiotics for suspected bacteremia pending susceptibility testing.

† Variability exists and serum levels should be monitored.

‡ Tobramycin has a spectrum and toxicity similar to gentamicin, except *Pseudomonas* is 2 to 4 times more susceptible to tobramycin. Dosage is the same as for gentamicin.

as nafcillin of oxacillin should be given in doses of 2 gm every 4 hours for 6 weeks. Serum bactericidal levels obtained just prior to the next dose of antibiotic should be at least ⅛. If the bactericidal dilution is less than this, indicating insufficient antibiotic blood levels, dosage should be increased or the drug given more frequently. The patient should receive 6 weeks of uninterrupted therapy. If the patient is allergic to penicillin, cephalosporins or vancomycin are alternatives. Gram-negative and fungal endocarditis may also require surgical intervention. Treat enterococci with high-dose aqueous penicillin G (3 million units every 3 hours) plus an aminoglycoside such as streptomycin (500 mg I.M. every 12 hours) or gentamicin (80 mg every 8 hours). Cephalosporins are not effective against enterococci even in combination with an aminoglycoside. Patients with enterococcal endocarditis who are allergic to penicillin should be given vancomycin (1 gm every 12 hours I.V.). Patients with underlying heart disease should receive antibiotic prophylaxis if undergoing a procedure likely to result in bacteremia.

ACUTE BACTERIAL MENINGITIS

CLINICAL FEATURES

Symptoms and signs of acute bacterial meningitis result from the non-specific manifestations of infection (chills, fever, malaise), increased intracranial pressure (headache, vomiting, papilledema), and meningeal inflammation (stiff neck, positive Kernig's and Brudzinski's signs). The classic triad of fever, nuchal rigidity, and alteration in mental status may be absent and diagnosis not as apparent, especially in the young, very old, chronically ill, or in those severely obtunded because of alcohol and other drugs. Fever is present in about two-thirds, confusion in one-half, and headache in one-third of adults with bacterial meningitis [16]. Minimal signs and symptoms of meningitis have also been reported in the immunosuppressed host, such as the renal transplant recipient [17]. The possibility of meningitis should be considered in all patients with pneumonia and an altered mental status, as well as in the alcoholic with "confusion." The benefit-risk ratio of doing a lumbar puncture far outweighs the potential harm of the procedure. About one-quarter of patients will have symptoms of 24 hours' or less duration. Most remaining patients will have symptoms of a week or longer duration, frequently associated with a respiratory illness. The classic petechial and purpuric lesions with meningococcal meningitis (50%) may occur in infections with ECHO virus type 9 [18] as well as with staphylococcal endocarditis [19].

CAUSES

The most frequent organisms causing meningitis are *Haemophilus influenzae*, *Streptococcus* (*Diplococcus*) *pneumoniae*, and *Neisseria meningitidis* [20]. Almost all cases of *H. influenzae* meningitis occur in children of less than 6 years of age. This organism infrequently causes meningitis in adults. Only 4 cases have been observed at the Boston City Hospital during 12 selected years [21]. Whereas a previous study suggested that most adults have bactericidal antibody to H. influenzae [22], a recent study reported only a 25% prevalence of antibody [23]. The low level of antibody may indicate that the incidence of this disease in adults will increase. Although the majority of cases of meningococcal meningitis occur in children of less than 6 years of age, this organism is still the leading cause during the 5- to 40-year age period. The majority of cases in adults over 40 years of age are due to Streptococcus (Diplococcus) pneumoniae. Pneumococcal pneumonia occurs in about half the patients with meningitis [16]. Other associated conditions are alcoholism, head trauma, otitis media, mastoiditis, and cerebrospinal fluid (CSF) rhinorrhea. Pneumococci are the commonest cause of recurrent bacterial meningitis. Gram-negative rods and staphylococci in adults are unusual causes and are usually associated with surgical procedures or direct trauma. The causes of meningitis in the immunosuppressed host include Streptococcus (Diplococcus) pneumoniae, gram-negative organisms such as Pseudomonas and E. coli, and fungi such as Cryptococcus and Aspergillus [24]. Cryptococcal meningitis occurs most commonly in patients with lymphoma. Tests for cryptococci include the Gram stain (gram-positive budding yeast), India ink preparation (yeast with large capsule), culture, and serology (cryptococcal antigen and antibody in cerebrospinal fluid and serum). Another cause of meningitis is Listeria monocytogenes, a gram-positive bacillus. This organism causes disease in patients with impaired cellular immunity such as the renal transplant recipient. Aerobic gram-positive rods isolated from the blood or cerebrospinal fluid should not all be called diphtheroids and labeled as contaminants.

DIAGNOSIS

The lumbar puncture and the CSF Gram stain and culture are the definitive tests to establish the diagnosis. Three tubes each containing at least 1.0 ml of fluid are collected. One tube is sent to the bacteriology laboratory. A second tube is sent to the biochemistry laboratory for glucose and protein analysis. After completing a cell count, the third tube should be centrifuged and the sediment examined for differential cell count, Gram stain, AFB stain, and India ink preparation. A Gram-stained smear of the centrifuged CSF identifies the causative agent in about 80% of patients in the absence of prior therapy. Culture of the CSF is positive in about 90% of patients. Demonstration of bacterial cell wall antigen by counterimmunoelectrophoresis is also useful [25]. Table 12-2 illustrates pressure, cell count, sugar, and protein findings in various types of meningitis. In about 50% of patients the CSF sugar will be less than 40 mg/100 ml or less than 40% of a simultaneously drawn blood sugar sample [20]. Blood cultures are positive in about 50% of patients. Occasionally, organisms will be present in the CSF in the absence of alterations in the other studies. Prior treatment with antibiotic drugs increases the number of negative Gram stains and cultures, but the characteristic CSF formula suggesting a bacterial cause is usually preserved [26]. If the initial CSF values are equivocal in differentiating between a bacterial and a viral cause, a repeat lumbar puncture after 8

TABLE 12-2 Initial Cerebrospinal Fluid Findings in Meningitis

Fluid	Pressure (mm H_2O)	Leukocytes (per mm³)	Protein (mg/100 ml)	Sugar (mg/100 ml)	Specific Findings
Normal	<200	0–5, lymphocytes	<45	>40	—
Acute bacterial	↑	Few thousand, polymorpho-nuclear leukocytes	↑	<40 or <½ of serum level	Positive Gram stain and culture in 90%
Partially treated bacterial	↑	Few to several thousand, lymphocytes or polymor-phonuclear leukocytes	↑	↓ or N1	Smear and culture frequently negative
Viral	N1 to ↑	<500 lymphocytes; 80% polymorphonuclear leukocytes early	N1 to ↑	N1 (↓ with mumps)	Virus isolation Rising antibody titer
Tuberculous	↑	25–500, lymphocytes	↑	→	Acid-fast organisms on smear of pellicle
Cryptococcal	↑	25–500, lymphocytes	↑	→	India ink positive Cryptococcal antigen
Parameningeal infection	↑	10–200, lymphocytes predominate	↑	N1	Polymorphonuclear leukocytes with acute bacterial endocarditis Smear and culture negative
Neoplastic	↑	Few to several hundred	↑	→	Abnormal cells on smear

hours of observation will usually show a change in cell type from predominantly polymorphonuclear to mononuclear cells [27]. However, individualization is crucial and antibiotic therapy should be started if bacterial meningitis is a reasonable possibility.

TREATMENT

The recommended antimicrobial therapy for meningitis in adults is detailed in Table 12-3. In meningitis, unlike endocarditis, a bactericidal antibiotic is not essential. In addition, clindamycin and the cephalosporins should not be used because of their poor CSF penetration. If the causative organism is a gram-negative rod susceptible only to gentamicin, systemic as well as intrathecal gentamicin is required. Antibiotic therapy should not be tapered as the patient improves. With antimicrobial therapy, inflammation decreases as well as penetration of the antibiotic through the blood-brain barrier. For example, in the early course of therapy, ampicillin achieves a CSF concentration which is 30% of the simultaneous serum concentration. Later, the CSF concentration may fall to 5% of the amount in the serum [28]. Therapy is continued until the CSF sugar is normal, the protein concentration is less than 50 mg/100 ml, the cell count shows 50 or fewer mononuclear cells, and the patient is afebrile for 5 days. Supportive therapy includes treatment of cerebral edema with glycerol or corticosteroids. If bleeding occurs secondary to disseminated intravascular coagulation, heparin therapy should be added. Fluids and oxygen are also important supportive measures. Central venous pressure should be monitored and hypotension treated. Although meningococcal meningitis is associated with intra-adrenal hemorrhage (Waterhouse-Friderichsen syndrome), adrenal insufficiency is not usually present.

Meningococcal prophylaxis should be given to household contacts and hospital personnel who report contact with the patient's oral secretions. If the organism is susceptible to sulfonamides, which is unlikely, adults

TABLE 12-3 Treatment of Acute Bacterial Meningitis in Adults

Organism	Drug and Dosage	Alternative
Streptococcus (Diplococcus) pneumoniae	Penicillin 2 million U q 2 h I.V.	Chloramphenicol 1 gm q 4 h I.V., or Erythromycin 1 gm q 4 h I.V.
Neisseria meningitidis	Penicillin 2 million U q 2 h I.V.	Chloramphenicol 1 gm q 4 h I.V.
Haemophilus influenzae	Ampicillin 2 gm q 4 h I.V.	Chloramphenicol 1 gm q 4 h I.V.
Gram-negative rod (resistant to ampicillin and chloramphenicol)	Gentamicin 1.6 mg/kg/q 8 h I.V., plus gentamicin, 8 mg q 24 h intrathecal	
Staphylococcus aureus	Nafcillin 2 gm q 3 h I.V.	Vancomycin (?) 500 mg q 6 h I.V.

should be given 1 gm twice a day for 3 days. Otherwise, rifampin, 600 mg, should be given every 12 hours for 2 days. In addition to prophylaxis, surveillance of close contacts for symptoms is vital.

BACTERIAL PNEUMONIA

Pneumonias remain a major cause of morbidity and mortality. Some patients with pneumococcal pneumonia die during the first 5 days of treatment, even with appropriate therapy [29]. However, overall mortality is still related to the cause and to the selection of an appropriate antibiotic. Common causes include bacteria, viruses, mycoplasma, and fungi. The differential diagnosis of infectious pneumonias is even broader if the patient is receiving immunosuppressive agents such as steroids or cytotoxic drugs. Epidemiologic data, such as animal exposure, occupation, illness in friends or family members, residence, and travel history are important [30]. This discussion will focus on the common bacterial pneumonias.

CLINICAL FEATURES

An abrupt onset of shaking chills with a fever, productive cough, dyspnea, and pleuritic chest pain are common. A history of upper respiratory illness is often present. Sputum is purulent and varies from rusty to bloody or yellow-greenish in color. Abdominal symptoms and signs may be prominent with lower lobe pneumonia. Signs of consolidation including increased tactile fremitus, dullness to percussion, and bronchial breath sounds should be differentiated from those of a pleural effusion.

Acute respiratory distress caused by aspiration of gastric contents may occur. This may be a presenting feature associated with alcoholic stupor, seizure, or drug overdose. Coma secondary to head trauma or cerebral vascular disease is also a frequent setting for acute aspiration pneumonia. All acutely ill and comatose patients are at high risk [31].

DIAGNOSIS

The key to the diagnosis of pneumonia is examination of the sputum. A specimen is obtained by expectoration, nasotracheal suction, or transtracheal aspiration. Sputum is readily contaminated with saliva and mouth flora. Transtracheal aspiration avoids this contamination [32]. In addition, the Gram stain helps one to identify an adequate sample. An adequate sputum sample contains bacteria along with sheets of polymorphonuclear leukocytes and lacks squamous epithelial cells. A culture is not a substitute but provides additional information. Blood cultures should also be obtained, because they are positive in about 30% of patients with pneumococcal pneumonia. Some evidence of pneumonia should be present on a chest x-ray even in dehydrated patients. Fluids will increase the likelihood of observing an x-ray abnormality in 12 to 24 hours. Leukocytosis with a left shift is usual, but leukopenia can occur with overwhelming infection in the elderly or alcoholic patient.

The site of an aspiration pneumonia depends on the patient's position at the time of aspiration. Upper lobe infiltrates, especially on the right, and lower lobe involvement are common [33]. Middle lobe infiltrates are rarely due to aspiration.

CAUSES

Streptococcus (*Diplococcus*) *pneumoniae* is still the most frequent cause of bacterial pneumonia at the Boston City Hospital and in other series, and accounts for more than half the cases [34]. Several problems exist in making this specific etiologic diagnosis. First, streptococci, which comprise the normal pharyngeal flora, appear quite similar to pneumococci on Gram stain. For this reason, several workers have revived the capsular swelling (Quelling) reaction using omnivalent pneumococcal antiserum as a means of differentiating pneumococci from streptococci in sputum [35]. Second, pneumococci are fastidious organisms and are usually cultured from the sputum in only half of patients with documented pneumococcal pneumonia [36]. Thus, a sputum culture report of "normal" flora by no means excludes this diagnosis.

Gram-negative organisms such as *Klebsiella pneumoniae, H. influenzae,* and less commonly *E. coli, Proteus,* Enterobacter, and *Pseudomonas* cause about 25 to 30% of cases of bacterial pneumonia [37, 38]. These pneumonias usually occur in middle-aged to older males in association with chronic obstructive pulmonary disease and alcoholism. The remaining community-acquired pneumonias are due to *Staphylococcus aureus* (2 to 10%) and rarely group A streptococci [34, 38, 39]. In contrast, nosocomial pneumonias are usually due to gram-negative bacteria. There is an increased frequency of staphylococcal pneumonia during influenza epidemics, but even then *Streptococcus* (*Diplococcus*) *pneumoniae* is still the leading cause [40].

Aspiration pneumonia acquired in the community is usually due to anaerobic bacteria. Aerobic as well as anaerobic bacteria have been isolated in hospital-acquired aspiration pneumonia [41].

TREATMENT

Penicillin is the drug of choice for pneumococcal pneumonia given in a dose of 1.2 to 2.4 million U per day. Treatment is continued for 3 to 5 days after the patient is afebrile. If the patient is allergic to penicillin, then either erythromycin, clindamycin, or a cephalosporin is an alternative. Cephalosporins should be avoided if the patient had a life-threatening reaction to penicillin. Tetracyclines should not be selected, because 10 to 20% of pneumococci are resistant. *H. influenzae* tracheobronchitis or pneumonia is treated with either ampicillin or a tetracycline. This organism is fairly resistant to the cephalosporins. Treat other aerobic gram-negative bacilli with either kanamycin or gentamicin, depending on antibiotic susceptibility testing. Combination therapy such as cephalothin plus kanamycin for *Klebsiella* or gentamicin plus carbenicillin for *Pseudomonas* is frequently used. However, there are no controlled studies showing superior outcome over an aminoglycoside used alone. Treat staphylococcal pneumonia with 12 gm/day of a semisynthetic penicillin like nafcillin or oxacillin. A cephalosporin, clindamycin, or erythromycin is a choice if the patient is allergic to penicillin. In addition to specific antibiotic therapy, vigorous chest physical therapy is essential. Dehydration and hypoxia should be corrected as well. Aspiration pneumonia secondary to anaerobic bacteria responds to penicillin. Corticosteroids have been used for aspiration, but controlled studies in man are lacking [42, 43]. Bronchoscopy is helpful for removing particulate material. The key is recognition of predisposing factors and prevention. Septic complications of pneumonia such as empyema, meningitis, endocarditis, pericarditis, and arthritis should be identified and treated. The challenge is to make an etiologic diagnosis and treat appropriately, recognizing that other diseases readily mimic bacterial pneumonia.

REFERENCES

1. McCabe, W. R., and Jackson, G. G.   Gram-negative bacteremia. *Arch. Intern. Med.* 110:847, 856, 1962.
2. DuPont, L., and Spink, W.   Infections due to gram-negative organisms: An analysis of 860 patients with bacteremia at the University of Minnesota Medical Center, 1958–1966. *Medicine* 48:307, 1969.
3. Myerowitz, R. L., Medeiros, A. A., and O'Brien, T. F.   Recent experience with bacillemia due to gram-negative organisms. *J. Infect. Dis.* 124: 239, 1971.
4. McCabe, W. R.   Gram-negative bacteremia. *D.M.* December 1973.
5. Stumacher, R. J., Kovnat, M. J., and McCabe, W. R.   Limitations of the usefulness of the limulus assay for endotoxin, *N. Engl. J. Med.* 288: 1261, 1973.
6. Soonattrokul, W., and Anderson, B. R.   Diagnostic accuracy of the nitroblue tetrazolium test. *Arch. Intern. Med.* 132:529, 1973.
7. McCabe, W. R.   Gram-negative bacteremia. Personal communication, 1975.
8. Louria, D. B., Hensle, T., and Rose, J.   The major medical complications of heroin addiction. *Ann. Intern. Med.* 67:1, 1967.
9. Ramey, R. G., Gunnar, R. M., and Tobin, J. R., Jr.   Endocarditis in the drug addict. *Am. J. Cardiol.* 25:608, 1970.
10. Bain, R. C., Edwards, J. E., Scheiffey, C. H., et al.   Right-sided bacterial endocarditis and endarteritis: Clinical and pathologic study. *Am. J. Med.* 24:98, 1958.
11. Weinstein, L.   Infective endocarditis: Past, present, and future. *J. R. Coll. Physicians Lond.* 6:161, 1972.
12. Cherubin, C. E., Baden, M., Kavaler, F., Lerner, S., and Cline, W.   Infective endocarditis in narcotic addicts. *Ann. Intern. Med.* 69:1091, 1968.
13. Dreyer, N. P., and Fields, B.   Heroin-associated infective endocarditis: A report of 28 cases. *Ann. Intern. Med.* 78:699, 1973.
14. Lerner, P. I., and Weinstein, L.   Infective endocarditis in the antibiotic era. *N. Engl. J. Med.* 274:199, 259, 323, 387, 1966.

15. Weinstein, L., and Rubin, R. H.   Infective endocarditis—1973. *Prog. Cardiovasc. Dis.* 16:239, 1973.
16. Carpenter, R. R., and Petersdorf, R. G.   The clinical spectrum of bacterial meningitis. *Am. J. Med.* 33:262, 1962.
17. Gantz, N. M., Myerowitz, R. L., Medeiros, A. A., Carrera, G. F., Wilson, R. E., and O'Brien, T. F.   Listeriosis in immunosuppressed patients. *Am. J. Med.* 58:637, 1975.
18. Lerner, A. M.   New viral exanthems. *Ann. Intern. Med.* 60:703, 1964.
19. Case Records of the Massachusetts General Hospital (Case 45212). *N. Engl. J. Med.* 260:1085, 1959.
20. Swartz, M. N., and Dodge, P. R.   Bacterial meningitis—A review of selected aspects. *N. Engl. J. Med.* 272:725, 779, 842, 898, 954, 1,003, 1965.
21. McGowan, J. E., Klein, J. D., Bratton, L., Barnes, M. W., and Finland, M.   Meningitis and bacteremia due to *Haemophilus influenzae*: Occurrence and mortality at Boston City Hospital. *J. Infect. Dis.* 130: 119, 1974.
22. Fothergill, L. D., and Wright, J.   Influenzal meningitis: The relation of age incidence to the bactericidal power of blood against the causal organism. *J. Immunol.* 24:273, 1933.
23. Norden, C. W.   Prevalence of bactericidal antibodies to *Haemophilus influenzae*, type b. *J. Infect. Dis.* 130:489, 1974.
24. Chernik, N. L., Armstrong, D., and Posner, J. B.   Central nervous system infections in patients with cancer. *Medicine* 52:563, 1973.
25. Coonrod, J. D., and Rytel, M. W.   Determination of aetiology of bacterial meningitis by counter-immunoelectrophoresis. *Lancet* 1:1154, 1972.
26. Lewin, E. G.   Partially treated meningitis. *Am. J. Dis. Child.* 128:145, 1974.
27. Feigin, R. D., and Shachelford, P. G.   Value of repeat lumbar puncture in differential diagnosis of meningitis. *N. Engl. J. Med.* 289:571, 1973.
28. Smith, D. H., Ingram, D. L., Smith, A. L., Gilles, F., and Bresnan, M. J.   Bacterial meningitis. *Pediatrics* 52:586, 1973.
29. Austrian, R., and Gold, J.   Pneumococcal bacteremia with especial reference to bacteremic pneumococcal pneumonia. *Ann. Intern. Med.* 60: 759, 1964.
30. Weinstein, L.   Common sense (clinical judgment) in the diagnosis and antibiotic therapy of etiologically undefined infections. *Pediatr. Clin. North Am.* 15:141, 1968.
31. Cameron, J. L., and Zuidema, G. D.   Aspiration pneumonia. *J.A.M.A.* 219:1194, 1972.
32. Ries, K., Levison, M. E., and Kaye, D.   Transtracheal aspiration in pulmonary infections. *Arch. Intern. Med.* 133:453, 1974.
33. Bernhard, W. F., Malcolm, J. A., and Wylie, R. H.   Lung abscess: A study of 148 cases due to aspiration. *Dis. Chest* 43:620, 1963.
34. Tillotson, J. R., and Finland, M.   Bacterial colonization and clinical superinfection of the respiratory tract complicating antibiotic treatment of pneumonia. *J. Infect. Dis.* 119:597, 1969.
35. Merrill, C. W., Gwaltney, J. M., Hendley, J. O., and Sande, M. A.   Rapid identification of pneumococci. Gram stain vs. Quelling reaction. *N. Engl. J. Med.* 288:510, 1973.
36. Barrett-Connor, E.   The nonvalue of sputum culture in the diagnosis of pneumococcal pneumonia. *Am. Rev. Respir. Dis.* 103:845, 1971.
37. Pierce, A. K., and Sanford, J. P.   Aerobic gram-negative bacillary pneumonias. *Am. Rev. Respir. Dis.* 110:647, 1974.

38. Sullivan, R. J., Jr., Dowdle, W. R., Marine, W. M., and Hiemholzer, J. C. Adult pneumonia in a general hospital. *Arch. Intern. Med.* 129: 935, 1972.
39. Shulman, J. A., Phillips, L. A., and Petersdorf, R. G. Errors and hazards in the diagnosis and treatment of bacterial pneumonias. *Ann. Intern. Med.* 62:41, 1965.
40. Schwarzmann, S. W., Adler, J. L., Sullivan, R. J., and Marine, W. M. Bacterial pneumonia during the Hong Kong influenza epidemic of 1968–1969. *Arch. Intern. Med.* 127:1037, 1971.
41. Lorber, B., and Swenson, R. M. Bacteriology of aspiration pneumonia. *Ann. Intern. Med.* 81:329, 1974.
42. Cameron, J. L., Mitchell, W. H., and Zuidema, G. D. Aspiration pneumonia. *Arch. Surg.* 106:49, 1973.
43. Dines, D. E., Titus, J. L., and Sessler, A. D. Aspiration pneumonitis. *Mayo Clin. Proc.* 45:347, 1970.

13

COMMONLY ENCOUNTERED
HEMATOLOGIC EMERGENCIES

MARK J. BRAUER

THERE ARE relatively few emergencies arising in hematology which require instantaneous diagnosis and treatment to thwart immediate fatal complications. In this report, frequently observed situations will be detailed with emphasis on clinical manifestations, rapid diagnostic maneuvers, treatment strategy, and unifying principles. When dealing with hematologic emergencies, split-second reaction is rarely required and undue haste may be detrimental. The urgent need to do something, whether on the emergency ward, in the operating room, in the delivery suite, or on the clinical wards, should always be tempered by an organized, thoughtful approach and plan of management.

BLOOD TRANSFUSION

Of all hematologic emergencies, the rapid replenishment of blood or blood volume deficit is the most acute. Although its execution has become formalized, the decision to transfuse blood involves far more than a hemoglobin or hematocrit determination. Understanding when and how much whole blood, packed cells, or plasma a patient requires entails knowledge of physiology, circulatory dynamics, immunology, coagulation mechanisms, and even forensic medicine. Properly administered, blood products save many who would otherwise die. Improperly employed, blood transfusions may kill.

There are three major indications for blood transfusion: (1) maintenance or restoration of an adequate circulating blood volume to prevent or combat shock; (2) continued delivery or improvement of the O^2 carrying capacity of the blood; (3) infusion of specific blood components such as plasma, albumin, or formed blood elements (red blood cells, platelets, leukocytes) because their absence produced or may produce clinical disease. In evaluating patients suffering from acute hemorrhage—spontaneous, surgical, or traumatic—the following observations will assist in deciding whether to transfuse. For a normal 70-kg man with a 5,000-ml total blood volume (slightly less in women), sudden loss of 10% (500 ml) of the circulating blood volume is not generally associated with any significant change in the circulation. A 20% loss (1,000 ml) may cause tachycardia with exercise and mild postural hypotension. A healthy adult can lose 2,000 ml of blood before developing clinical shock. Symptoms of hypoxemia are noted to develop when 50% of the blood volume is lost associated with intractable shock and death (Table 13-1). Although a normal healthy adult can tolerate a rapid significant loss of blood volume, a person with atherosclerosis may experience organ ischemia with as little as a 30% fall in circulatory volume.

Great emphasis is placed upon the physical examination of patients with acute blood loss because determination of the hemoglobin level or hematocrit is not a reliable method for assessing the amount of blood to replace. Hours to days (36 hours) may elapse before the plasma volume is replenished and hemodilution occurs, reflecting the true extent of blood deficiency. On the other hand, a reduced hemoglobin level and hematocrit within 6 hours of a hemorrhage strongly suggest a substantial drop in blood volume. Fingertip blood drawn from vasoconstricted vessels in patients with shock or preshock may give falsely elevated hemoglobin values and hematocrits because of stasis and hemoconcentration. Finally, rough estimates of blood loss during surgical procedures are usually off by 25%. It is for these reasons that sound clinical judgment is so critical in deciding whether to transfuse.

Acute blood loss is best managed by replacement with whole blood equivalent to the estimated volume shortage (Table 13-2). In a previously healthy person, when whole blood is not immediately available, plasma, saline, or "plasma protein" solutions may be used to restore the blood volume. Patients with a history of cardiovascular disease and the elderly must be managed more carefully; packed red blood cells are preferred. Transfusions following acute hemorrhage should be monitored by measuring the central venous pressure and observing its return to normal. If this is not possible, the blood pressure, pulse, and signs of peripheral perfusion may be utilized. When massive transfusions of blood

TABLE 13-1 Clinical Response to Gradations of Blood Loss*

Blood Volume Lost (%)	Loss (ml)	Signs and Symptoms
5–15	250–750	None
15–20	750–1,000	Exercise tachycardia, postural hypotension
20–35	1,000–1,750	Borderline shock
35–40	1,750–2,000	True shock
>40	>2,000	Death 50%

* Adult 70-kg male: 5,000 ml = total blood volume.

TABLE 13-2 Indications for Appropriate Use of Blood and Components

Component	Indications
Whole blood	Surgery or severe, acute blood loss
Packed cells	All other hemoglobin needs, wherever overload anticipated
Platelet concentrate	Platelet count less than 30,000
Plasma protein fraction	Volume expansion, shock
Serum albumin	Protein depletion, burns
Cryoprecipitate, fresh frozen plasma, concentrates	Clotting factors

(>10 units) are given, then the age of the blood becomes important in terms of coagulation factors, platelets, and the oxygen transport mechanisms (e.g., 2,3-diphosphoglycerate level).

The rate of infusion of blood depends upon the clinical condition of the patient and the product being transfused. Most patients who are not in congestive heart failure or in danger from fluid overload tolerate the infusion of one unit of whole blood or packed cells in 1 to 2 hours. Under extreme conditions, blood is given as quickly as it is lost. It is very important to be familiar with the blood bank's regulations regarding samples for ordering blood, correct labeling, and especially procedures for immediate acquisition of blood. Pretransfusion testing of the recipient requires a clotted sample not less than 48 hours old for the purpose of typing and cross matching.

Finally, rapid administration of large quantities of blood under emergency conditions may occasionally cause a variety of transfusion reactions (Table 13-3). Patients may complain of chills, fever, back pain, severe myalgia, and experience hypotension or even cardiac arrest. The transfusion must be stopped and the patient supported by volume expanders until the blood bank has reanalyzed the blood for compatibility. If blood is not stopped, you must bear full legal responsibility for all sequelae. Only after clearance from the blood bank can blood be given again. One of the most important maneuvers is personally notifying the blood bank or transfusion service of your problems and anticipated needs so as to enlist their expertise.

TABLE 13-3 Common Transfusion Reactions

Reaction	Cause	Frequency
Febrile	Leukoagglutinins	1–5%
Circulatory overload	Volume overexpansion	Occasional
Intravascular hemolysis	Mismatched blood	<0.1%
Hyperkalemia Hypocalcemia Thrombocytopenia	Massive transfusion (>12 units rapidly)	Rare
Cardiac arrest	Cold blood given rapidly	Occasional

DRUG-INDUCED HEMOLYTIC CRISIS

Although hemolysis is not usually thought of as a medical emergency, instances of hemolysis secondary to drug ingestion constitute a unique and serious group of disorders. Two of the most commonly encountered types are (1) glucose 6-phosphate dehydrogenase deficiency and (2) Coombs' test positivity secondary to drugs (Table 13-4).

GLUCOSE 6-PHOSPHATE DEHYDROGENASE DEFICIENCY

No rigid protocol for the study of patients with a suspected hereditary hemolytic disorder can be prescribed. As with all problems in medicine, a thorough history often can provide essential clues that lead to the proper diagnosis: (1) lifelong anemia with or without transfusions; (2) anemia at birth; (3) recurrent episodes of jaundice; (4) symptomatic episodes secondary to drug ingestion; (5) aplastic crisis after minor infections; (6) pigment gallstones; and (7) a history of leg ulcers. A family history may reveal clinical disease seen predominantly in hemizygous males.

Glucose 6-phosphate dehydrogenase (G6PD) deficiency is the most frequently recognized human erythrocyte enzyme deficiency. More than 80 different variants have been recognized, and it is estimated to occur in

TABLE 13-4 Drugs Associated with Hemolytic Anemia

Agent	Pathogenesis
	Immunologic mechanism (Coombs' test positive)
1. Alphamethyl dopa, L-dopa	1. Autoimmune antibody to erythrocyte
2. Penicillin	2. Membrane fixation of drug to erythrocyte
3. Cephalothin	3. Plasma protein adherence to membrane of erythrocyte induced by drug
4. Stibophen	4. Complement fixation to erythrocyte surface mediated by IgM
	Nonimmunologic mechanism (Heinz-body formation)
1. Acetanilid Chloramphenicol Naphthalene Nitrofurantoin Phenylhydrazine Primaquine Sulfonamides	1. Glucose 6-phosphate dehydrogenase deficiency
2. Sulfonamides	2. Unstable hemoglobins (e.g., Zurich)
3. Dapsone, phenacetin phenothiazine	3. Unknown mechanism

3% of the world's population. Hemolysis secondary to G6PD deficiency following ingestion of drugs is seen most often in males who have received the antimalarial drugs primaquine and pamaquine, sulfonamides, nitrofurantoin, naphthalene, or acetanilid. Milder hemolysis may be observed in affected females. Extreme hyperbilirubinemia and stormy clinical courses have been observed in G6PD-deficient subjects with hepatitis or other infections. Red blood cell inclusions called Heinz bodies can be demonstrated in blood smears by supravital staining with methyl violet. They represent denatured intracellular hemoglobin and are seen during drug-induced hemolytic episodes with G6PD deficiency.

A deficiency in G6PD is not always associated with a shortened red blood cell survival. Chronic hemolysis, if present, is usually quite mild in the most common types: Gd^{A-} (hemizygous black males) and $Gd^{Mediterranean}$ (usually white persons of the Mediterranean group). Under normal circumstances, the common types of G6PD deficiency are silent. Literally millions of individuals carry one or another of these deficits without any awareness of it. Nor could they be detected without specific screening tests.

Intravascular hemolysis occurs after drug ingestion in G6PD-deficient cells because of "redox stress." Depending upon the nature of the offending agent and the character of the person's enzyme deficiency, hemolysis may be brisk enough to be fatal. The difference between the extreme deficiency in the Gd^{Med} and the less severe Gd^{A-} accounts for the difference in intensity of episodes. Gd^{A-} attacks may be dramatic but are characteristically self-limited (Table 13-5).

Hemolysis occurs from 2 to 3 hours to days after offending drugs are ingested. Episodes are characterized by intravascular hemolysis with hemoglobinemia, hemoglobinuria, jaundice, and the appearance of "pinched" erythrocytes in the peripheral blood. Favism is beyond the scope of this presentation but continues to be a problem restricted to Gd^{Med} individuals. Finally, it should be emphasized that G6PD deficiency in a newborn may predispose to neonatal jaundice, and a drug history late in pregnancy must be sought from the mother. In most instances, removal of the offending agent or medication will abort the acute hemolytic process. In the case of some individuals of Mediter-

TABLE 13-5 Clinical Distinctions Between Gd^{A-} and Gd^{Med} Individuals During Drug-Induced Hemolytic Crisis

Course and Events	Gd^{A-} (Afro-American Black)	Gd^{Med}
Onset	24–36 hr	3–12 hr
Hemoglobinemia	Only with precipitant agent	Constant (worse with drug)
Anemia	Moderate	Profound
Duration	Self-limited	Continuous if drug present
Therapy	Simple drug discontinuation	Stop drug, transfusion as needed

ranean ancestry (Gd^{Med}), because of the severity and abruptness of anemia, blood transfusion may be required without delay. No other therapy is of proved effectiveness.

THE COOMBS' POSITIVE DRUG SYNDROMES

Autoimmune hemolytic anemia, whether idiopathic or drug-induced, presents the clinician with a formidable problem, especially if blood transfusion should be required. Because of the presence of autoantibodies to the person's own erythrocytes, the Coombs' test is uniformly positive. Although occasionally one can demonstrate specificity for known red blood cell antigens, most often these antibodies are panagglutinins causing all donor blood available for transfusion to be incompatible. For this reason—inability to find compatible blood for urgent transfusion—Coombs' positive hemolytic anemia can evolve into a major medical crisis.

The antihypertensive drug methyldopate hydrochloride (Aldomet) was reported by Carstairs in 1966 to cause a positive Coombs' test. Subsequently, it has been shown that from 10% to 30% of patients treated continuously with methyldopate hydrochloride in high dosage, 1 to 2 gm/day or more, may have a positive Coombs' test after 3 to 12 months. When use of the drug is discontinued, the Coombs' test eventually becomes negative a few months to over a year later. Recent studies of patients receiving L-dopa for the treatment of Parkinson's disease have revealed positive Coombs' test and hemolytic anemia, caused by similar if not identical antibodies.

Most patients receiving methyldopate hydrochloride in whom a positive Coombs' test occurs do not develop severe clinical hemolysis or anemia. The incidence of anemia in all patients receiving methyldopate hydrochloride is less than 0.1%. However, when hemolysis does occur it is indistinguishable from idiopathic autoimmune hemolytic anemia. All the features are present, including indirect hyperbilirubinemia, reticulocytosis, shortened red blood cell survival, positive Coombs' test, and splenic enlargement. In general, patients improve within weeks when use of the drug is discontinued. In instances where hemolysis has been exceptionally severe, corticosteroids may be successfully employed for short periods in moderate dose.

Transfusion therapy becomes a difficult decision. One may be dealing with a desperately ill patient whose hematocrit is below 10%. The blood bank will report a positive Coombs' test and a total absence of compatible blood. Even ABO and RH typing of the patient may be impossible because of autoagglutination. Choosing the "most compatible" blood is of doubtful value. One must weigh the risk of a transfusion reaction against the risk of death from hypovolemic and hypoxic shock, always keeping in mind that the transfused blood will be hemolyzed exactly as are the recipient's own cells. O RH-negative packed cells are considered to be the best choice for immediate transfusion.

Other drugs (Table 13-4) have been reported to cause Coombs' positivity and rarely hemolytic anemia. Penicillin has been implicated by a mechanism similar to quinidine-induced thrombocytopenia. Antibodies are directed at penicillin which is fixed to the erythrocyte membrane. The reaction depends upon the dose of penicillin the patient is receiving (usually 10 or more million units) and is reversible if use of the drug is stopped.

DISSEMINATED INTRAVASCULAR COAGULATION

Over the last several years, disseminated intravascular coagulation (DIC) has been an increasingly described pathophysiological condition. Observed in association with a number of disease states (Table 13-6), it is not always apparent whether DIC is a precipitating event or a secondary complication of a primary disease. Acute DIC constitutes one of the major medical emergencies physicians must currently contend with, be able to diagnose, and manage. The range of disorders with which DIC has been associated includes generalized infection, abruptio placentae, shock, amniotic fluid embolus, acute hemolysis of blood transfusion reactions, malaria, anaphylactic reactions, burns, snakebite, trauma, intoxications, and a variety of other conditions.

For the house officer observing this bleeding diathesis for the first time, the paradox of hemorrhage resulting from excessive blood coagulation is conceptually difficult, since bleeding and clotting are usually regarded as actively opposed phenomena. Indeed, coagulation and fibrinolysis are in constant equilibrium to maintain vascular integrity and blood flow. Acceleration of coagulation, with secondary activation of fibrinolysis, is responsible for the syndrome of DIC, which may be defined as acceleration of the coagulation process in the dynamic circulation with the consumption of clotting factors and platelets, possible obstruction of the microvasculature, and the secondary activation of fibrinolysis. Procoagulant material such as tissue or red blood cell thromboplastin, bacteria, antigen-antibody complexes, proteolytic enzymes (snake venom), and tissues (abruptio placentae) enter the circulation to initiate the process. Flow abnormalities, as observed in shock, prevent their clearance

TABLE 13-6 Conditions Frequently Associated with Disseminated Intravascular Coagulation

1. Infections
   a. Viral
   b. Bacterial (esp. gram-negative)
   c. Sepsis with asplenia
2. Abruptio placentae; amniotic fluid embolus
3. Malignancy
4. Snakebite
5. Heat stroke
6. Intravascular hemolysis (cardiac surgery, transfusion reactions)

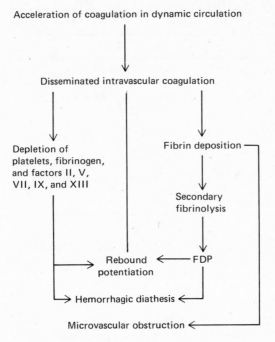

FIGURE 13-1   Pathophysiology of disseminated intravascular coagulation.

and aggravate the situation. Once the syndrome is triggered, the basic pathophysiology is fibrin deposition, microvascular obstruction, hemorrhagic diathesis caused by consumption of clotting factors, secondary fibrinolysis with its attendant split products, and hypofibrinogenemia. The acuteness or chronicity of the process depends upon interplay of these factors (Fig. 13-1).

The possibility of DIC should be considered in any patient with unexplained bleeding or signs of systemic thrombotic process. Clinically, the depletion of coagulation factors may be shown by major or minor bleeding at any site, although indeed this can be absent. Laboratory coagulation studies (Table 13-7) usually show a reduction in coagulation factors, especially fibrinogen, a low platelet count, and prolongation of the prothrombin time and partial thromboplastin time. The determination of fibrin monomers and fibrin degradation products by means of the protamine sulfate test and staphylococcal clumping may be of value. Formed as fibrinogen converts to fibrin and as a result of fibrinolysis, fibrin monomers and soluble fibrin polymers are readily detected in DIC. Traumatization of red blood cells by their passage across partially obstructed blood vessels can cause anemia, which in turn causes fragments or helmet cells to appear on peripheral smear of the blood. The diagnosis of DIC is therefore based upon a composite of the clinical circumstances associated with corresponding laboratory data. The differential diagnosis is in general between entities causing low levels of certain clotting factors, most commonly platelets and fibrinogen. It may not be possible to

TABLE 13-7 Laboratory Studies Helpful in Diagnosis of Disseminated Intravascular Coagulation

Test	Result
Simple observation for whole blood clot lysis	Often rapid (1 hr)
Examination of blood smear	Fragmented erythrocytes, decreased platelets
Prothrombin time (NL 12 sec)	Prolonged
Thrombin time (NL 15 sec)	Prolonged
Fibrinogen level	Usually depressed
Tests for fibrin breakdown products Protamine sulfate Staphylococcal clumping	Often positive

distinguish DIC with secondary fibrinolysis from the rare case of primary fibrinolysis (e.g., caused by cancer of the prostate). In liver disease, however, fibrin split products are usually not increased.

TREATMENT

Initially, treatment of DIC should include supportive measures to combat shock and acidosis, as well as efforts to establish a diagnosis of the underlying illness for which specific therapy should be rapidly instituted. In many instances of acute DIC, by the time the diagnosis is made, the acute event has passed and specific therapy for DIC is no longer needed. In the past, specific therapy for DIC has included anticoagulants, epsilon-aminocaproic acid (EACA), and fibrinogen. The latter is no longer used because it carries the risk of supplying more substrate for further intravascular clotting as well as the hazard of transmitting hepatitis. EACA should be reserved for primary fibrinolysis, more often in combination with heparin for secondary fibrinolysis.

It is now generally agreed that when specific therapy for DIC is indicated, rapid anticoagulation is the treatment of choice. In severe forms of DIC, intravenous heparin is given continuously, 1,000 U/hr by I.V. drip or pump, and monitored by coagulation tests such as the activated partial thromboplastin time (APTT) or the whole blood clotting time. The APTT should be 1½ to 2 times over a control of 30 seconds, the whole blood clotting time 25 to 30 minutes. Improvement of the fibrinogen level or shortening of the prothrombin time may herald clinical improvement. Therapy with heparin should be used only in patients with acute DIC accompanied by acidosis or shock, in subacute DIC, and when it is unclear whether an episode of DIC has subsided. The majority of patients with manifestations of mild DIC should not be treated. Special consideration must be given before administration of anticoagulants to patients suffering from active liver disease with DIC. They might show more improvement if given fresh frozen plasma and platelet concentrates. Before treatment of any patient with DIC, a careful review of pathophysiologic mechanisms is mandatory.

ACUTE SICKLE CELL SYNDROMES

Sickle cell anemia is a chronic disorder which can cause acute illness in persons of all ages. Crises come suddenly, and the patient can neither prevent nor abort them. Between crises, anemia may compromise normal function, and during crisis patients may be totally disabled from days to weeks. The patient's age to a large extent determines these problems and their management. Parents must be alerted to potential problems in young children such as meningitis and pneumonia; in adolescence, the inability to compete with peers often leads to poor performance in school. Older patients have multisystem involvement, and treatment becomes increasingly complex and difficult.

Certain hemoglobin abnormalities, notably HbS, C, and thalassemia, exist in a relatively high frequency in certain populations, owing to a selective advantage of the heterozygous (carrier) state. Heterozygotes (traits) tend to be asymptomatic. One notable exception is hematuria, not infrequently observed in Hb AS (sickle trait). Clinical manifestations occur in homozygous individuals or when variants are present in the heterozygous state in combination with other hemoglobin variants, e.g., hemoglobin sickle cell disease, sickle-thalassemia (S-thal).

The clinical manifestations of the sickling disorders ultimately can be attributed to the intraerythrocytic polymerization of deoxygenated HbS (Table 13-8). The factors that determine sickling include the concentration of HbS in the red blood cell, hemoglobins that potentiate (e.g., HbC) or ameliorate (e.g., HbF) sickling, the oxygen tension, oxygen affinity of the hemoglobin, and the time of exposure to hypoxia. Fluid and electrolyte loss secondary to fever, diarrhea, vomiting, and dehydration associated with the polyuria of sickle state causes increased blood viscosity, stasis, and vascular occlusion. Pneumonia and pregnancy not infrequently are precipitating factors.

In order to treat acute sickle cell syndromes, the differential diagnosis usually must be resolved in the hospital emergency room. Crises may mimic more treatable disorders or can be triggered by them. Frequently, crisis and precipitant coexist, and both need treatment. Infection must be excluded in all patients. *Streptococcus (Diplococcus) pneumoniae* and *Salmonella* infections occur with unusual incidence in sickle cell anemia. Infections can precipitate both painful and aplastic crisis.

Patients with sickle cell disease and fever should always have a reticulocyte count. Streptococcal pharyngitis requires prompt antibiotic treatment. Pneumococcal disease can include pneumonia and meningitis which can only be confirmed by early lumbar puncture. Pulmonary infiltrations associated with fever and called pneumonia not infrequently represent pulmonary infarction caused by marrow emboli or intravascular thrombosis. Arterial oxygen pressure (P_{O_2}) should be measured in all patients with lung infiltrations. If the P_{O_2} is less than 70 mHg, oxygen should be given. Should oxygen not improve the P_{O_2}, immediate partial exchange transfusion is an important consideration.

Painful crises are the most dramatic emergencies observed in sickling

TABLE 13-8 Correlations Between Symptoms in Sickling Syndromes, Organ Involvement, and Pathogenesis

Symptom or Complaint	Organ Involved	Pathogenesis
Hematuria	Kidney	Occlusion vasa recta
Acute monocular blindness	Eye, retina	Retinal infarct with detachment
Limp, hip pain, acute inset	Femoral head	Aseptic necrosis of head of femur
Priapism	Penis	Engorgement, stasis corpora cavernosa
Acute respiratory distress with dyspnea, pain, splinting, hemoptysis, and fever	(1) lung paren- chyma (2) pulmonary vessels	Pneumonia Thrombosis
"Hand-foot syndrome," dactylitis	(1) dorsum of hands, feet in children	Medullary bone infarction with bone destruction
Hemolytic jaundice with high incidence of pig- ment, gallstones	(1) blood (2) biliary tree	Shortened red cell survival Pigment stones
Acute hemiplegia	Brain	Fat embolism secondary to marrow infarct
Aplastic anemia	Bone marrow (erythroid series)	Marrow failure secondary to viral infection
Sudden death	Blood	Massive intravascular sickling

syndromes. Pain is probably due to infarction, ischemia, or vascular engorgement. Fever implies tissue necrosis. At best, treatment can relieve ischemia and vascular engorgement and can prevent further infarction. Treatment of pain is very difficult to evaluate, especially because pain may abate spontaneously with the passage of time.

Initially, precipitating causes must be sought out and treated. Analgesic drugs should be given liberally, and the patient rehydrated. Acidosis must be corrected. An almost endless list of agents, including dextran, phenothiazines, bicarbonate, urea solutions, vasodilators, steroids, and antithyroid agents, have been employed with inconsistent results. Partial exchange transfusion may have a role in treatment of severe unremitting pain, but occsasionally blood transfusions have made painful crises worse. Any discussion of sodium cyanate in prevention of painful crisis is beyond the scope of this presentation, except to say that preliminary trials are now being conducted and its role is currently controversial.

Of all therapeutic measures, the factor that already has prolonged survival for patients with sickling syndromes has been improvement in general medical care. The next obvious step is improvement in care of the painful crisis and a better understanding of its pathogenesis.

SELECTED READINGS

Blood Transfusion

Diethrich, E. B. Evaluation of blood transfusion therapy. *Transfusion* 5:82, 1965.

Duke, M., Herbert, V. D., and Abelman, W. H. Hemodynamic effects of blood transfusion in chronic anemia. *N. Engl. J. Med.* 271:975, 1964.

Mollison, P. L. *Blood Transfusion in Clinical Medicine.* 5th ed. Oxford: Blackwell Scientific Publications, 1972.

Moyer, C. Blood adjuncts in the treatment of hemorrhagic hypovolemias or shock. Conference on blood groups and blood transfusions. In *Blood Transfusion*, vol. 2. New York: Better Bellevue Association, 1967.

Drug-induced Hemolytic Crisis

Beutler, E. Drug-induced hemolytic anemia. *Pharmacol. Rev.* 21:73, 1969.

Carstairs, K. C., Breckenridge, A., and Dollery, C. T. Incidence of a positive Coombs' test in a patient on alpha methyldopa. *Lancet* 2:113, 1966.

Fraser, I. M., and Vessell, E. S. Effects of drugs and drug metabolites in erythrocytes from normal and glucose 6-phosphate dehydrogenase deficient individuals. *Ann. N.Y. Acad. Sci.* 151:777, 1968.

Garrity, J., and Petz, L. D. Drug-induced immune hemolytic anemia. *Am. J. Med.* 58:398, 1975.

LoBuglio, A. F., and Jandl, J. H. The nature of the alpha methyldopa red cell antibody. *N. Engl. J. Med.* 276:658, 1967.

Disseminated Intravascular Coagulation

Bisno, A. L., and Freeman, J. C. The syndrome of asplenia, pneumonoccal sepsis and disseminated intravascular coagulation. *Am. Intern. Med.* 72:389, 1970.

Deykin, D. The clinical challenge of disseminated intravascular coagulation. *N. Engl. J. Med.* 283:636, 1970.

Kirsker, C. T., and Rush, R. Detection of intravascular coagulation. *J. Clin. Invest.* 50:2234, 1971.

Kwaan, H. C. Disseminated intravascular coagulation. *Med. Clin. North Am.* 56:177, 1972.

Mirskey, C. Defibrination syndrome or . . . ? *Blood* 41:599, 1973.

Whaun, J. H., and Oski, F. A. Experience with disseminated intravascular coagulation in a children's hospital. *Can. Med. Assoc. J.* 107:963, 1972.

Sickling Syndromes

Finch, J. T. Structure of sickled erythrocytes and sickle cell hemoglobin fibers. *Proc. Natl. Acad. Sci. U.S.A.* 70:718, 1973.

Gillette, D. N., and Cerami, A. Sodium cyanate as a potential treatment for sickle cell disease. *N. Engl. J. Med.* 290:654, 1974.

Lessin, L. S., and Jensen, W. N. Sickle cell symposium. *Arch. Intern. Med.* 133:529, 1974.

Ranney, H. M. Sickle cell disease. *Blood* 39:433, 1972.

14

DIAGNOSIS AND MANAGEMENT OF ACUTE GASTROINTESTINAL BLEEDING

Charles Michael Bliss

ACUTE GASTROINTESTINAL (GI) bleeding may be a life-threatening condition which necessitates immediate assessment of the extent and source of the blood loss. Only in this fashion can a rational plan of therapy be formulated and proper treatment instituted.

INITIAL ASSESSMENT AND THERAPY

A key question in a patient in whom gastrointestinal bleeding is suspected is, "Is the patient in shock?" A systolic blood pressure of less than 90 to 100 mHg or a significantly lowered blood pressure in a patient with known hypertension, together with classic signs and symptoms such as pallor, cold clammy extremities, chilliness, restlessness, dyspnea, or faintness, suggests shock. However, to differentiate hypovolemic shock caused by blood loss from other forms of shock, one should always look for postural hypotension or an increase in pulse rate (20 to 30 beats per minute) when the patient is raised to a sitting position.

If the patient is in hypovolemic shock, replacement therapy should begin immediately, preferably by a central venous pressure (CVP) line. In all patients with gastrointestinal bleeding, a large-bore (18-gauge) intravenous line should be inserted. If the patient is in severe shock, two lines with attached pressure cuffs are frequently necessary. The central venous pressure line is especially important in elderly patients to avoid pulmonary edema from overexpansion of the blood volume. The central venous pressure does not always accurately reflect hypovolemia; thus, a trial of rapid infusion of saline solution may be necessary. If there is no change in the CVP, the patient is hypovolemic. Normal saline solution can be used temporarily, but typed and cross-matched whole blood should be available within 20 to 30 minutes. If shock is severe, type O RH-negative blood may be used for life-saving immediate transfusion. Blood can be transfused rapidly if the shock is severe—500 ml every 30 minutes, if necessary. After 4 units of blood have been transfused, fresh blood is preferable to bank blood. If fresh blood is not available, 1 unit of fresh frozen plasma and platelets should be added to provide coagulation factors. Thereafter, 1 unit of fresh frozen plasma and platelets should be added to every 4 units of bank blood.

Nasal oxygen is useful in overcoming the ischemic effects of hypovolemia, especially in elderly persons or in patients with known coronary artery disease. An electrocardiogram should always be performed, since secondary acute myocardial ischemia is always a threat.

The other important part of the initial assessment of the patient is the extent of blood loss. If the patient has been vomiting, how much has he vomited, how frequently, and what does the vomitus look like? A few flecks of dark blood are of quite different significance from three or four cupfuls of bright red blood with clots. Does the stool show simply bright red blood, maroon color mixed with feces, black sticky melena, etc.? A nasogastric tube is an invaluable diagnostic aid. A large tube, i.e., 18 French (size in millimeters in circumference), should be inserted into the stomach, aspiration performed, volume estimated, and irrigation begun with iced tap water (saline solution is not necessary, especially in patients who may have sodium overload caused by liver disease, with ascites, edema, etc.). Manual irrigation to clear the stomach of clots is more successful than intermittent suction. One may introduce 50 ml of iced tap water, and if less than 40 ml is returned, the tube should be repositioned and aspiration performed again. If clots or food continue to plug the tube, one should switch to a larger Ewald tube. Nasogastric suction should be maintained for a minimum of 24 hours if the patient has been actively bleeding. The tube serves two purposes: (1) it maintains surveillance of bleeding activity; (2) it is therapeutic in patients with peptic ulcer disease.

The early hematocrit and hemoglobin determinations are useful primarily as a baseline, because in acute bleeding the hematocrit will not reflect blood loss for up to 6 hours [1, 2]. Coagulation studies, such as prothrombin time, partial thromboplastin time, and platelet counts, should also be initiated early. If these are abnormal, appropriate therapy should be instituted, such as vitamin K or platelet transfusions.

DETERMINATION OF CAUSE

Once the magnitude of blood loss has been determined and steps have been taken to correct hypovolemia, the etiology of the blood loss should be determined. A history and physical examination should be done at this point to determine the sequence of events that led the patient to seek aid, the character of the bleeding, any history of previous bleeding, other associated symptoms, associated disease (such as peptic ulcer, liver disease, alcoholism, etc.), and drug use. Symptoms and signs that may suggest a bleeding site are outlined in Table 14-1.

When the patient vomits blood or obviously has blood in the nasogastric aspirate, the differentiation of upper versus lower GI bleeding is not a problem. However, some patients with upper GI lesions may have

TABLE 14-1 Symptoms and Signs in Common Upper GI Tract Bleeding Lesions

Diagnosis	Characteristic Symptoms	Characteristic Findings on Physical Examination
Esophagitis	Reflux, heartburn	None
Esophageal varices	Sudden vomiting	Spider angiomata, hepatomegaly, ascites
Cardioesophageal tears	Retching followed by hematemesis	None
Gastric erosions	Stress-CNS, burns, aspirin, steroids, other drugs	None
Diffuse gastritis	Alcohol abuse, retching	Chronic liver disease, abdominal tenderness
Gastric ulcer	Peptic ulcer symptoms*	Epigastric tenderness
Gastric cancer	Malaise, anorexia, abdominal pain	Abdominal mass, cachexia
Marginal ulcer	Gastric surgery, peptic ulcer symptoms*	Epigastric tenderness
Duodenal ulcer	Peptic ulcer symptoms*	Epigastric tenderness

* Peptic ulcer symptoms include postprandial epigastric pain or indigestion, accompanied by nausea or vomiting. The pain may be relieved by antacids or food.

stopped bleeding prior to gastric aspiration, or duodenal contents may not have refluxed into the stomach. The stool examination may then be helpful in distinguishing upper from lower GI lesions. Possible bleeding sites are outlined in Table 14-2. In general, the shorter the time blood stays in the GI tract, the brighter the color of the blood. Thus, bleeding from the upper GI tract usually produces melena, and colonic bleeding usually consists of bright red blood. However, exceptions may occur, since it is possible with very rapid transit to pass a bloody stool containing predominantly bright red blood from a massive upper GI tract hemorrhage, whereas bleeding from the cecum may produce melena if the transit time is slow enough [3, 4].

The black color of melena is produced when the iron in the heme molecule is oxidized from the ferro-divalent state to the ferri-trivalent state, producing hemin or acid hematin. Oxidation can be accomplished by acid, i.e., the HCl secreted by the stomach, or by bacteria in the gut [5].

DIAGNOSIS

If upper GI bleeding is suspected, emergency fiberoptic endoscopy of the esophagus, stomach, and duodenum is now recognized as the best procedure, in most instances, for determining the bleeding site [6]. Ideally, endoscopy is done in an alert, cooperative patient who has been stabi-

TABLE 14-2 Stool Characteristics in GI Bleeding

Stool Color	Possible Bleeding Site
Bright red blood	
Blood only	Rectum and lower sigmoid
Mixed with stool	Below midtransverse colon
On stool surface	Rectum and lower sigmoid
Maroon with diarrhea	Above midtransverse colon
Melena with diarrhea	Above ligament of Treitz
Melena without diarrhea	Above midtransverse colon
Blood and stool mixed with pus	Inflammatory disease of the colon
Occult blood	Anywhere in GI or upper respiratory tracts

lized and whose stomach has been well washed out with iced tap water. It can be diagnostic not only in identifying the specific type of pathology but also in identifying which of multiple lesions is actually bleeding. Our recent experience at the Boston City Hospital illustrates this point (Table 14-3). Of 136 patients admitted with acute upper GI bleeding, 100 had endoscopy within the first 24 hours. Of a total of 152 lesions seen, only about half were actively bleeding at the time of examination. This low rate applied particularly to esophageal varices, where in only 5 of 26 patients with varices was this the observable bleeding site.

Endoscopy as a diagnostic procedure is more accurate than an upper GI series in determining the site of bleeding when the bleeding is due to esophageal varices, cardioesophageal tears (Mallory-Weiss syndrome), diffuse gastritis, gastric erosions, or chronic duodenal ulcer disease [6] (Table 14-4).

TABLE 14-3 Acute Upper GI Bleeding: Boston City Hospital Endoscopic Experience

Diagnosis	Actively Bleeding	Not Bleeding	Total
Diffuse gastritis	24	11	35
Acute gastric erosions	16	11	27
Esophageal varices	5	21	26
Gastric ulcer	12	7	19
Esophagitis	5	9	14
Duodenal ulcer	4	7	11
Duodenitis	1	9	10
Marginal ulcer	3	1	4
Esophageal tear	2	0	2
Gastric carcinoma	1	1	2
Gastric polyps	0	2	2
Normal examination			11
Total diagnosis	73	79	152

TABLE 14-4 Sources of Upper Gastrointestinal Hemorrhage

Source	No. of Cases	Identified by: Endoscopy	Identified by: Gastro-intestinal Series
Esophagus			
Esophageal varices	16	16/16[a]	6/12
Esophagitis	13	13/13	1/13
Mallory-Weiss	8	8/8	0/7
Stomach			
Gastric ulcer, total	15		
Gastric ulcer, deep	12	12/12	5/11
Gastric ulcer, shallow	3[b]	1/3	0/1
Erosive gastritis	9	9/9	0/9
Gastric carcinoma	2	2/2	2/2
Marginal ulcer	6	6/6	2/5
Pyloroduodenal ulcer	3	3/3	2/3
Duodenal ulcer	23	21/23	8/22[c]
Duodenal diverticulum	1	1/1	1/1
Unknown	4	0/4	0/4
Total	100	92/100	27/90

[a] Number of attempts.
[b] Two cases diagnosed at emergency surgery (acute gastric fundal ulcer).
[c] Three cases reported as deformity, 2 as duodenitis (in addition to the 8 ulcers).

Source: From Katon, R. M., and Smith, F. W. *Gastroenterology* 65:728, 1973.

Although endoscopy is a very useful tool, there are contraindications to it (Table 14-5). The risk of perforation, and/or aspiration, is greater in uncooperative patients, in patients who are unresponsive, or in patients who have potential esophageal obstruction. The endoscope increases airway resistance and has been reported to produce cardiac arrhythmias [7]. In addition, on busy services, several endoscopes may be necessary, because the endoscope cannot be steam sterilized. Thus, gas sterilization is required—a procedure which takes 3 days. However, these are relative contraindications in the sense that if emergency operation is contemplated to control bleeding, important positive and negative information can be rapidly obtained which can greatly aid the surgeon in the proper approach, and thus reduce surgical mortality.

An emergency upper GI series has been the standard approach for many years and is complementary to endoscopy. It is often very helpful if endoscopy was refused, was unsuccessful for technical reasons, or was nondiagnostic [1].

Emergency arteriography is particularly useful for massive bleeding, because selective cannulation of the bleeding artery may demonstrate effusion of contrast medium from a specific site into the lumen of the gut [8]. If arteriography is indicated, it should always be done before the barium studies, because the barium obscures the arteriogram. Arteriogra-

TABLE 14-5 Relative Contraindications to UGI Endoscopy

1. Uncooperative or unwilling patients, i.e., in delirium tremens, coma
2. Significant cardiorespiratory disease, pulmonary edema, respiratory or cardiac failure, cardiac arrhythmias, acute myocardial infarction
3. Obstructive esophageal disease
4. Active tuberculosis or serum positive for hepatitis-associated antigen
5. Severe shock
6. Suspected perforation

phy may also be therapeutic in controlling hemorrhage when the bleeding artery is perfused with pitressin [9]. In variceal bleeding, the superior mesenteric artery may be perfused with pitressin to reduce portal pressure and, in this fashion, bleeding may be controlled. These patients should be followed in an intensive care unit where perfusion may be continued for up to 48 hours. Arterial perfusion is the preferred way to control variceal bleeding rather than by inflation of the Sengstaken-Blakemore tube, because the complication rate is lower [9].

Besides the commoner causes of bleeding outlined in Tables 14-3 and 14-4, gastrointestinal bleeding may also be associated with rarer disorders which primarily affect blood vessels [Table 14-6]. Many of these disorders have skin manifestations which should be carefully sought out.

In lower GI bleeding, sigmoidoscopy should always be performed and is often diagnostic. In acute inflammatory bowel disease (ulcerative colitis, granulomatous colitis), the mucosa is red, edematous, friable, and bleeds easily. Often the mucosa in ischemic colitis has a dusky blue cast. Internal hemorrhoids with overlying proctitis can be differentiated from ulcerating adenocarcinoma.

A flat plate of the abdomen may show the edema of the bowel wall as "thumbprints" in ischemic colitis, or the rough serrated margins of acute inflammatory bowel disease.

If there is massive lower GI bleeding, or if ischemic bowel disease is suspected, an arteriogram of the superior and inferior mesenteric arteries may be able to pinpoint the lesion. If the sigmoidoscopy and arteriogram are not diagnostic, in massive bleeding an emergency barium enema may be therapeutic in controlling bleeding from diverticula·of the colon. However, a barium enema is contraindicated in acute ulcerative colitis, for it may precipitate toxic megacolon and perforation of the colon.

REASSESSMENT

Patients with GI bleeding need to be followed carefully to ensure that vital signs are stable and that blood volume has returned to normal. One must check that the nasogastric tube remains patent and urinary output is adequate. The amount of nasogastric aspirate and the frequency and character of bowel motions must be monitored. Hyperactive bowel sounds are common if the gut is distended by blood, and thus ausculta-

TABLE 14-6 Rare Causes of Gastrointestinal Bleeding

Vascular lesions
  1. Aortic aneurysms
  2. Ruptured vascular suture lines following an aortic homograft repair
  3. Aneurysms of the gastric or splenic arteries
  4. Hepatic or portal biliary fistula producing hemobilia (usually following trauma to the liver, in the remote or recent past)

Mucocutaneous or related disorders associated with GI bleeding
  1. Hereditary hemorrhagic telangiectasia
  2. Universal angiomatosis
  3. Blue rubber bleb nevus syndrome
  4. Multiple phlebectasia
  5. Pseudoxanthoma elasticum
  6. Ehlers-Danlos syndrome
  7. Homocystinuria
  8. Polyarteritis nodosa
  9. Atrophying papulosis of Degos
 10. Neurofibromatosis
 11. Kaposi's sarcoma
 12. Peutz-Jeghers syndrome
 13. Carcinoid syndrome

tion of the abdomen is another nonspecific method used to assess potential continued bleeding. One should try to bring the hematocrit to above 30, especially in elderly patients, who tolerate anemia poorly. Extra blood should be available at all times in case bleeding occurs again.

Early surgical consultation is very important so that the surgeon can follow the patient's course as well. The necessity and timing of operation depend on the source and quantity of the bleeding. Early operation is recommended for recurrent bleeding peptic ulcers, especially if the patient has had repeated bleeding in the hospital or has silent ulcer disease. For diffuse gastritis one would prefer to delay surgery, for the most effective surgery is total gastrectomy, although vagotomy and pyloroplasty sometimes are effective [1].

Variceal bleeding is a much more difficult problem, since recent prospective studies demonstrate that emergency (while the patient is actively bleeding), prophylactic (varices present but have never bled), and therapeutic (varices have bled but are controlled) portocaval shunts are not helpful in reducing morbidity and mortality in alcoholic liver disease [10]. The selective splenorenal shunt has recently been proposed as beneficial, but further evaluation is necessary. The ligation of varices has been shown to be, at best, a temporary measure.

Age itself is generally not a factor in assessing surgical risk. More important are other concomitant problems, such as cardiopulmonary disease, active liver disease, and acute delirium tremens.

In summary, management of massive GI bleeding should include:

1. Frequent monitoring of vital signs
2. Establishment of large-bore central venous line(s)
3. Blood sample for type and cross match, blood urea nitrogen, electrolytes, coagulation studies, and complete blood cell count
4. Intravenous infusion of normal saline solution, followed by type-specific whole blood (O RH-negative if time is short)
5. Continuous nasogastric aspiration and gastric wash with iced tap water for upper GI bleeding
6. Nasal oxygen and an ECG
7. Endoscopic evaluation, or if bleeding is uncontrollable, radiology consultation for emergency arteriography and pitressin infusion
8. Surgical consultation

REFERENCES

1. Gordon, H. E. Diagnosis and management of gastrointestinal bleeding. *Ann. Intern. Med.* 71:993–1011, 1969.
2. Palmer, E. D. The vigorous approach to upper gastrointestinal tract hemorrhage. *J.A.M.A.* 207:1477–1480, 1969.
3. Schiff, L., Stevens, R. J., Shapiro, N., and Goodman, S. Observations on the oral administration of citrated blood in man. II. The effect on the stools. *Am. J. Med. Sci.* 203:409–412, 1942.
4. Hilsman, J. H. The color of blood-containing feces following the instillation of citrated blood at various levels of the small intestine. *Gastroenterology* 15:131–134, 1950.
5. White, A., Handler, P., Smith, E. L., and Stetten, D., Jr. *Principles of Biochemistry.* 2d ed. New York: McGraw Hill, 1959. Pp. 202–204.
6. Katon, R. M., and Smith, F. W. Panendoscopy in the early diagnosis of acute upper gastrointestinal bleeding. *Gastroenterology* 65:728–734, 1973.
7. Silvis, S. E., Nebel, O., Rogers, G., Sugawa, C., and Mandelstam, P. Endoscopic complications. Results of the 1974 American Society for Gastrointestinal Endoscopy survey. *J.A.M.A.* 235:928–930, 1976.
8. Baum, S., Stein, G. N., Nusbaum, M., and Chait, A. Selective arteriography in the diagnosis of hemorrhage in the gastrointestinal tract. *Radiol. Clin. North Am.* 7:131–145, 1969.
9. Conn, H. O., Ramsby, G. R., Storer, E. H., Mutchnick, M. G., et al. Intraarterial vasopressin in the treatment of upper gastrointestinal hemorrhage: A prospective, controlled clinical trial. *Gastroenterology* 68: 211–221, 1975.
10. Resnick, R. H., Iber, F. L., Ishihara, A. M., Chalmers, T. C., et al. A controlled study of the therapeutic portacaval shunt. *Gastroenterology* 67:843–857, 1974.

Raymond S. Koff

THE TERM *hepatic failure* is often used to describe a number of clinical manifestations which may occur independently or in combination in patients with advanced or extensive liver disease. These include jaundice, variceal hemorrhage, ascites, hepatic encephalopathy, disturbances of blood coagulation, and the oliguric renal failure of liver disease (the hepatorenal syndrome). The prognostic importance of these manifestations of liver failure and the therapeutic response they elicit are dependent upon both the specific problem and the clinical circumstances in which it arises.

Only a few of these conditions may be considered emergencies. Variceal hemorrhage, which is discussed in Chapter 14, on gastrointestinal bleeding, and hepatic encephalopathy, which will be discussed in this chapter, fall into this category. In contrast, urgent intervention for ascites is best limited to two specific complications of ascites. Although neither the coagulation disorders associated with liver disease nor the hepatorenal syndrome is frequently life-threatening in itself, both conditions appear to contribute to the death of the patient with hepatic failure and will therefore be discussed briefly.

In adult patients jaundice per se cannot be considered an emergency. Although the intensity of jaundice tends to reflect the severity of hepatic disease, there is no convincing evidence that hyperbilirubinemia contributes to hepatic failure. Specific treatment aimed at lowering bilirubin levels is unnecessary for all except neonates with rising serum levels of unconjugated bilirubin, in whom exchange transfusion or phototherapy is mandatory to prevent the development of kernicterus (bilirubin encephalopathy).

ASCITES

The accumulation of free peritoneal fluid in patients with advanced liver disease is the result of an abnormality of the hepatic vasculature leading to increased portal venous pressure, leakage of hepatic lymph, and hypoalbuminemia caused by impaired hepatic synthetic function and direct transfer of newly formed albumin from the liver to the peritoneal space. A variety of secondary mechanisms lead to striking renal sodium retention, which contributes to the development and perpetuation of the ascites.

In the majority of patients improvement of hepatic function per se will result in spontaneous diuresis and diminution in ascites. Urgent or aggressive therapy is rarely necessary and may, in fact, be harmful. There are, however, two circumstances in which ascites may precipitate catastrophic events: rupture of an umbilical hernia and severe respiratory embarrassment. In the former the typical patient is cirrhotic, with progressively increasing and tense ascites. The increased pressure within the peritoneal space expands the umbilical sac, with thinning of the overlying skin. Ulceration, weeping, necrosis, and infection of the abdominal wall may precede rupture. Should rupture ensue and loss of peritoneal fluid be extensive, which is usually the case, then intravascular volume depletion, hepatic encephalopathy, and renal failure may be expected. This sequence usually ends in the death of the patient.

Severe respiratory embarrassment usually occurs in a similar setting, i.e., a cirrhotic patient with tense ascites complicated by extensive bilateral pleural effusions. Arterial hypoxemia is not uncommon in cirrhotic patients who may have portopulmonary or intrapulmonary arteriovenous shunting, an abnormality of the oxyhemoglobin dissociation curve, and a defect in closing volume. Hydrothorax may impair ventilation severely and contribute further to life-threatening hypoxemia.

To prevent these potentially catastrophic sequences immediate therapeutic paracentesis with removal of 1 to 2 liters of fluid may be necessary. Subsequently management with a sodium-restricted diet is undertaken. Aggressive therapeutic paracentesis, in an attempt to dry out an ascitic cirrhotic patient, is contraindicated, for such therapy may replicate the dreaded consequences of spontaneous rupture of an umbilical hernia. On the other hand, paracentesis for diagnostic purposes, with removal of 50 to 100 ml, should be a nearly routine procedure in the management of ascites. It is clearly mandatory in the study of unexplained fever, abdominal pain, or encephalopathy in the cirrhotic patient with ascites.

HEPATIC ENCEPHALOPATHY

Hepatic encephalopathy, also known as hepatic coma and portal-systemic encephalopathy, is characterized by alterations of consciousness, a flapping tremor (asterixis), and an abnormal electroencephalogram, which in the presence of extensive or advanced liver disease signal the existence of hepatic failure. Inappropriate behavior, agitation, and disordered sleep patterns may be the first features, but progressive obtundation almost invariably develops. Hepatic encephalopathy may be a manifestation of either massive hepatic necrosis or advanced chronic liver disease with portal-systemic venous admixture.

Mechanism of Encephalopathy

A number of factors have been implicated in the mechanism of hepatic encephalopathy in both massive hepatic necrosis and advanced chronic liver disease. Ammonia, which may be more intimately involved in the latter than in the former, may interfere with the Krebs (citric acid) cycle in brain. Unfortunately, the correlation of blood ammonia levels with encephalopathy is far from perfect. Ammonia, derived chiefly from exogenous gut protein and endogenously from the kidney, is normally detoxified by the formation of urea in the liver. At physiological pH almost all ammonia is in the form of ammonium ion. With alkalosis the equilibrium favors free ammonia, which can cross the blood-brain barrier. Regardless of whether ammonia is contributory, treatment aimed at reducing ammonia formation often corrects encephalopathy in advanced liver disease. Removal or reduction of ammonia appears to be less effective in reversing encephalopathy in massive hepatic necrosis.

Elevated serum levels of short- and medium-chain fatty acids have also been implicated and may act as depressants of neuronal membranes. High levels of methanethiol (methylmercaptan), derived from methionine, may be present and act synergistically with ammonia and short-chain fatty acids in the production of encephalopathy. Another potential causative factor is alpha-ketoglutaramate, a glutamine derivative formed by transamination, which is found in high concentrations in the cerebrospinal fluid of patients with hepatic encephalopathy and which may interfere with neurotransmission. In addition, phenylethylamines, formed from phenylalanine and tyrosine, may displace or inhibit production of norepinephrine and act as false neurotransmitters in the central nervous system (CNS). Elevated plasma levels of aromatic amino acids associated with depressed branched-chain amino acids have also been implicated in the pathogenesis. Hypoglycemia is present in about 5% of patients with massive hepatic necrosis and may also contribute to encephalopathy. Although similar metabolic disturbances may be involved in the pathogenesis of encephalopathy in massive hepatic necrosis and advanced chronic liver disease, differences in prognosis are striking and discussion of therapy requires, for the present, separation of the two clinical entities.

Massive Hepatic Necrosis

The syndrome of massive hepatic necrosis, symptoms of which are fulminant hepatitis and acute yellow atrophy, can be defined as acute necrosis of sufficient severity to produce alterations of mental status and behavior. Diminution in liver size and progressive jaundice are characteristic but are not required for diagnosis. The chief causes of massive hepatic necrosis are acute viral hepatitis (hepatitis A, B, etc.), drug hepatotoxic reactions, e.g., halothane hepatitis and mushroom poisoning, hypoperfusion syndromes, and, infrequently, chronic active hepatitis. A similar clinical picture has been observed in Reye's syndrome in children, acute fatty liver of pregnancy, and tetracycline-induced liver disease. In

TABLE 15-1 Staging of Hepatic Encephalopathy in Massive Hepatic Necrosis

State	Mental Status	Asterixis	EEG	Survival Rate (%)
I	Euphoria/depression Mild confusion Slurred speech Disordered sleep	±	Usually normal	
II	Lethargy/confusion	+	Abnormal	75
III	Sleeping but rousable Incoherent speech Marked confusion	+	Abnormal	
IV	Coma; may or may not respond to noxious stimuli	−	Abnormal	10–35

these disorders examination of liver tissue reveals hepatic fatty accumulation rather than extensive necrosis.

Prognosis in massive hepatic necrosis may be determined by staging. The criteria shown in Table 15-1 have been useful. The survival rate with conventional therapy in stages I to III is approximately 75%. In contrast, only 10 to 35% of patients who reach stage IV are likely to survive. Age also influences recovery rates, because only 5 to 10% of patients over 40 years of age will recover from stage IV encephalopathy. Recent studies suggest that early liver biopsy with estimation of liver cell mass may be of value in estimating the prognosis and probability of regeneration. The bleeding diathesis usually present in these patients makes this procedure quite hazardous in inexperienced hands without superb hemostasis backup. Alpha-fetoprotein levels may be elevated during hepatic regeneration, but their utility as a prognostic marker is not yet certain.

A number of complications may contribute importantly to mortality in massive hepatic necrosis. Cerebral edema has been observed in patients with or without assisted ventilation. Sepsis and peptic ulceration with bleeding and/or perforation have been noted in patients treated with corticosteroids, although this complication has also occurred in the absence of corticosteroid therapy. Hemostasis disturbances, including impaired synthesis of clotting factors, abnormal platelet function, thrombocytopenia, and disseminated intravascular coagulation (DIC), may result in overt bleeding. Renal and respiratory failure are commonly noted, and aspiration may be the *coup de grace*.

ADVANCED CHRONIC LIVER DISEASE WITH PORTAL-SYSTEMIC VENOUS ADMIXTURE

Hepatic encephalopathy in advanced chronic liver disease with portal-systemic venous admixture may be acute, chronic, or both. Approximately 20 to 33% of patients with surgically constructed portacaval anastomosis may develop chronic hepatic encephalopathy or recurrent acute encephalopathy.

Although chronic or acute hepatic encephalopathy may be a feature of progressive, end-stage liver disease (alcoholic cirrhosis, postnecrotic cirrhosis), more often than not acute encephalopathy is precipitated by exogenous factors. Important precipitants which appear to increase intestinal ammonia production include gastrointestinal bleeding, excessive protein ingestion, constipation, and azotemia. Diuretic therapy, hypokalemia, and alkalosis are common identifiable factors which may act by altering ammonia production and distribution.

Administration of sedative and hypnotic agents which depress the CNS is a notorious precipitant, for the half-lives of these agents are usually prolonged in patients with liver disease and more free drug will be available in the presence of hypoalbuminemia. Encephalopathy may be provoked by local or systemic infection, dehydration, hypotension, overzealous therapeutic paracentesis, minor surgical procedures, and general anesthesia. The prognosis of any single episode of hepatic encephalopathy precipitated by such factors is considerably better than that of encephalopathy in massive hepatic necrosis. Furthermore, the prognosis in patients with an identified precipitating event is better than that of patients without such a precipitant.

Therapy of Hepatic Encephalopathy in Massive Hepatic Necrosis

The goal of treatment in this setting is to sustain vital functions while awaiting regeneration and repair of the damaged liver. Concomitantly with maintaining life functions, one attempts to avoid or treat promptly those complications which may impair the chances of survival.

Specific Measures of Therapy Hospitalization in an intensive care unit is highly desirable. Good nursing care requirements include maintenance of an open airway, frequent turning of the patient, and scrupulous care of intravenous infusion sites.

Protein ingestion is halted. Protein-free nourishment may be provided orally or by nasogastric tube (thin diameter) with 20% glucose or protein-free, carbohydrate-rich commercial preparations. Intravenous glucose will be necessary for the patient in deep coma or when hypoglycemia occurs. Multivitamins, especially thiamine, should be given parenterally. Presently available hyperalimentation fluid preparations have not been helpful. Newer formulations, varying the amino acid composition or employing alpha-keto precursors of amino acids which trap ammonia, are under study. Cathartics or bowel cleansing agents should be given to remove protein from the bowel. Oils are avoided because of the risk of aspiration.

Intravenous fluids and electrolytes are given as needed to maintain fluid and electrolyte balance. Functional renal failure (the hepatorenal syndrome) may develop in approximately a third of patients. Osmotic loading and diuretic agents are best avoided in these patients. Infrequently, severe metabolic acidosis, usually caused by lactic acidosis, may require therapy with bicarbonate. Hypernatremia may result from injudicious intravenous administration of large quantities of fresh frozen plasma or hypertonic glucose. Frequent monitoring of serum sodium concentration is necessary.

Minimally absorbed antibiotics are used to suppress intestinal bacteria. Neomycin may be given orally or by a thin-diameter nasogastric tube, in a dose of 4 to 8 gm daily. It may be given rectally as a 1% retention enema; however, this is not recommended, for poor retention and penetration are common and may impede the antibiotic's efficacy. Adverse reactions are uncommon with short-term therapy in massive hepatic necrosis. Paromomycin in a dose of 50 to 75 mg/kg (in divided doses) may be used but has no decided advantage over neomycin. Experience with lactulose (see below) is very limited.

Unproved Drug Treatment Corticosteroids have been used for over 20 years in the treatment of massive hepatic necrosis. They are usually administered intravenously in large doses (0.5 to 1.0 gm of hydrocortisone daily) and may be responsible for some complications. Their efficacy remains uncertain. A randomized prospective trial of corticosteroid therapy in massive hepatic necrosis caused by viral and drug-induced hepatitis is underway.

L-Dopa has been used in daily oral doses of 2 to 12 gm. In a few patients hepatic encephalopathy was transiently reversed, presumably because L-dopa replaces false neurotransmitter amines or serves as the CNS precursor of norepinephrine. The general experience with this agent has, however, been disappointing, and the drug may induce gastric erosions and bleeding.

Infusion of plasma containing high titers of antibody to the hepatitis B surface antigen has been shown not to affect survival in patients with massive hepatic necrosis due to hepatitis B.

Massive hepatic necrosis caused by ingestion of poisonous mushrooms may respond to treatment with thioctic (alpha-lipoic) acid (presently available only through the National Institutes of Health, Bethesda, Maryland). Controlled trials of this agent are not yet available.

Dramatic Therapy A number of dramatic measures have been used in heroic attempts to halt or reverse encephalopathy in massive hepatic necrosis. Exchange transfusion; plasmapheresis; cross-circulation with human volunteers, nonhuman primates, or the perfused livers of other mammals; hemodialysis or peritoneal dialysis; asanguineous total body washout with hypothermia; and most recently hemoperfusion over charcoal have all had their advocates. A single randomized trial of exchange transfusion indicated no therapeutic value for this method (see Table 15-2). The other forms of therapy have not yet been critically assessed by carefully controlled prospective studies.

Therapy of Hepatic Encephalopathy in Advanced Chronic Liver Disease with Portal-Systemic Admixture

The goal of therapy in this clinical setting is to restore the patient to his or her optimal pre-encephalopathy state. The major initial effort should

TABLE 15-2 Exchange Transfusion in Massive Hepatic Necrosis

Randomization Group	No. Patients	Survivors	
		No.	%
Exchange transfusion	15	1	7
Actually performed	8	0	0
Not performed	7	1	14
No exchange transfusion	13	4	31

Adapted from Redeker, A. G., and Yamahiro, H. S. Controlled trial of exchange transfusion therapy in fulminant hepatitis. *Lancet* 1:3–6, 1973.

be directed toward identification and correction of factors which may have precipitated encephalopathy, e.g., gastrointestinal bleeding or hypokalemia.

As in massive necrosis, excellent nursing care is a necessity, although it is often not practical to treat each patient in an intensive care unit. Patients with profuse gastrointestinal hemorrhage or stage IV encephalopathy may do better in such a unit. Regardless of where therapy is undertaken, prevention of aspiration and of sepsis are mandatory.

Dietary treatment includes discontinuation of protein but maintenance of adequate calories and vitamins with carbohydrate preparations and multivitamins. With improvement of clinical status, protein intake may be increased slowly in 10-gm increments. Purgatives and enemas are given to diminish the protein content in the gut. Electrolyte and fluid balance are maintained with care to avoid severe dilutional hyponatremia or hypernatremia, both with adverse cerebral consequences. Functional renal failure is treated conservatively without either tubular or osmotic diuretics.

Neomycin is given orally in a daily dose of 1 to 4 gm. Long-term neomycin therapy may be associated with malabsorption, particularly of vitamin K, which should be given parenterally. Because 1 to 3% of orally or rectally administered neomycin is absorbed, one must be aware of the possibility of renal toxicity (check creatinine and urinalysis) and sensorineural hearing loss caused by neomycin-induced ototoxicity. Renal excretion of absorbed neomycin may produce a sterile urine despite signs of urinary tract infection. In a very few patients bacterial resistance to neomycin may be responsible for therapeutic failure. Paromomycin may be used in lieu of neomycin as previously indicated.

A synthetic disaccharide, lactulose, consisting of galactose and fructose, may be given orally, instead of the aminoglycoside antibiotics, in a dose of 15 to 30 ml 4 times daily. Because man has no disaccharidase capable of splitting lactulose, lactulose is broken down by bacterial enzymatic activity in the terminal ileum and colon, producing an acidic diarrhea. Lactulose appears to be as effective as neomycin with fewer side effects. The mechanism of action of lactulose is not completely understood.

The role of L-dopa in the treatment of encephalopathy in advanced liver disease is uncertain. Although corticosteroids have been reported in one study to be effective in encephalopathy associated with alcoholic hepatitis, in four other studies no evidence of efficacy was obtained. Their use is not recommended.

Dramatic measures in the treatment of encephalopathy in advanced liver disease are impractical and probably ineffective, although studies are extremely limited at present.

Practical Management in Hepatic Encephalopathy

It is important to avoid potential CNS-depressant drugs in patients with liver disease. If treatment with such an agent is absolutely necessary, it should be given in small doses with careful reevaluation before repeated administration.

The patient with encephalopathy should have, at least twice a day, a carefully performed and recorded examination of mental status, including serial-seven subtraction, recording of handwriting, and simple constructional tasks, to assess the efficacy of treatment.

Assessment of electrolytes, weight alteration, and hydration must be performed on a regular basis. Each stool specimen and nasogastric aspirate collected in the encephalopathic patient should be examined for evidence of gastrointestinal bleeding. Frequent examination for occult infection is mandatory. In the patient with encephalopathy and ascites, spontaneous bacterial peritonitis is not unusual, and clinical signs of infection may be minimal.

Avoidance of overvigorous diuresis and paracentesis is necessary to prevent the development of encephalopathy in ascitic cirrhotic patients. Therapeutic paracentesis should be limited to 1 to 2 liters and reserved, as indicated above, for patients with impending umbilical hernia rupture or severe respiratory embarrassment.

COAGULATION DISTURBANCES

Impaired hemostasis may contribute to the bleeding episodes frequently complicating hepatic failure. Decreased synthesis of clotting factors in the liver is common, but only rarely is it so profound as to be considered of major importance. In these instances infusion of fresh frozen plasma may restore hemostasis.

Laboratory evidence of DIC, presumably caused by impaired clearance of activated coagulation factors, has been obtained in some patients with massive hepatic necrosis as well as in patients with advanced liver disease. In most, but not all, patients, the DIC associated with liver disease is self-limiting and asymptomatic. When DIC appears to be contributing to clinical deterioration and the diagnosis of DIC is unequivocal, emergency treatment with heparin may be attempted. The effectiveness of heparin for DIC associated with hepatic failure is unknown.

Fibrinolytic activity is often increased in patients with liver disease. This is generally believed to be a compensatory response to accelerated coagulation. In a few patients fibrinolysis may be primary. Treatment of these rare persons remains controversial, and heparin is often administered before antifibrinolytic agents.

Thrombocytopenia, caused by consumption or hypersplenism and defective platelet aggregation, may contribute further to the impaired hemostasis of the patient with liver disease. Platelet concentrates may provide temporary control of bleeding in some instances.

HEPATORENAL SYNDROME

The development of functional oliguric renal failure in patients with liver disease is ominous. The diagnosis of the hepatorenal syndrome is dependent, at present, on the exclusion of other forms of reversible renal failure. A trial of volume expansion may be attempted judiciously with monitoring of central venous pressure, in order to exclude prerenal azotemia due to diminished "effective" blood volume. Volume expansion may precipitate gastrointestinal hemorrhage and should be continued only in those patients who respond favorably. Treatment for nonresponders is unsettled, and their prognosis is dismal. Hemodynamically appropriate, but transient, effects have been claimed following treatment of the hepatorenal syndrome with L-dopa, corticosteroids, dopamine, Dibenzyline, metaraminol, and phenylalanine-vasopressin, but their efficacy remains undefined by controlled clinical trials.

SELECTED READINGS

Conn, H. O. A rational approach to the hepatorenal syndrome. *Gastroenterology* 65:321–340, 1973.

Conn, H. O. The Rational Management of Ascites. In Popper, H., and Schaffner, F. (Eds.), *Progress in Liver Diseases*. New York: Grune & Stratton, 1974. Pp. 269–288.

Fischer, J. E., Yoshimura, N., Aguirre, A., et al. Plasma amino acids in patients with hepatic encephalopathy: Effects of amino acid infusions. *Am. J. Surg.* 127:40–47, 1974.

Redeker, A. G., and Yamahiro, H. S. Controlled trial of exchange-transfusion therapy in fulminant hepatitis. *Lancet* 1:3–6, 1973.

Schenker, S., Breen, K. J., and Hoyumpa, A. M. Hepatic encephalopathy: Current status. *Gastroenterology* 66:121–151, 1974.

Scotto, J., Opolon, P., Étévé, J., et al. Liver biopsy and prognosis in acute liver failure. *Gut* 14:927–933, 1973.

Vergara, F., Plum, F., and Duffy, T. E. α-Ketoglutaramate: Increased concentrations in the cerebrospinal fluid of patients in hepatic coma. *Science* 183:81–83, 1974.

Wilkinson, S. P., Blendis, L. M., and Williams, R. Frequency and type of renal and electrolyte disorders in fulminant hepatic failure. *Br. Med. J.* 1:186–189, 1974.

Zimmerman, H. J. Hepatic Failure. In Gall, E. A., and Mostofi, F. K. (Eds.), *The Liver*. Baltimore: Williams & Wilkins, 1973. Pp. 384–405.

16

PSYCHIATRIC EMERGENCIES

Ethan Samuel Rofman

FEW CRISES are more capable of disrupting the normal activity of a well-run emergency unit than those precipitated by a psychiatric emergency. House officers who treat ventricular fibrillation with assurance and speed often find themselves withdrawing when confronted with an acute schizophrenic psychosis. The tendency to avoid mentally disturbed or disturbing patients often arises because staff have usually received little training in practical emergency psychiatry. In this discussion, the most common types of psychiatric emergencies will be outlined, drugs commonly used in their management will be discussed, and some general psychiatric interviewing principles will be presented.

The common types of psychiatric emergencies can be divided into six categories: those in which (1) the patient's behavior is a potential hazard to himself and others; (2) the patient's disordered thinking produces abnormal behavior; (3) the patient's affect is a source of concern; (4) a toxic substance has been ingested; (5) the patient is elderly; and (6) legal concerns lead to psychiatric intervention.

THE PATIENT'S BEHAVIOR IS A POTENTIAL HAZARD TO HIMSELF AND OTHERS

Much of the fear associated with psychiatric emergencies derives from the violent, assaultive, or destructive patient, although the actual number of these patients is often exaggerated. Violent behavior is not peculiar to any one type of diagnosis, although it is most commonly associated with metabolic toxicity, character disorder, or paranoid schizophrenia. It must consequently be approached from both a psychodynamic and an organic point of view.

Psychodynamically, violent behavior can be viewed as a defense mechanism by means of which the individual protects himself from unbearable inner feelings of helplessness and fragility. Organically, it can be viewed as a disorder of a specific cerebral anatomic structure and/or electrical and metabolic function. The former approach eventually leads to a search for events, feelings, and conflicts which may help to explain seemingly unintelligible aggressive outbursts. The latter leads to a search for head injury, electrical disturbances of the brain (especially temporal lobe epilepsy), and metabolic abnormalities such as barbiturate or alcohol use or withdrawal, electrolyte imbalance, or hypoxia. For most patients, a combined psychodynamic and organic approach is most useful.

On an emergency service certain methods of management may need to be instituted before psychodynamic or organic diagnosis can be established. Patients who are so agitated and out of control that they will not respond to reasonable attempts at verbal or pharmacological control may have to be brought to a horizontal position on the floor by no less than four or five security men or attendants, in order to ensure safety to both patient and staff. Advance planning in such cases is necessary so that no one gets hurt. It is useful to have a mattress or soft carpet already on the floor. Action, when taken by the staff, should be quick and decisive, rather than ambivalent. Spectators should be cleared from the area, for they seldom understand and usually misinterpret what is happening. One man for each extremity and one to hold the head generally prevents injury. A stretcher can be placed under the patient and sheet or cuff restraints employed to maintain secure control. No person should ever attempt to subdue a violent patient without help.

The physician should not actively involve himself in the physical handling of the patient, for it will hamper later attempts at interviewing. After securing the patient in a horizontal position, medication should be offered to help him maintain his own control. By offering a choice of oral or injected medication, the physician can begin the process of asking the patient to assume control of himself and of his behavior. Once the patient is securely restrained and medicated, it is useful to speak with him alone. The physician should convey the attitude that he believes the patient to be a decent fellow human being who is struggling to control difficult thoughts and feelings. After the physician's assurance that he will not let any harm come to the patient nor let anyone else be harmed by the patient, neutral questions should be asked, such as, "What is your name?" and "Where are you from?" This should be done in order to establish a basis from which to proceed to the issues which produced the agitation. It is useful to acknowledge the patient's power and ask him what happened to make him want to give up control, while always maintaining an impartial and nonthreatening attitude oneself.

A most frightening situation is one in which a patient produces a weapon, especially a gun. If this happens, and it is impossible to get out of the area quickly and safely, one may try saying such things as, "You can do a lot of harm if you want to, even without that gun. You look frightened and I feel frightened. I'd like to help you, but I'm concerned that you might do something you can't take back with that gun. Could you please put it down or let me hold it for you until we can finish talking about what is troubling you?" Above all, one should keep on talking, allow no prolonged silences to develop, and make no abrupt movements. If the patient is psychotic, one should ask if he is hearing frightening voices and offer help in testing them against reality. If the patient will not give up his weapon, he may at least be willing to put it into his pocket or into a nearby desk drawer.

Where the physician stands in a room is important, as the patient may feel comfortable and cooperative or trapped and cornered. He should be offered free access to the exit and he should be asked if he would feel better leaving the room or staying there. If he leaves, the physician should warn personnel to clear the area and call for police help.

After any restraining of or altercation with a violent patient, a meeting of all staff concerned is a necessity. A chance to air feelings about what was done and explain why it was done is the minimum support needed by all persons involved. A similar opportunity should be provided to the patient if he can be seen in a follow-up visit.

THE PATIENT'S DISORDERED THINKING PRODUCES ABNORMAL BEHAVIOR

THE FIRST BREAK SCHIZOPHRENIC

Schizophrenia usually occurs in a young person between the ages of 16 and 30. Flat affect, loosening of associations, delusions that thoughts, moods, or actions are mysteriously influenced by other people or strange forces, hallucinations of thoughts being broadcast or spoken aloud, the delusion that others know what the patient is thinking, as well as specific catatonic symptoms such as rigidity, waxy flexibility, and posturing, when present, make the diagnosis of schizophrenia extremely likely. Apathy, inappropriate affect, autism, auditory hallucinations, bodily hallucinations, and catatonic excitement and stupor are less specific for a diagnosis of schizophrenia but are very common and, when present, make the diagnosis very likely. Other symptoms of schizophrenia are also frequently seen in other conditions. These include paranoid delusions, ideas of reference, inappropriate behavior, extreme social isolation, markedly unstable interpersonal relationships, poor academic and occupational adjustment, and excessive concern with physical symptoms. Visual hallucinations, disorientation as to time, place, and person, and fecal or urinary incontinence rarely occur in schizophrenia and should lead the physician to think of neurological disorders such as brain tumor, delirium tremens, or toxic psychosis as possible causes. If the patient is clearly schizophrenic and relatively cooperative, the ideal plan is to have him transported to a psychiatric hospital without medication. This gives the admitting physician at the psychiatric facility a chance to observe the patient's pathology more clearly. It is frustrating for the admitting psychiatrist to interview a new patient who is sleepy from too much medication. Often the family can be enlisted to transport the patient, eliminating the need for medication or an ambulance. If medication is required, which is frequently the case, haloperidol (Haldol) is an excellent choice. If pregnancy is suspected, however, chlorpromazine (Thorazine) is preferable.

In most states it is worthwhile to send a request form for involuntary hospitalization with the patient even if he seems willing to enter the psychiatric hospital voluntarily. In Massachusetts an opportunity to sign a voluntary admission paper must, in any case, be offered to all patients before admission. The involuntary form may be of great assistance to the psychiatric institution if admission is resisted at the last minute. In Massachusetts any licensed physician may fill out a request for 10-day temporary involuntary hospitalization.

The Chronic Schizophrenic

Since the advent of community psychiatry in the late 1960s, a large number of patients formerly housed in the back wards of state mental hospitals have been discharged into foster homes or directly into the community. Unfortunately, their follow-up treatment may not be comprehensive. From time to time, these patients may stop taking their medication, their therapists may go away, or they may not have a therapist at all. These circumstances commonly lead to decompensation and abnormal behavior indistinguishable in symptoms from acute schizophrenia. If this behavior is observed in a public place, such persons are likely to be brought to the emergency service by the police. Occasionally, they will wander into the emergency room on their own or be brought by other agents, such as relatives, nurses, or foster home care personnel.

The problem facing the emergency room physician is whether to hospitalize or to send the patient back to his community placement. A fivefold assessment similar to that suggested by Anderson and Kuehnle may prove useful (Table 16-1). First, one should determine if the exacerbation is due to a physical illness requiring medical treatment. It is common for schizophrenic people to exhibit more psychopathology when they become physically ill. This usually improves once they are hospitalized for medical or psychiatric purposes. Second, one should assess the degree to which the patient is suicidal or homicidal. If he is dangerous to himself

TABLE 16-1 Evaluation of the Chronic Schizophrenic Patient

Question	Action
Is exacerbation due to physical illness?	Hospitalize for care of medical illness
Is patient suicidal or homicidal?	Hospitalize in psychiatric hospital with temporary commitment if necessary
What medication does patient take and who prescribes it?	Reinstitute medication. Add antiparkinsonian agent if necessary. Contact physician who prescribes medication for patient, both to find out what patient is taking and to inform him of what you plan to do
Is patient able to reality-test his symptoms?	If patient cannot see the unrealistic quality of his symptoms he needs rehospitalization
What is the nature of patient's social and family support?	Contact family and social agents to obtain information and to inform them of your thinking and plans

or others, he should be rehospitalized. Third, one should determine what medication the patient has been receiving, who gives it to him, and if he has recently stopped taking it. If the patient receives weekly injections of fluphenazine enanthate (Prolixin enanthate) he may be experiencing an extrapyramidal reaction. In these cases, institution or reinstitution of antiparkinsonian medication quickly relieves the symptoms and prevents rehospitalization. If cessation of antipsychotic medication has led to the exacerbation, it is often possible to reinstitute pharmacotherapy without rehospitalizing the patient. Fourth, one should evaluate the patient's contact with reality. Does he know he is talking to a doctor? Has he come to the emergency room for help? Does he behave appropriately in the hospital? When answered positively, these questions usually indicate relatively good reality testing. If the patient "knows" that the physician is the devil and that he wishes to deprive him of his sexual powers, if he thinks that the emergency room is basically a massage parlor, then his reality testing is poor. Delusional or hallucinating patients often can disregard their symptoms and participate in their evaluation in an appropriate way. They will say they are deluded or hearing voices, but that they have learned not to pay attention to these inner commands and beliefs. Patients unable to ignore the dictates of their hallucinations or delusions most often need rehospitalization. Finally, one should assess what family or social supports the patient actually has. If he is living in a foster home or cooperative apartment, and the person in charge can be reached, this will greatly aid in deciding whether the patient can return there or must be sent to a hospital. If adequate community follow-up cannot be arranged, he probably should be sent to the hospital and not back into the community.

THE PATIENT'S AFFECT IS A SOURCE OF CONCERN

DEPRESSION

When a patient comes to the emergency service and says that he is depressed, it is useful to ask him what he means. People who say they are depressed may actually be very angry and unable to say so; they may be medically ill and not realize it; or they may indeed be depressed. If they are depressed, it is sometimes hard for them to know or to say whether they are having a reactive, event-related depression or an endogenous depression unrelated to events. The differentiation between these two syndromes is difficult and frequently not precise. It is useful for the emergency room physician to distinguish those patients with severe psychomotor retardation from those who are potentially suicidal and from those who can be referred for continued treatment on an outpatient basis.

If the patient is barely communicative, has slowed, painful speech, mentions trouble with concentration and memory, feels terribly guilty about inconsequential occurrences, describes worthlessness, has severe insomnia of any type, as well as constipation, weight loss, and a diminished interest in sexual activity in the face of a completely unrevealing medical study for mimicking organic diseases, the most likely diagnosis is severe depressive illness. Psychiatric hospitalization in such cases should definitely be discussed with the family and realistically considered. Vigorous treatment is indicated for this condition, either with antidepressant medication or electroconvulsive therapy (ECT), and is best instituted on an inpatient basis.

All depressed patients should be questioned regarding previous suicide attempts, as well as current thoughts, plans, and actions. Family history of suicide makes it a less forbidden form of action and should be asked about specifically. In general, the questions outlined in the next section on suicide risk evaluation should be asked where suicidal ideation is suspected. Despite common fears, direct questioning about suicidal thoughts or plans seldom precipitates the action.

For the patient who has recently separated from a loved one, failed an examination, lost a job, or is suffering from any other recent disappointment, the best policy is to allow time for ventilation, offer a sympathetic ear, and refer the patient for further psychiatric treatment as seems necessary. Reassurance that most depressions are self-limited and do improve with time is useful. Many patients who are depressed come to the accident floor simply because they do not know how one goes about finding a psychiatrist. Your job then is to see that the patient has a reasonable referral.

A patient's depression may manifest itself mainly in physical complaints. For any patient with persistent puzzling physical symptoms with normal medical studies, depression should be considered as one possible underlying cause.

SUICIDE RISK

One needs to evaluate the degree of true risk of suicide in a patient who is threatening suicide or who has made an unsuccessful suicide attempt. The techniques employed in doing this have evolved from statistical studies and clinical experience. There is no simple, reliable test which can be given to make this difficult clinical judgment. It is best to err on the conservative side—when in doubt, hospitalize.

At the Boston City Hospital residents are encouraged to ask the following questions, similar to those suggested by Stengel, of patients who have made recent suicide attempts:

1. What were the circumstances (social adjustment, work and financial adjustment, sexual and marital adjustment, emotional tone, recent losses) which led up to your attempt?
2. What were your motives for the attempt?
3. How were you feeling at the time of the attempt?
4. Did you really wish to die?
5. What do you think being dead would be like?
6. What do you think the reactions of your friends and relatives will be like?
7. Was a note left, and what did it contain?
8. Has the attempt changed in any way the factors which brought it about?

9. Have any people, who you feel care about you, visited you since the attempt and what have their reactions been?
10. What are your plans for the future?
11. In retrospect, how do you feel about the attempt?

In an effort to develop criteria for utilization review of treatment for suicide attempters, Kirstein lists 9 criteria which, in the opinion of several experts, ought to lead to psychiatric hospitalization of a patient who has made a recent suicide attempt. These criteria are:

1. A clear lethal suicide *plan*
2. A recent *history* of medically serious suicide attempts
3. The presence of suicidal thoughts, gestures, or attempts in association with a *thought disorder*
4. A *recent progression in the seriousness* of suicidal thoughts, to the point of action
5. An *expectation of hospitalization* which cannot be changed during the interview
6. The presence of *high-risk circumstances,* such as severe depression, social isolation, recent loss, alcoholism, or painful chronic disease
7. A *current, clear* suicide attempt
8. The expression of strong suicidal thoughts with intent and *without seeing any other way out*
9. The *expectation of change in behavior* of significant others due to suicidal behavior is *not met;* change cannot be accomplished appropriately

Although some experts feel that the presence of any one of these criteria should lead to psychiatric hospitalization, the 4 operationalized criteria which were most important to determine disposition in actual clinical practice were:

1. The risk of suicidal behavior by the patient in the near future
2. Motivations based on a thought disorder
3. The seriousness of the patient's intent to kill himself
4. The seriousness of the major medical effects of the attempt

Another essential criterion requiring assessment is the patient's perception of the availability of people who really care about whether he lives or dies. The importance of evaluating the patient's subjective view, rather than the physician's objective assessment, is stressed here. A person may have loving relatives or friends, but the severity of his depression or impaired thinking may result in his feeling that they are unavailable to him.

Aside from the case of the immediate suicide risk, it is sometimes worthwhile to hospitalize a patient with a less serious suicide attempt. This is done when the person involved could benefit from establishing a relationship with a psychiatrist but would not usually find making such a contact acceptable.

Hypochondriacal Panic Reactions

The prototypical patient with a hypochrondriacal panic reaction is the person with chest pain who fears he is dying of a heart attack. The first step in managing such a patient is a careful medical history, physical examination, and laboratory assessment. If the physician is unsure of his diagnosis, the patient will pick up the uncertainty and become more anxious. The taking of the pulse, the percussion of the chest, and the use of the stethoscope usually provide rapid, if only partial, relief of the patient's fright.

An approach which is frequently helpful is to ask the patient, "What do you think this pain means?" or "What are you afraid of and how would you like us to help you?" If the physician understands the patient's fears, he can address his diagnostic efforts in a manner which will tend to reduce them.

Assuming that myocardial infarction and medical conditions which mimic it have been ruled out, the physician must then provide the patient with an alternative explanation for the pain. Acid reflux into the esophagus followed by spasm of the cardiac sphincter is an explanation which is usually acceptable. Once the physical symptom is explained, the panic can then be explored separately with a question such as, "What could be going on in your life right now that might cause you to fear your symptoms so much?" The principle here is to avoid a contest with the patient over the reality of his symptoms while trying to elicit his participation in an introspective inquiry. If depression is suspected, one might say, "Are there some reasons, other than heart attack, which could cause you to fear not living?" Taking a history of recent losses, deaths, family illnesses, and anniversaries may reveal otherwise hidden precipitants.

The physician must acknowledge the existence of the patient's discomfort. To minimize the symptoms may exacerbate the panic reaction. Without denying the pain, the physician needs to reassure the patient that the symptoms are not caused by anything serious or life-threatening. After doing this, the physician may offer an alternative explanation. It is important that the patient explicitly accept his explanation. If he does not, he will probably return to the emergency room or seek care elsewhere.

If medication is required, the minor tranquilizers are preferred. Hospitalization of these patients is seldom necessary. A follow-up visit to the psychiatry outpatient department is usually indicated.

Hyperventilation Syndrome

The symptoms of air hunger, panicky fear, numbness and tingling of the extremities, muscular twitching and spasms, and lightheadedness characteristic of the hyperventilation syndrome are frequently encountered by the emergency room physician. The syndrome arises as a symptom either of primary anxiety or of anxiety secondary to physical disorder, such as angina pectoris, gallbladder colic, or asthma. It is useful to think of the syndrome as a response to physical pain coupled with great fear.

The simplest treatment for hyperventilation is to have the patient re-breathe into a paper bag. This relieves the symptoms which result from loss of carbon dioxide and accompanying alkalosis and gives the patient a task which distracts his thinking from the original source of pain and fear. Again, it is often useful to spend some time taking the pulse while calmly trying to take a history. Minor tranquilizers may prove useful as a means of sedation.

Once the patient is sufficiently calm to talk, it is important to uncover and make efforts to treat the emotional stress which usually has triggered the episode. It is common to hear about phobic reactions and fears of death, dying, and loss when one listens to the associations of these patients. Hyperventilation is also a frequent symptom of grief, mourning, and separation. When the patient himself cannot clearly identify his feelings and relate them to the events in his life, a family member can often provide useful additional information.

A TOXIC SUBSTANCE HAS BEEN INGESTED

ALCOHOL INTOXICATION

The confusional state produced by acute alcohol intoxication is one of the most difficult problems for the house officer to treat. He must be wary of medical complications, such as delirium tremens, subdural hematoma, seizures, and hepatic coma. At the same time, he must contend with a patient whose emotional controls are distorted by alcohol. Drunkenness itself produces moroseness on top of depression, combativeness on top of anger.

Boston City Hospital is fortunate to have a special area where patients suspected of being confused owing to alcohol ingestion can be controlled and observed for several hours under medical supervision. Watchful waiting without unnecessary active intervention is the safest and most desirable procedure to follow in the management of intoxicated patients. This is true both medically and psychiatrically. Time and again, we have seen assaultive and suicidal patients leave the accident floor in a cooperative, apologetic state. The history which then emerges is far different from the despair and urgency expressed during the period of intoxication.

No acutely intoxicated patient should leave an accident floor without an evaluation of the circumstances which led to his intoxication and the overall pattern of his alcohol use. If chronic alcoholism is a problem, appropriate referral should be made. Having alcoholism counselors on the accident floor greatly improves the possibility of an alcoholic person entering a treatment program. If the patient is not an alcoholic, psychiatric referral may be indicated for an underlying emotional problem. If sedation of an extremely belligerent patient is required, we find that one dose of haloperidol (Haldol), 1 to 2 mg I.M., is a very effective tranquilizer. Medication must, however, be used with extreme caution in patients with very high blood alcohol levels, as it may cause respiratory depression and coma.

ALCOHOLIC HALLUCINATIONS

Acute alcoholic hallucinosis exists on a continuum with delirium tremens and is a serious psychiatric emergency. Frank delirium tremens often occurs after several hours or days of hallucinosis. Because these patients are often oriented to time, place, and person and are not tremulous, it is important to distinguish them from schizophrenics. The former require prompt and careful medical observation, whereas the latter are best treated in a psychiatric facility. Illusions and visual hallucinations can usually be noted in those patients with delirium tremens or alcoholic hallucinosis, if they are carefully interviewed. Auditory hallucinations and delusions, when present, are almost always of the paranoid type.

Patients with delirium tremens or alcoholic hallucinosis should be treated as if they were suicidal, even when they deny self-destructive feelings. They may hang themselves from pipes in the bathroom, run out into the street in front of cars, or jump from windows in an attempt to escape from terrifying auditory or visual hallucinations. In these patients, suicide is often an occurrence difficult to predict. It may happen despite improving physical and mental status.

PSYCHIATRIC PROBLEMS RELATED TO DRUG ABUSE

With the current use and abuse of drugs in our society, the emergency room physician has frequent contact with several drug-related psychiatric problems in addition to the medical problems discussed in Chapter 1. Some of the most commonly encountered are psychotometic drug reaction, barbiturate-type overdose with or without withdrawal, and simulation of medical and psychiatric illness in order to manipulate drugs from the unwary physician.

The "bad trip" from lysergic acid diethylamide (LSD) seen commonly in the late sixties is still an occasional occurrence. If not too severe, it usually responds to a supportive protective environment and "talking the patient down." Phenothiazines, or preferably haloperidol (Haldol), may be used to calm the patient as well. If the patient cannot be watched closely by supportive family or friends until the panic clears, hospitalization is indicated.

Barbiturate addiction is an increasingly familiar drug problem. Other sedatives and minor tranquilizers, such as glutethimide (Doriden), methyprylon (Noludar), meprobamate (Miltown), chlordiazepoxide (Librium), and diazepam (Valium), also produce barbiturate-type dependence to a milder degree. Lateral gaze nystagmus, dysarthria, ataxia, decreased alertness, confusion, memory disruption, disorientation, and emotional instability are seen in patients intoxicated, but not yet comatose, from barbiturates. The emotional instability these patients manifest often has a paranoid aggressive character. Hospitalization of such patients in a medical environment is indicated to observe the progression of their symptoms. If symptoms increase, the patient may progress to coma and require supportive medical treatment. If they lessen, and the patient is addicted to barbiturates, prompt attention to the barbiturate withdrawal syndrome is imperative, because abrupt abstinence may lead to hallucinations or life-threatening status epilepticus. Patients who show signs of barbiturate withdrawal should be hospitalized for barbiturate tolerance testing and subsequent gradual withdrawal, as outlined by Wikler (see Selected Readings).

When known heroin overdose brings the patient to the hospital, naloxone hydrochloride (Narcan), 0.4 mg I.M., is the narcotic antagonist of choice, because it produces no respiratory depression of its own. If addiction is suspected, but denied by the patient, a test dose of naloxone, 0.4 mg, will rapidly produce withdrawal symptoms if the patient is lying.

Many patients addicted to heroin or maintained on methadone appear at the emergency service in order to obtain extra drugs, such as the benzodiazapines or barbiturates. Most have access to the *Physicians' Desk Reference* and medical texts and are able to simulate various syndromes in order to manipulate a prescription from the unsuspecting physician. A patient may believe that if he becomes unpleasant or anxious enough, the physician will give him a prescription just to get rid of him. Unfortunately, there is no clearly definable way to separate the manipulator from other patients, which is why manipulative patients cause their physicians to feel considerable uncertainty, anger, and guilt.

THE PATIENT IS ELDERLY

It is common for local nursing homes and family to bring in elderly confused men and women when their behavior becomes intolerable to others. Sometimes such people arrive on the accident floor with fungating tumors and then refuse treatment with a statement such as, "I don't want to stay in this sex den of a motel." No matter what the diagnosis (and diagnosis is usually by no means certain), these patients are the senior citizens whom no one seems to want.

Close examination, however, reveals that few have ever had even a minimal basic dementia examination. Many need medical or neurological admission to rule out the treatable causes of dementia and to allow for rational management and disposition if they cannot be treated. If diagnosis is determined and sedation is required, thioridazine (Mellaril), 10 mg p.o. t.i.d., or haloperidol (Haldol), 1 to 2 mg p.o. b.i.d., may be used. One must beware of hypotension with thioridazine, and of parkinsonian side effects with haloperidol.

LEGAL CONCERNS LEAD TO PSYCHIATRIC INTERVENTION

COMPETENCY

The psychiatrist is frequently called to the accident floor to determine the mental competency of a patient refusing treatment or desirous of leaving the hospital against medical advice. When this occurs, it is important to keep in mind that courts, and not physicians, determine competency. Furthermore, competency is never determined globally, but always with respect to the performance of a particular act or function.

Competency to sign out of a hospital against medical advice requires a different determination from competency to drive an automobile. The general principle to follow is that people are presumed competent unless specific evidence is presented to prove they are not. Whenever a physician admits or treats a patient against his will, and without the appointment of a legal guardian by the probate court, the physician does so at his own risk. He should clearly document his observations in the chart which support the conclusion that the patient requires urgent, life-saving emergency treatment. If the medical problem is not immediately life-threatening one should wait for the court to decide competency and appoint a guardian.

If the physician decides to treat without patient or guardian consent, a carefully documented mental status examination, with particular attention to the sphere of judgment, is more important than a statement about the patient's competence. When dealing with patients refusing treatment or wishing to sign out against medical advice, the questions "Does the patient grasp the nature and extent of his illness?" and "Does the patient grasp and understand the consequences of his refusing treatment?" must be clearly answered and the answers documented. It is also important to make a statement as to the immediate life-threatening nature of the medical problem.

It should be noted, however, that many times difficulties between doctors and patients masquerade as competency problems. The physician's inability to speak the language of his patient, his inability to spend enough time with his patient, and his inability to understand the dynamic meaning of a particular illness for a particular patient are but three examples of problems in the doctor-patient relationship which come to the surface in requests for a "competency" evaluation. When these and similar problems occur, they are best handled nonlegally.

MEDICATION

The use of medication to assist in the management of the agitated, assaultive, or acutely psychotic patient must be considered in relation to the diagnostic assessment, whenever possible. The drugs of choice for acute catatonic, paranoid, or manic excitements are the butyrophenones (haloperidol, Haldol) or the aliphatic phenothiazines (chlorpromazine, Thorazine). When postictal state, delirium tremens, or other cerebral dysfunction is suspected, it is more prudent to employ adequate doses of the benzodiazepines.

There are several unusual conditions which respond best to specific nontranquilizing medications. The atropine-like psychosis induced most often by an overdose of proprietary sleeping medications containing scopolamine or tricyclic antidepressants responds best to cholinesterase blockers which cross the blood-brain barrier, such as physostigmine salicylate (Antilirium). Acute agitation owing to oculogyric crisis or other acute parkinsonian side effects, usually secondary to ingestion of phenothiazines, responds best to treatment with intramuscular diphenhydramine hydrochloride (Benadryl) or benztropine mesylate (Cogentin).

The Boston City Hospital experience suggests that a rapid tranquilization technique using haloperidol is the safest and most effective pharmacologic method of controlling the general target symptoms of severe agitation, psychomotor hyperactivity, assaultiveness, and mania. Before medicating a patient, the diagnosis of manic depressive psychosis or schizophrenia should be established. This can be done by means of the interview and mental status examination, by consulting hospital records, and by talking with relatives, friends, or police. If diagnostic certainty is not possible, the difficult and always risky decision to medicate a patient without a clear-cut diagnosis must be carefully weighed.

The rapid tranquilization technique involves the administration of 2.5 or 5 mg I.M. of haloperidol at 30-minute intervals until the disturbed behavior is brought under control. We have found this technique to be far safer than the older method which employed chlorpromazine (Thorazine) and which often led to hypotension. Control of symptoms generally occurs between total doses of 15 and 40 mg/day of haloperidol. The total daily dosage should generally not exceed 40 mg/day. Hypotensive reactions with haloperidol are rare, but patients do occasionally develop parkinsonian side effects several days after receiving and then continuing to receive haloperidol. These side effects must be recognized and treated rapidly with benztropine mesylate should they occur.

If pregnancy is a reality or a possibility, one should not use haloperidol, because of potential teratogenicity. Chlorpromazine and prochlorperazine (Compazine) have had the most extensive use of all the antipsychotics in pregnant women. Their advantages should be weighed against possible risks to the fetus. If chlorpromazine is used in a patient not cuurrently taking phenothiazines, a 25- to 50-mg test dose should be carefully monitored for the production of severe postural hypotension. If reasonable blood pressure is maintained after 30 minutes, an additional 50 to 75 mg may then be administered every hour until behavior is controlled or total dosage reaches 600 mg. Lying and standing blood pressure should be monitored before each dose.

Table 16-2 lists the drugs most commonly used in the pharmacologic treatment of psychiatric emergencies.

GENERAL MANAGEMENT PRINCIPLES

1. Allow sufficient time for the interview. It is impossible to do a psychiatric interview in a hurry. An adequate psychiatric interview generally takes 30 to 60 minutes. It is unwise to start unless you have set aside sufficient time to sit down and talk with the patient, free from interruptions and distractions. Failure to do so is a frequent cause of unnecessary misunderstanding and subsequent aggressive or other difficult behavior on the part of the patient. Taking sufficient time at the outset can save considerable time in the end.

2. Do not interview a patient in a setting which makes you or the patient anxious. In order to make an objective assessment, you must not fear the patient's violent or self-destructive acting out. If violent behavior

TABLE 16-2 Parenteral Drugs in the Treatment of Psychiatric Emergencies

Drug	Initial I.M. Adult Dose (mg)	Subsequent I.M. Dose (mg)	Maximum Initial Daily Dose (mg)	Frequent Initial Side Effects	Infrequent Initial Side Effects	Contraindications	Major Use
Antipsychotic Agents							
Haloperidol (Haldol)	0.5–5.0	0.5–5.0 q 30–60 min	40	Extrapyramidal	Hypotension with alpha blockade Lowered seizure threshold Cholinergic blocking Somnolence	Pregnancy Hypersensitivity Narrow angle glaucoma CNS depression Severe cardiac disease with arrhythmia	Acute schizophrenia Alcoholic hallucinosis Sedation with uncertain diagnosis
Chlorpromazine (Thorazine)	25–50	25–100 q 1–2 h	600	Hypotension with alpha blockade Somnolence Cholinergic blocking	Extrapyramidal Lowered seizure threshold	Hypersensitivity Narrow angle glaucoma CNS depression Severe cardiac disease with arrhythmia	Acute schizophrenia when considerable sedation required
Antianxiety Agents							
Chlordiazepoxide (Librium)	25–50	25–100 q 1–2 h	300	Drowsiness Ataxia	Confusion Paradoxical excitement Hypotension Prolonged sedation Impotence	Hypersensitivity	Severe neurotic anxiety and agitation Impending delirium tremens Sedation with uncertain diagnosis
Diazepam (Valium)	5–10	5–10 q 1–2 h	60	Drowsiness Ataxia	Confusion Paradoxical excitement Hypotension Prolonged sedation Impotence	Hypersensitivity	Severe neurotic anxiety and agitation Impending delirium tremens Sedation with uncertain diagnosis

Drug						
Antihistamines						
Hydroxyzine hydrochloride (Atarax, Vistaril)	25–100	25–100 q 4–6h	400	Drowsiness, Ataxia, Dry mouth	Confusion, Hypotension, Cholinergic blocking	Hypersensitivity, Narrow angle glaucoma	Treatment of severe anxiety agitation when benzodiazepines or major tranquilizers are not desirable
Diphenhydramine hydrochloride (Benadryl)	25–50	25–50 q 4–6h	400	Drowsiness, Ataxia, Dry mouth, Blurred vision	Confusion, Hypotension, Cholinergic blocking	Hypersensitivity, Narrow angle glaucoma	Drug-induced extrapyramidal reactions
Antiparkinsonian Agents						
Benztropine mesylate (Cogentin)	1–2	1–2 p.r.n.	6	Cholinergic blocking, Dry mouth, Blurred vision	Toxic psychosis	Hypersensitivity, Narrow angle glaucoma	Drug-induced dystonic reactions
Acetylcholinesterase Inhibitors						
Physostigmine salicylate (Antilirium)	0.5–2	0.5–2 q ½–2 h p.r.n. titrate	8	Lacrimation, rhinorrhea, and other signs of cholinergic excess are indications for stopping drug		Cardiac disease, Hypersensitivity, Asthma, Gangrene, Diabetes	Anticholinergic psychosis
Narcotic Antagonists						
Naloxone hydrochloride (Narcan)	0.4	0.4 q 3 min	2	Acute opioid withdrawal syndrome	Syndrome of interstitial or alveolar pulmonary congestion	Hypersensitivity, Known severe narcotic dependency	A test for narcotic addiction, To counteract narcotic overdose

is possible, be sure to have help immediately available. If there is any question of a weapon, insist that the patient be searched prior to any interview. This can also be accomplished by asking the patient to change into an examining gown with his clothes kept some distance from him. If this is done in a matter of fact way, it reduces the embarrassment surrounding a search.

It is important that neither the patient nor the doctor feels cornered. Ideally, there should be a two-door room available from which the doctor or the patient can exit quickly, if either feels the necessity to leave. To be sure a patient does not escape, security guards should be ready to stop him after he leaves the room.

It is important not to interview patients in corridors, parking lots, or crowded public places. The lack of structure and the surrounding distraction contribute to both doctor and patient anxiety. Remember, one cannot be objective if one fears for one's own life.

3. Talk with the patient alone first, if at all possible, but do not neglect family and friends. It is usually a good idea to make one attempt to interview the patient by himself before consulting with relatives, friends, or other agents accompanying him to the accident floor. Try to be the first, and not the twelfth, person to interview the patient. If the patient is actually psychotic, the initial interview may be short, and the most productive use of your time may involve meeting with accompanying persons. If possible, it is a good idea to have the patient present while talking with others, although sometimes the patient is so out of control that this is not possible. If medication is used to control the patient, the time it takes to work can be used productively in talking with family, friends, or others.

Because families are most often frightened and worried, they need reassurance and support. Their positive understanding of what is happening on the emergency service contributes to the long-range treatment and recovery of the patient. As allies, they may help calm and transport an otherwise unmanageable patient and later assist in his treatment. As adversaries, they may become involved with the patient in a way which encourages loss of control and aggression and sabotages all efforts at both current and later treatment.

Having the family in the interview room makes it harder for them to deny the patient's illness. A general principle to follow is that if the family wants a sick patient out of the hospital, every effort should be made to have them in the room; if they are trying to force an unwilling patient into the hospital, they are best kept out. Remember that the police, ambulance drivers, and other social agents often file reports which provide valuable information about the patient and his present illness. These reports provide the address where the patient was picked up, which is useful if hospitalization becomes necessary. They should be sought out when they are available. A call to the local police station about a patient may also help to clarify diagnosis and aid in disposition.

4. Find out what is going on now, not what happened when the patient was five years old. The physician should try to focus on a patient's illness and its precipitant. He should try to trace both the behavioral and emotional events immediately prior to admission. Obtaining a history

of these events often relieves the anxiety of the patient and clarifies the meaning of his behavior, both to you and to him, which is of use therapeutically as well as diagnostically.

Focusing on the present is harder to do than is at first apparent. Asking, "Why are you here today at this time?" may be too threatening an approach for an agitated patient. In these difficult cases, a tangential approach may yield better information than a direct frontal assault. Ask questions, such as "Where are you from?" or "Who brought you to the hospital?" Try to start from neutral ground and gingerly approach affectively charged territory.

Psychiatric emergencies may be as life-threatening as their medical counterparts. Their adequate management can provide a challenge and a source of satisfaction for the medical house officer. The early phases of psychiatric treatment are of critical importance to patients and may often set the tone for later treatment success or failure.

SELECTED READINGS

Ames, F.   The hyperventilation syndrome. *J. Ment. Sci.* 101:466–525, 1955.

Anderson, W. H., and Kuehnle, J. C.   Strategies for the treatment of acute psychosis. *J.A.M.A.* 229:1884–1889, 1974.

Ayd, F. J.   Haloperidol: Fifteen years of clinical experience. *Dis. Nerv. Syst.* 33:459–469, 1972.

Cole, J. O., and Hollister, L. E.   *Schizophrenia.* New York: Medcom, 1970.

Granacher, R. P., and Baldessarini, R. J.   Physostigmine. *Arch. Gen. Psychiatry* 32:375–380, 1975.

Heiser, J. F., and Gillin, J. C.   The reversal of anticholinergic drug-induced delirium and coma with physostigmine. *Am. J. Psychiatry* 127:1050–1054, 1971.

Kirstein, L., et al.   Utilization review of treatment for suicide attempters. *Am. J. Psychiatry* 132:22–27, 1975.

Lion, J. R.   *Evaluation and Management of the Violent Patient.* Springfield, Ill.: Thomas, 1972.

MacKinnon, R. A., and Michels, R.   *The Psychiatric Interview.* Philadelphia: Saunders, 1971. Pp. 401–427.

Man, P., and Chen, C. H.   Rapid tranquilization of acutely psychotic patients with intramuscular haloperidol and chlorpromazine. *Psychosomatics* 14:59–69, 1973.

Schwab, J. J.   *Handbook of Psychiatric Consultation.* New York: Appleton-Century-Crofts, 1968.

Shader, R. I.   *Manual of Psychiatric Therapeutics.* Boston: Little, Brown, 1975.

Stengel, E., and Cook, N. G.   *Attempted Suicide: Its Social Significance and Effects.* London: Oxford University Press, 1958.

Wikler, A.   Diagnosis and treatment of drug dependence of the barbiturate type. *Am. J. Psychiatry* 125:758–765, 1968.

17

ARTHRITIS AS A
MEDICAL EMERGENCY

Don L. Goldenberg
Alan S. Cohen

DESPITE THE FACT that many forms of arthritis are chronic and indolent in nature, certain rheumatic diseases may represent acute medical emergencies. We therefore will review in some detail the single most common and serious form of acute arthritis, septic arthritis, and highlight some of the more important acute complications which may occur in other rheumatic illnesses.

SEPTIC ARTHRITIS

Although many diseases may cause an acute arthritis, acute infectious arthritis is the most common, serious rheumatic disease requiring immediate diagnosis and therapy. To evaluate properly a patient with possible septic arthritis, one must first determine that a true arthritis is present, because periarticular inflammation such as phlebitis, tendonitis, bursitis, cellulitis, and osteomyelitis may also cause acute inflammation about the joints. The cardinal signs of an acute arthritis are pain, swelling, heat, and erythema of the joint. These signs may all be present with periarticular inflammation, although the swelling is not confined to the joint space. Similarly, the peripheral blood leukocyte count, the patient's temperature, and joint x-rays are seldom helpful in differentiating acute arthritis and periarthritis. Thus it is often impossible to distinguish a joint effusion from periarticular swelling prior to needle aspiration of the joint. An arthrocentesis is necessary whenever acute arthritis develops and the cause of the arthritis is not perfectly clear. Indeed, the diagnosis of a septic arthritis can be made with certainty only after recovery of the microorganisms from the synovial fluid.

The arthrocentesis should be done under sterile conditions. Although fluid can be removed from any joint without too much difficulty, the knee is most often aspirated. A large-gauge (18 to 20) needle is used after anesthetizing the skin and subcutaneous tissue with Xylocaine 1 to 2%. (For technique see [1, 2].) As much fluid as possible should be withdrawn into sterile syringes. It is important to place a portion of the fluid (0.5 ml) into sterile tubes for culture and other appropriate bacteriologic tests, and another portion into a heparinized tube for cytologic study. All essential tests can be performed on a small quantity of synovial fluid placed in the tube with anticoagulant; however, when larger amounts of synovial fluid are removed, a more complete synovianalysis may be performed (Table 17-1) and culture and smears are more likely to be positive. While culture results are awaited, synovial fluid findings may enable a presumptive diagnosis of a joint infection or make the diagnosis unlikely (Table 17-2). For example, the demonstration of monosodium urate or calcium pyrophosphate crystals in the synovial fluid assures the diagnosis of gout or pseudogout. The cell count is often a helpful clue in the differential diagnosis of an acute arthritis. In septic joints, synovial fluid leukocyte counts may vary from less than 10,000 to greater than 200,000/mm^3. Although leukocyte counts greater than 25,000 are seen in many rheumatic illnesses, the higher the cell count and the greater the percentage of polymorphonuclear leukocytes, the greater the likelihood of infection. A synovial fluid count of greater than 50,000/mm^3 always suggests septic arthritis until proved otherwise. Fasting synovial fluid glucose values are often less than one-half the simultaneous blood glucose in patients with infectious arthritis. Unfortunately, Gram-stain smears of the joint fluid reveal organisms in only 50% of patients with definite bacterial arthritis. In addition, false-positive Gram stains may occur, since mucin aggregates may stain positively and resemble organisms.

As noted above, the cardinal features of acute arthritis are pain, swelling, heat, and erythema. Although these symptoms are almost always found in a patient with septic arthritis, they are present also in most

TABLE 17-1 Collection and Analysis of Synovial Fluid

Tube	Procedure	Comments
1	Culture using sterile tubes containing heparin. Culture aerobically and anaerobically. If gonoccal arthritis is suspected, immediately inoculate on chocolate agar or Thayer-Martin media. If TB is suspected add several more ml for guinea pig inoculation	All synovial fluids should be routinely cultured
2	Nonsterile tube with heparin, for cytology. Mix well	If necessary, can use for mucin determination and examination for crystals
3	Nonsterile with no anticoagulant for analysis of mucin determination, clot, and examination for crystals	May also be used for rheumatoid factor, complement, protein, lipid studies
4	Nonsterile with potassium oxalate for sugar analysis	Requires simultaneous blood sample for synovial fluid–blood glucose differential

Table 17-2 Synovial Fluid Analysis for Differential Diagnosis (Average Findings)

Diagnosis	Appearance	Total WBC/mm³ Average (Range)	Polymorphonuclear Leukocytes (%)	Mucin Test	Crystals	Synovial Fluid–Blood Glucose Differential (mg/100 ml)
Normal	Clear yellow	200 (0–200)	7	Good	–	0
Group I: Noninflammatory Effusions						
Traumatic arthritis	Clear or bloody	1,500 (50–6,500)	20	Good	–	5
Degenerative joint disease	Clear or turbid	600 (50–3,750)	13	Good	–	5
Group II: Noninfectious Mild Inflammatory Effusions						
Systemic lupus erythematosus	Clear or slightly turbid	2,860 (0–8,600)	30	Good	–	22
Group III: Noninfectious Severe Inflammatory Effusions						
Gout	Turbid	21,500 (100–160,000)	70	Poor	Na urate	11
Pseudogout	Slightly turbid	14,200 (50–75,000)	68	Fair	Ca pyrophosphate	5
Rheumatic fever	Slightly turbid	17,800 (0–60,000)	50	Good–Fair	–	6
Rheumatoid arthritis	Turbid	19,000 (250–80,000)	66	Fair–Poor	–	30
Group IV: Infectious Inflammatory Effusions						
Reiters	Turbid	18,500 (100–43,000)	60	Poor	–	16
Acute bacterial	Very turbid	80,000 (150–250,000)	90	Poor	–	91
Tuberculous	Turbid	20,000 (2,500–100,000)	60	Poor	–	70

From Cohen [1]. For more detailed analysis regarding viscosity, clot, cellular inclusions, total protein, complement, e.g., values, see [1, 2].

other types of acute arthritis. The clinical pattern of joint involvement is also not specific. Acute monoarthritis of large joints, especially the knee, is a common symptom of septic arthritis, yet is frequently observed in gout, pseudogout, rheumatoid arthritis, and Reiter's disease. Metatarsophalangeal arthritis (acute podagra) is often a clue to the diagnosis of gout, but it can also be caused by infection, rheumatoid arthritis, and other rheumatic diseases. Extra-articular signs and laboratory tests often are of limited diagnostic aid. Fever may be low grade and transient in septic arthritis as in gout, rheumatoid arthritis, etc. Leukocytosis (peripheral blood leukocyte count greater than $10,000/mm^3$) is present in only about 60% of patients with septic arthritis. X-rays of the infected joint usually demonstrate only soft-tissue swelling and are of little diagnostic aid other than demonstrating the absence of radiologic features of rheumatoid arthritis, gout, pseudogout, etc. However, x-rays of the affected joint must be obtained in the initial evaluation of a patient with septic arthritis to rule out a contiguous focus of osteomyelitis.

It is essential to maintain a high index of suspicion regarding joint infection, even in patients with underlying rheumatic disease. This is particularly true in view of the fact that bacterial arthritis may complicate rheumatoid arthritis. Anti-inflammatory and immunosuppressive medications may mask the local and systemic response to infection; in addition, the physician may believe that the synovitis is merely a local flare-up of rheumatoid arthritis. Any microorganism can cause septic arthritis, and viral, fungal, and tuberculous arthritis are well recognized. However, acute bacterial arthritis is the most common and most rapidly destructive form of septic arthritis. Between 1965 and 1972, 74 patients with definite acute bacterial arthritis (i.e., organisms were recovered from the synovial fluid) were hospitalized at Boston City Hospital and University Hospital. In addition, more than 30 patients were treated for presumed bacterial arthritis, not confirmed by synovial fluid culture results, during those eight years.

The bacteria we have recovered most frequently from the synovial fluid have been gram-positive cocci and *Neisseria gonorrhoeae* (Table 17-3). However, the gonococcus is difficult to isolate from synovial fluid [3, 4], and therefore these figures underestimate the true incidence of gonococcal arthritis. For example, 10 patients were treated for gonococcal arthritis who had negative synovial fluid but positive blood cultures (Table 17-3). In addition, at least 25 patients had presumed gonococcal arthritis which responded to antibiotics, but had negative blood and synovial fluid cultures.

Patients with gonococcal arthritis may show a distinctive clinical picture [3, 4, 5]. Tenosynovitis and purulent arthritis frequently involve multiple joints. Characteristic skin lesions may develop, and rarely the organism may be recovered from the erythematous pustules. Patients with gonococcemia may not have positive synovial fluid cultures at the time of their bacteremia [5]. Of patients with proved staphylococcal arthritis, 39%, and of patients with streptococcal arthritis, 57%, had corresponding positive blood and synovial fluid cultures, whereas only 5% of our patients with gonococcal arthritis had positive blood and synovial fluid cultures. Unlike patients with gonococcal arthritis, the

TABLE 17-3 Bacteria Recovered from Synovial Fluid in 74 Patients (1965–1972)

Bacteria	No. Patients
Staphylococcus aureus	19
Streptococcus hemolyticus	16
Neisseria gonorrhoeae	15*
Streptococcus (Diplococcus) pneumoniae	7
Hemophilus influenzae	6
Escherichia coli	6
Proteus mirabilis	4
Salmonella choleraesuis	1
Salmonella typhimurium	1
Pseudomonas aeruginosa	1
Serratia marcescens	1
	77†

* Ten additional patients had presumed septic arthritis with gonococcal bacteremia but negative synovial fluid culture.
† Three patients were infected with 2 kinds of bacteria in the same joint.

patients with arthritis caused by gram-positive cocci or gram-negative bacilli had no distinctive findings. The only uniform finding was an acutely inflamed joint, extremely painful to active or passive motion.

Our data suggest that septic arthritis caused by gram-negative bacilli is more common in recent years (see Table 17-3), reflecting the increased incidence of gram-negative bacteremia, especially in hospitalized and immunosuppressed patients. The organism recovered from synovial fluid varies with the patient's age. Thus, in children less than 6 years old, Hemophilus influenzae and Staphylococcus aureus are the most frequent offenders. In young, healthy adults, Neisseria gonorrhoeae is usually responsible for bacterial arthritis. On the other hand, arthritis caused by gram-negative bacilli usually occurs in the compromised host [6] or in users of intravenous drugs [7]. In our 13 patients with gram-negative bacillary arthritis (see Table 17-3), two had associated malignancy, one had diabetes mellitus, one had sickle cell anemia, and two had been receiving immunosuppressive drugs prior to the development of septic arthritis. Thus, the patient's age and medical condition may often give a clue as to the bacterial agent involved while the physician is awaiting the culture reports.

Septic arthritis usually results from hematogenous infection with spread to the synovium and synovial fluid. Occasionally, a penetrating wound, a contiguous focus of osteomyelitis, or prior corticosteroid injection may be the primary source of joint infections. Despite the fact that bacteremia is presumed to be the cause of most cases of septic arthritis, positive blood cultures at the time of diagnosis are found in only 50% of patients. However, extra-articular sites will frequently yield cultures positive for the same bacteria recovered from the synovial fluid; i.e., not infrequently the same agent is recovered from a common extra-articular site [6]. For example, most patients with staphylococcal or streptococcal arthritis have concurrent skin or upper respiratory tract infections. Patients with pneumococcal arthritis frequently have documented pneumococcal pneumonia, and patients with arthritis caused by gram-negative bacilli often have urinary tract infections.

Once septic arthritis is suspected, it becomes critically important to complete all diagnostic studies and immediately start therapy while awaiting definite culture results. Blood agar should be used for routine cultures, but chocolate agar or other similar suitable media must be used in suspected gonococcal arthritis (see Table 17-1). All possible extra-articular sites of infection must be cultured, and in suspected gonococcal infections, these should include the skin, anal, and pharyngeal lesions, as well as the blood and genitourinary sites. In selected cases, especially in patients with gram-negative bacillary arthritis, further bacteriologic evaluation is needed. A tube dilution assay of serum and synovial fluid may be done to assure that bactericidal levels in the synovial fluid have been achieved [8].

The longer the duration of the joint infection prior to treatment, the less chance there is for complete recovery [9]. A rational choice of initial antibiotic therapy depends on the Gram-stain smear results and the age and medical condition of the patient (Table 17-4). When the Gram-stain smear is positive, the antibiotic initially chosen can be expected to closely approximate definitive antimicrobial therapy. However, when the Gram-stain smear is negative, the antibiotic chosen depends solely on the underlying medical condition of the host and the presumed route of the infection. Thus, because of the prevalence of gonococcal arthritis in healthy young patients, penicillin is the initial drug recommended; however, immunosuppressed patients or intravenous drug users must be initially treated with antibiotics that will cover staphylococcal and gram-negative bacilli joint infections. Antibiotics should initially be administered parenterally.

In addition to appropriate antibiotic therapy, successful treatment of septic arthritis requires the removal of fibrin clots and purulent exudates which may retard antibiotic penetration and which by nature of enzymatic release and intra-articular pressure may result in cartilage destruction [10]. Surgical drainage is necessary in patients with a contiguous osteomyelitis who have sequestrae and in most cases of septic arthritis of the hip. In other patients, the joint should be initially drained by closed needle aspiration. This should be repeated daily or more often until the joint fluid is no longer grossly purulent and not reaccumulating in large quantities [9]. If there is little improvement after one week of medical therapy, surgical drainage should be considered. In the early treatment of septic arthritis, immobilization with splints may be necessary to maintain proper functional position and joint exercise should be limited to muscle setting. The extent of articular damage following septic arthritis thus depends not only on the virulence of the organism and on the host defenses but also on the rapidity of initiation of therapy as well as the proper use of antibiotics and joint drainage. Therefore, septic arthritis is a rheumatologic illness which indeed requires prompt diagnosis and treatment.

TABLE 17-4 Recommended Initial Antibiotic Therapy Prior to Microbial Identification

Finding on Gram-Stain Smear	Drug of Choice	Initial Dosage	Alternate Treatment*
Gram-positive cocci	Penicillinase-resistant penicillin (nafcillin, methcillin, etc.)	8–10 gm daily I.V.	Cephalothin, erythromycin
Gram-negative cocci	Penicillin G	2–6 million U daily I.V.	Erythromycin, tetracycline
Gram-negative bacilli	Gentamicin and carbenecillin	3 mg/kg/day I.M.; if normal renal function 30 gm daily I.V.	Carbenecillin and cephalothin
Smear negative			
Young healthy patient	Penicillin G	4–10 million U daily I.V.	Erythromycin, cephalothin
Patient on immunosuppressive drugs with cancer, intravenous drug user, etc.	Penicillinase-resistant penicillin (nafcillin) Gentamicin	10 gm daily I.V. 3 mg/kg daily	Carbenecillin and cephalothin
Children below 6 years	Ampicillin Penicillinase-resistant penicillin	50 mg/kg q 6 h 8–10 gm daily I.V.	Chloramphenicol, cephalothin

* Use when history of allergy or intolerance to the first drug.

RHEUMATOID ARTHRITIS

Rheumatoid arthritis is a common medical condition rarely requiring immediate diagnostic evaluation or treatment. However, cervical myelopathy complicating rheumatoid arthritis may be a medical emergency. Radiologic evidence of cervical spine involvement in long-standing rheumatoid arthritis is common [11]. Frequently this involvement consists of atlantoaxial subluxation, defined radiologically as a distance of greater than 2.5 mm in females and 3.0 mm in males between the posterior aspect of the anterior arch of the atlas and the anterior surface of the odontoid process during a lateral view of the cervical spine in full flexion.

Despite its frequent occurrence radiologically in patients with chronic rheumatoid arthritis, atlantoaxial subluxation rarely produces clinical symptoms [12]. However, destruction of the transverse ligament of the atlas and the anterior atlantoaxial ligament may eventually allow the dens to move posteriorly into the spinal canal, resulting in cord compression. Symptoms may then be insidious, with chronic, aching pain in the upper cervical and occipital regions, aggravated or precipitated by neck motion. This chronic myelopathy may produce muscle atrophy and loss of deep tendon reflexes. However, symptoms may develop acutely, and any neurological signs that occur in patients with rheumatoid arthritis should bring to mind the possibility of impending cord compression associated with cervical arthritis. These symptoms commonly include headache with neck pain, paresthesias, diminished vibration sense, flexor spasms, urinary retention or other bladder disturbances, unexplained "giving way" of the knee, and Babinski's sign.

Quadriparesis and death may result if continued cord compression is untreated. However, clinical symptoms usually respond to gentle collar immobilization. Rarely, patients are first seen with signs of acute severe cord compression, especially when vertebral subluxation involves C3–C4 or other lower vertebrae. These patients must undergo emergency operative intervention. In most other cases, conservative therapy will result in complete recovery. The aim of treatment is limitation of anterior flexion and prevention of unexpected accidental flexion.

ACUTE VASCULITIS

Rarely, rheumatoid arthritis, but more commonly systemic lupus erythematosus (SLE), may require immediate medical attention because of an acute vasculitis. For example, patients with chronic severe rheumatoid arthritis may develop inflammation of the vasa nervorum and other vessels resulting in polyneuropathy, digital gangrene, or, rarely, visceral ischemia, including intestinal infarction [13]. Such acute arteritis occurs more often in patients with SLE. Cerebral vasculitis may result in an acute psychosis or an organic brain syndrome which can be difficult to differentiate from corticosteroid toxicity. Many other central nervous system (CNS) manifestations, including epilepsy, aseptic meningitis, transverse myelitis, and paraplegia, may develop suddenly [14]. It thus becomes important to differentiate cerebral vasculitis from steroid psychosis, infection, etc., in patients with SLE. Unfortunately, neurological and cerebrospinal fluid examination are of little help in the diagnosis of cerebral vasculitis. Brain scans may be of some aid in differentiating CNS lupus from other syndromes, and recent reports indicate that depressed cerebrospinal fluid complement (especially C4) may be helpful in the diagnosis [15]. Some manifestations of CNS lupus appear to respond to corticosteroids, although the role of high-dose corticosteroid therapy in these patients must be further evaluated [16].

Temporal (giant cell) arteritis may be seen as an acute medical and ophthalmologic emergency. This vascular inflammation, usually confined to the cranial arteries, almost invariably occurs in patients older than 55 years [17]. Local symptoms include unilateral or bilateral temporal headaches, burning of the scalp, and jaw claudication. Often the temporal artery appears prominent, tortuous, red, and tender. Constitutional symptoms such as fever, malaise, and weight loss are common. Polymyalgia rheumatica, a syndrome in elderly patients manifested by pain and stiffness of the proximal muscles without marked weakness, is often associated with temporal arteritis. In fact, Fauchald and others [17] were unable clinically or histologically to distinguish patients with polymyalgia rheumatica from those with temporal arteritis. In their series, 49 patients had myalgias without local findings in the temporal region, yet 20 of these patients had histologic evidence of temporal arteritis.

Ocular involvement occurs in 50% of patients with temporal arteritis, and sudden loss of vision caused by vascular occlusion is the most common and most catastrophic complication. Ischemic optic neuritis may occur abruptly, but frequently early diagnosis may prevent permanent blindness. Often, prodromal symptoms such as temporal headache or tender temporal arteries alert the physician to the possibility of temporal arteritis. Laboratory tests are of little specific help, although the erythrocyte sedimentation rate is invariably markedly elevated. Thus, temporal artery biopsy followed by a thorough histologic examination of the vessel, in view of the segmental nature of the arteritis, is the only definitive way to make the diagnosis. If the patient has abrupt onset of severe local findings or if the patient has any visual symptoms, high-dose corticosteroid therapy (60 to 80 mg prednisone per day) should be promptly started while awaiting the results of the biopsy.

In summary, although most rheumatic diseases are chronic in nature, acute arteritis may complicate any connective tissue disease. In addition, bacterial arthritis continues to be a common rheumatic illness requiring immediate diagnosis and treatment.

REFERENCES

1. Cohen, A. S. (Ed.). *Laboratory Diagnostic Procedures in the Rheumatic Diseases*. 2d ed. Boston: Little, Brown, 1975.
2. Hollander, J. L., and McCarty, D. J., Jr. (Eds.). *Arthritis and Allied Conditions*. 8th ed. Philadelphia: Lea & Febiger, 1972.
3. Holmes, K. K., Counts, G. W., and Beaty, A. N. Disseminated gonococcal infection. *Ann. Intern. Med.* 74:979, 1972.
4. Lightfoot, R. W., and Gotschlich, E. C. Gonococcal disease. *Am. J. Med.* 56:347, 1974.
5. Brandt, K. D., Cathcart, E. S., and Cohen, A. S. Gonococcal arthritis: Clinical features correlated with blood, synovial fluid and genitourinary cultures. *Arthritis Rheum.* 17:503, 1974.
6. Goldenberg, D. L., Brandt, K. D., Cathcart, E. S., and Cohen, A. S. Acute arthritis caused by gram negative bacilli: A clinical characterization. *Medicine* 53:197, 1974.
7. Tindel, J. R., and Crowder, J. G. Septic arthritis due to *Pseudomonas aeruginosa*. *J.A.M.A.* 218:559, 1971.
8. Parker, R. H., and Schmid, R. R. Antibacterial activity of synovial fluid during therapy of septic arthritis. *Arthritis Rheum.* 14:96, 1971.
9. Goldenberg, D. L., Brandt, K. D., Cohen, A. S., and Cathcart, E. S. Treatment of septic arthritis: A comparison of needle aspiration and surgery as initial modes of joint drainage. *Arthritis Rheum.* 18:83, 1975.
10. Curtiss, P. H., and Klein, L. Destruction of articular cartilage in septic arthritis. *J. Bone Joint Surg.* 45a:797, 1963.
11. Bland, J. H., Davis, P. H., London, M. G., et al. Rheumatoid arthritis of the cervical spine. *Arch. Intern. Med.* 112:893, 1963.

12. Isdale, I. C., and Conlon, P. W.   Atlanto-axial subluxation, a six-year follow up. *Ann. Rheum. Dis.* 30:387, 1971.
13. Schmid, F. R., Cooper, N. S., Ziff, M., and McEwen, C.   Arteritis in rheumatoid arthritis. *Am. J. Med.* 30:56, 1961.
14. Johnson, R. T., and Richardson, E. P.   The neurological manifestations of systemic lupus erythematosus. *Medicine* 47:337, 1968.
15. Hadler, N. W., Gerawin, R. D., Frank, M. M., et al.   The fourth component of complement (C4) in the cerebrospinal fluid (CSF) in systemic lupus erythematosus (SLE). *Arthritis Rheum.* 16:507, 1973.
16. Sergent, J. S., Lockshin, M. D., Klempner, M. S., and Lipsky, B. A.   Central nervous systemic disease in systemic lupus erythematosus. *Am. J. Med.* 58:644, 1975.
17. Fauchald, P., Rygrold, O., and Oystese, B.   Temporal arteritis and polymyalgia rheumatica: Clinical and biopsy findings. *Ann. Intern. Med.* 77:845, 1972.

18

EMERGENCY MEDICAL SERVICES — AN OVERVIEW

Michael W. Pozen

EMERGENCY MEDICAL SERVICES (EMS) communications networks, ambulances, and emergency rooms are conduits for each of the medical emergencies discussed in the preceding chapters. The importance of these EMS components has either explicitly or implicitly been stressed by the other authors of this text in their emphasis on early, effective, and closely monitored medical interventions for these patients.

The EMS system in which patients with these medical emergencies find themselves is quite variable, as a result of differences in local interest, finances, geography, and medical resources. Despite these differences, the political and medical community's consensus in 1973 that the public was demanding increased services and that advanced technology was applicable to EMS resulted in the first comprehensive federal EMS legislation [1]. With this impetus, responsible medical and civic organizations at all levels have become concerned with the purpose, organization, and effectiveness of EMS. In the present developmental stage of EMS, it is essential that physicians and house officers treating medical emergencies be aware of these issues, both to appreciate the larger context in which they provide emergency medical services and to encourage their involvement in formulating the direction and goals of the EMS system.

PURPOSE OF EMS

Only about 10% of emergency room (ER) visits are for true emergencies, while one-half to two-thirds are for nonurgent conditions, with the remainder for "urgent" conditions [2, 3, 4]. The annual 10% increase of ER visits to more than 50 million per year is principally due to this high proportion of nonurgent visits, especially among the nonwhite, poor, poorly educated, and urban populations [5].

The four principal objectives of the EMS system for patients with true emergencies remain airway establishment, hemodynamic stabilization, diagnosis, and triage [6]. The prevailing concept has been to shift these four activities as close to the emergency event as possible. The operationalization of this concept has taken many forms: public dissemination of first aid education, including cardiopulmonary resuscitation (CPR) and seizure control, especially among public servants such as policemen and firefighters; life-support stations in loci of high-density populations (e.g., airports, shopping malls, football stadiums); and emergency vehicles which carry trained staff and advanced equipment to the scene of the emergency. Efforts within emergency rooms have been to optimize the performance of activities related to these four objectives by providing appropriate training and support services and to standardize minimum criteria for meeting these objectives.

ORGANIZATION

The organization of EMS varies widely in goals, structure, size, membership, and stage of development. Six federal agencies [7], many state offices, and at least five local service organizations are involved with EMS. With the assistance of operations research science and the impetus of the federal EMS Act of 1973, the Health Services Administration has developed a model for EMS containing 5 subsystems, with a total of 45 component parts to integrate these efforts [8]. Figure 18-1 outlines the essentials.

SPECIALIZATION

Recent developments in a number of these components should be cited. Early resistance to specialization of emergency facilities has been overcome by the development of standard criteria [9] which designate emer-

Facilities
Staff
Categorization of ERs
Equipment

Communications
911 central telephone
Screening personnel
Interorganizational linkage
Command center

Management
Access mechanisms
Finances
Citizen participation
Standardized records
Program evaluation
Disaster plan

Transportation
Staff
Vehicles
Interorganizational arrangements

Training
Professional staff
Allied health personnel

Public Education
Knowledge of access
First aid training

FIGURE 18-1 Essential components of emergency medical services.

gency services as comprehensive (I), major (II), general (III), or basic (IV) on the basis of (1) scope of capability—immediate care and type of emergency; (2) staffing—director, nurses, physicians; (3) support services—consultants, blood bank, laboratory services, radiology, angiography, operating and recovery rooms; and (4) intensive care units. Regionalizing these specialized services to maximize accessibility and cost effectiveness of EMS is now the task of the local medical and civic organizations.

VEHICLES

Vehicles for EMS transportation have benefited from modern technology. Helicopters designed for the Indochina war have been used for transporting patients from rural areas to medical centers and from distant highway accidents to trauma units, and for taking newborns in distress to regional neonatal intensive care units. Mobile coronary units with electrocardiographic (ECG) telemetry have been claimed to significantly reduce the 60% out-of-hospital myocardial infarction mortality rate [10], though some conflicting reports have recently appeared [11].

ALLIED HEALTH PERSONNEL

Allied health personnel, often called "physician extenders," are being trained in increasing numbers. They have been employed in EMS systems in many capacities: EMTs (emergency medical technicians following an 81-hour course of instruction) on ambulances; advanced EMTs (with up to 490 hours of training), for specialized mobile units in which they perform intubation and defibrillation, start intravenous transfusions, and give drugs; nurse practitioners and health associates, who triage ER patients and, in some locales, diagnose and treat minor problems with the use of algorithms (clinical decision trees) [12]; and patient advocates, who pursue the needs and assure the rights of patients.

PUBLIC EDUCATION

The scope of public education has continued to broaden. Beyond knowledge of accessibility and availability of EMS through central 911 telephone numbers, programs have been instituted to educate the public about prodromata of life-threatening illness (e.g., myocardial infarction), first aid measures (e.g., for trauma and accidental overdoses), and early, preventive detection of potential emergency situations (e.g., faulty electrical wiring, falls). Public education has resulted in increased awareness of patients' rights and informed consent.

EVALUATION

Evaluation efforts have not kept pace with other EMS advancements. The post-World War II thrust in EMS has been preoccupied with developing and making operational a minimum set of standards across all regions of the country. Lack of a uniform data base, interdisciplinary research cooperation, discriminating medical care measurements, and resources has also hampered these endeavors. The 1973 EMS Act and the possibility of a national health insurance plan, however, now mandate close scrutiny of EMS in order to maximize the cost effectiveness of the system. In a recent article, Gibson has suggested a strategy for this activity which incorporates basic and applied research [13]: (1) epidemiological description of *EMS needs*; (2) operational evaluation of *EMS structure*; (3) understanding of the determinants of *EMS demand process* and their effects on the individual and the system; and (4) development of practical and sensitive *EMS outcome* measurements. He explains the ultimate aim of such a model:

The model to be aimed at here is a set of regression equations that from knowledge of the population base and environmental factors can predict the nature and quantity of EMS-related medical incidents, the tasks they generate, and the manpower mix needed to care for them optimally. Thus, if it is known that Community X will generate Y auto accidents producing Z fractures of known geographic, temporal, and severity distributions, an EMS system can estimate the need for ambulance evacuation, the orthopedic coverage needed in emergency rooms, and how many emergency rooms are required with what kind of manpower mix. Clearly, such predictive equations need series much larger and more representative than 674 abused children in Los Angeles or 182 pedestrian fatalities in Baltimore or 142 attempted suicides in East Harlem. Nationwide cooperative studies and trauma registries—probably the only means of generating this kind of data—should therefore receive high priority at the national level [13].

In instances where popular notions about EMS have been examined, a number of revealing findings have already been translated into practical programs. The fact that lay ambulance staff read ECG rhythm with a high degree of accuracy [14] has stimulated their use in lieu of physicians on mobile coronary care units. Differential mortality rates for trauma in various types of ERs [16] have led to their specialization. The success of physician extenders in diagnosis and treatment of certain conditions [16] has encouraged their involvement in ER triage and basic care. Obviously, these research findings are not related to these changes in a direct, causal manner. Rather, they have provided EMS physicians and administrators with data to make the most rational decisions possible.

With the contemplated vast increase in expenditures in EMS, there is increased urgency and importance for such research, and new, more sophisticated measures of effectiveness will have to be developed. Not only will costs have to be related in a meaningful manner to outcomes but the definition of outcomes and relationship of process of care (i.e., interventions) to the outcome of care will have to be explored [17]. Traditional outcome measures such as mortality and length of hospital stay should be supplemented by levels of residual symptoms, psychosocial disruptions, and capacity for employment. Commonly held dogma that measures such as lidocaine for premature ventricular contractions after myocardial infarction [18] and a 5 : 1 cardiac compression-ventilation ratio for cardiopulmonary resuscitation needs reexamination in terms of the outcomes observed.

CONCLUSION

Emergency Medical Services have come a long way in recent years: a concept of common purpose which includes ambulatory care is beginning to emerge, multiple organizational inputs into the EMS system are beginning to unify, and a framework for EMS evaluation is actively developing. The public's expectations for fast, effective, and inexpensive personalized emergency medical services, however, are outstripping the system's capacity to respond. It is folly to believe that mere application of technology and cost controls will be successful in answering these unfulfilled demands. Public expectations will undoubtedly have to change. Physicians will have to become increasingly aware of the fiscal, political, and organizational context in which they deliver emergency medical services. And, most important, it should be clear that with appropriate levels of public, legislative, and medical commitment to EMS, the goals of humane, cost-effective, and quality emergency medical services are realizable in this generation.

REFERENCES

1. Public Law 93–154. The Emergency Medical Services Systems Act of 1973.
2. Kirkpatrick, J. R., and Tabenhaus, L. J. The non-urgent patient on the emergency floor. *Med. Care* 5:19, 1967.
3. Lee, S. S., Solon, A., and Sheps, C. G. How new patterns of medical care affect the emergency unit. *Mod. Hosp.* 94:97, 1960.
4. Lavenhar, M. A., Ratner, R. S., and Weinerman, E. R. Social class and medical care: Indices of non-urgency in use of hospital emergency services. *Med. Care* 6:368, 1968.
5. *Hospitals* Guide Issue, Aug. 1, 1955, and Aug. 1, 1971.
6. Carpenter, C. C. I., and Voigt, G. C. Medical Emergencies–Cardiac Arrest. In Harvey, A. M., Johns, R. J., Owens, A. H., and Ross, R. S. (Eds.), *The Principles and Practice of Medicine*. 18th ed. New York: Appleton-Century-Crofts, 1972.
7. Senate Report No. 93–135, May 3, 1973, p. 42.
8. *A Model for Assessing EMS System Adequacy*. Health Resources Administration, Department of Health, Education and Welfare, Rockville, Md., 1975.
9. Public Law 93–154.
10. Pantridge, J., and Adgey, J. Pre-hospital coronary care. The mobile coronary care unit. *Am. J. Cardiol.* 24:666–673, 1969.
11. Pozen, M., Barrett, D., Voigt, G., and Lindsay, L. Ambulance telemetry evaluation—methodological considerations. Paper presented at 47th Scientific Sessions, American Health Association Meetings, Nov. 18–21, 1974, Dallas, Texas.
12. Sherman, H., and Komaroff, A. Ambulatory Care Project II. Progress Report 8A. Oct. 1, 1973. Public Health Service, Department of Health, Education, and Welfare, Washington, D.C.

13. Gibson, G.   Emergency medical service: The research gaps. *Health Serv. Res.* 9:6–21, 1974.
14. White, N., Parker, W., Binning, R., Dember, E., Ead, H., and Chamberlain, D.   Mobile coronary care provided by ambulance personnel. *Br. Med. J.* 3:618–622, 1973.
15. Gerner, H. R., Baker, S. P., Rutherford, R. B., and Spitz, W. U.   Evaluation of the management of vehicular fatalities secondary to abdominal injury. *J. Trauma* 12:425–431, 1972.
16. Sims, N. H., Seidel, H. M., and Cooke, R. E.   A structured approach to the use of physician extenders in well-child evaluations. *J. Pediatr.* 79:151–163, 1971.
17. Donnabedian, A.   Evaluating the quality of medical care. *Milbank Mem. Fund Q.* 44:166–206, 1966.
18. Marriott, H., and Myerbury, R.   Recognition and Treatment of Cardiac Arrhythmias and Conduction Disturbances. In Hurst, J. W. (Ed.), *The Heart.* 3d ed. New York: McGraw-Hill, 1974. Pp. 502–558.
19. McCall, M.   Cardiopulmonary Resuscitation. In Hurst, J. W. (Ed.), *The Heart.* 3d ed. New York: McGraw-Hill, 1974. Pp. 591–599.